ANTICANCER AND INTERFERON AGENTS

DRUGS AND THE PHARMACEUTICAL SCIENCES

A Series of Textbooks and Monographs

Edited by

James Swarbrick
School of Pharmacy
University of North Carolina
Chapel Hill, North Carolina

Volume 1. PHARMACOKINETICS, *Milo Gibaldi and Donald Perrier* (out of print)

Volume 2. GOOD MANUFACTURING PRACTICES FOR PHARMACEUTICALS: A PLAN FOR TOTAL QUALITY CONTROL, *Sidney H. Willig, Murray M. Tuckerman, and William S. Hitchings IV* (out of print)

Volume 3. MICROENCAPSULATION, *edited by J. R. Nixon*

Volume 4. DRUG METABOLISM: CHEMICAL AND BIOCHEMICAL ASPECTS, *Bernard Testa and Peter Jenner*

Volume 5. NEW DRUGS: DISCOVERY AND DEVELOPMENT, *edited by Alan A. Rubin*

Volume 6. SUSTAINED AND CONTROLLED RELEASE DRUG DELIVERY SYSTEMS, *edited by Joseph R. Robinson*

Volume 7. MODERN PHARMACEUTICS, *edited by Gilbert S. Banker and Christopher T. Rhodes*

Volume 8. PRESCRIPTION DRUGS IN SHORT SUPPLY: CASE HISTORIES, *Michael A. Schwartz*

Volume 9. ACTIVATED CHARCOAL: ANTIDOTAL AND OTHER MEDICAL USES, *David O. Cooney*

Volume 10. CONCEPTS IN DRUG METABOLISM (in two parts), *edited by Peter Jenner and Bernard Testa*

Volume 11. PHARMACEUTICAL ANALYSIS: MODERN METHODS (in two parts), *edited by James W. Munson*

Volume 12. TECHNIQUES OF SOLUBILIZATION OF DRUGS, *edited by Samuel H. Yalkowsky*

Volume 13. ORPHAN DRUGS, *edited by Fred E. Karch*

Volume 14. NOVEL DRUG DELIVERY SYSTEMS: FUNDAMENTALS, DEVELOPMENTAL CONCEPTS, BIOMEDICAL ASSESSMENTS, *edited by Yie W. Chien*

Volume 15. PHARMACOKINETICS, Second Edition, Revised and Expanded, *Milo Gibaldi and Donald Perrier*

Volume 16. GOOD MANUFACTURING PRACTICES FOR PHARMACEUTICALS: A PLAN FOR TOTAL QUALITY CONTROL, Second Edition, Revised and Expanded, *Sidney H. Willig, Murray M. Tuckerman, and William S. Hitchings IV*

Volume 17. FORMULATION OF VETERINARY DOSAGE FORMS, *edited by Jack Blodinger*

Volume 18. DERMATOLOGICAL FORMULATIONS: PERCUTANEOUS ABSORPTION, *Brian W. Barry*

Volume 19. THE CLINICAL RESEARCH PROCESS IN THE PHARMACEUTICAL INDUSTRY, *edited by Gary M. Matoren*

Volume 20. MICROENCAPSULATION AND RELATED DRUG PROCESSES, *Patrick B. Deasy*

Volume 21. DRUGS AND NUTRIENTS: THE INTERACTIVE EFFECTS, *edited by Daphne A. Roe and T. Colin Campbell*

Volume 22. BIOTECHNOLOGY OF INDUSTRIAL ANTIBIOTICS, *Erick J. Vandamme*

Volume 23. PHARMACEUTICAL PROCESS VALIDATION, *edited by Bernard T. Loftus and Robert A. Nash*

Volume 24. ANTICANCER AND INTERFERON AGENTS: SYNTHESIS AND PROPERTIES, *edited by Raphael M. Ottenbrite and George B. Butler*

Other Volumes in Preparation

ANTICANCER AND INTERFERON AGENTS

SYNTHESIS AND PROPERTIES

Edited by

RAPHAEL M. OTTENBRITE
Department of Chemistry, and Massey Cancer Center
Virginia Commonwealth University
Richmond, Virginia

GEORGE B. BUTLER
Center for Macromolecular Science
University of Florida
Gainesville, Florida

RC271
C5
A66
1984

MARCEL DEKKER, INC. New York and Basel

Library of Congress Cataloging in Publication Data
Main entry under title:

Anticancer and interferon agents.

(Drugs and the pharmaceutical sciences ; v. 24)
Includes index.
1. Antineoplastic agents--Testing. 2. Cancer--Chemotherapy. 3. Interferon--Testing. I. Ottenbrite, Raphael M. II. Butler, George B., [date]
III. Series. [DNLM: 1. Antineoplastic agents.
2. Interferons. W1 DR893B v.24 / QV 269 A6295]
RC271.C5A66 1984 616.99'4061 84-7006
ISBN 0-8247-7189-3

COPYRIGHT © 1984 by MARCEL DEKKER, INC.
ALL RIGHTS RESERVED

Neither this book nor any part may be reproduced or transmitted in any form or by any means, electronic or mechanical, including photocopying, microfilming, and recording, or by any information storage and retrieval system, without permission in writing from the publisher.

MARCEL DEKKER, INC.
270 Madison Avenue, New York, New York 10016

Current printing (last digit):
10 9 8 7 6 5 4 3 2 1

PRINTED IN THE UNITED STATES OF AMERICA

This book is dedicated to our wives, Nancy
and Josephine, and to our families

PREFACE

The human body is awesomely and wonderfully designed to carry out the functions of life as we know them. Unfortunately, this body is subject to disease and genetic problems which are the product of environmental conditions and/or mutagenic changes. One of the currently most devastating afflictions faced by humankind is cancer. Through the centuries many approaches have been developed to stem the tide of this ever-increasing menace—with little success. It has been only in the last few years that a better understanding of the disease and better methods of treatment have been developed.

It has become apparent that one of the most successful anticancer modalities is chemotherapy. These chemical agents have evolved from natural products and synthetic materials. Unfortunately, most chemists are unaware of the potentially active anticancer and interferon agents: thus, this book has been compiled to familiarize chemical scientists with cancer treatment, anticancer drug evaluation, anticancer drug administration, anticancer drug design, and research.

The first chaper deals, at a basic level, with tumor biology and the present chemotherapeutic treatment. The next chapter describes in detail the search and screening of new materials, the types of compounds that are of interest, and the specific tests available for evaluating drug potential. The third chapter deals with the pharmacology of the more potent materials: how they are administered and evaluated for anticancer efficacy. The ensuing chapters relate to the research presently being carried out with some of the more effective chemotherapeutic agents. The final chapter deals with interferon as a clinical agent, its present potential, and its possibilities for the future.

It is hoped that readers of this book will attain a better understanding of anticancer agents and their potential. It is also hoped that the book will stimulate more chemists to become involved in the research for the necessary elements to curb this dreadful disease.

Raphael M. Ottenbrite
George B. Butler

CONTENTS

CONTRIBUTORS

WILLIAM E. ANTHOLINE* *University of Wisconsin-Milwaukee, Milwaukee, Wisconsin*

GEORGE B. BUTLER *Center for Macromolecular Science, University of Florida, Gainesville, Florida*

PAUL E. CAME† *HEM Research Incorporated, Rockville, Maryland*

WILLIAM A. CARTER *Herbert L. Orlowitz Institute for Cancer and Blood Diseases, Hahnemann University of the Health Sciences, Philadelphia, Pennsylvania*

ROBERT B. DIASIO *Departments of Medicine and Pharmacology, Medical College of Virginia, Virginia Commonwealth University, Richmond, Virginia*

RUTH I. GERAN‡ *Developmental Therapeutics Program, Division of Cancer Treatment, National Cancer Institute, National Institutes of Health, Bethesda, Maryland*

JOHN W. KUSIAK *Macromolecular Chemistry Section, National Institute on Aging, Baltimore City Hospitals, Baltimore, Maryland*

Present affiliations:
* The Medical College of Wisconsin, Milwaukee, Wisconsin
† Heidrick and Struggles, Inc., Chicago, Illinois
‡ Retired

RAPHAEL M. OTTENBRITE *Department of Chemistry, and Massey Cancer Center, Virginia Commonwealth University, Richmond, Virginia*

DAVID H. PETERING *Department of Chemistry, University of Wisconsin-Milwaukee, Milwaukee, Wisconsin*

JOSEF PITHA *Macromolecular Chemistry Section, National Institute on Aging, Baltimore City Hospitals, Baltimore, Maryland*

DONALD J. REED *Department of Biochemistry and Biophysics, Oregon State University, Corvallis, Oregon*

LEON A. SARYAN *Laboratory for Molecular Biomedical Research, Department of Chemistry, University of Wisconsin-Milwaukee, Milwaukee, Wisconsin*

ALBERT T. SNEDEN *Department of Chemistry, Virginia Commonwealth University, Richmond, Virginia*

ROBERT J. SPIEGEL* *Department of Medicine, New York University Medical Center, New York, New York*

PAUL F. TORRENCE *Laboratory of Chemistry, National Institute of Arthritis, Diabetes, and Digestive and Kidney Diseases, National Institutes of Health, Bethesda, Maryland*

*Present affiliation: Department of Oncology, Clinical Research, Schering-Plough Corporation, Kenilworth, New Jersey

ANTICANCER AND INTERFERON AGENTS

1

PRINCIPLES OF CHEMOTHERAPY AND IMMUNOTHERAPY

ROBERT J. SPIEGEL*

New York University Medical Center, New York, New York

I. INTRODUCTION

Until the middle of this century, the conventional therapeutic approach to most cancers was simply the surgical excision of visible tumor. The predominant premise of tumor biology was that cancer progressed primarily by local invasion, secondarily by the spread of malignant cells to contiguous structures and lymph nodes, and only in a late phase into the bloodstream and to distant sites. This dictated the principles of radical cancer surgery which were developed in the late nineteenth and early twentieth centuries.

*Present affiliation: Department of Oncology, Clinical Research, Schering-Plough Corporation, Kenilworth, New Jersey

However, the effectiveness of surgery alone plateaued and despite remarkable improvements in antibiotic therapy, anesthesia, and other surgical advances, today the cure rate for many types of cancer following surgery remains the same as at the turn of the century. The advent of modern radiation therapy provided the first realistic alternative to surgery and was soon widely utilized to complement the surgical approach. Many tumors are "radiosensitive" and cytotoxic doses of radiation can result in prompt shrinkage of gross tumor. Radiation can also be applied to a wide field surrounding the visible tumor and thus eradicate the local microscopic spread of malignant cells. Furthermore, radiation can be used as an "adjuvant" to surgery, that is, to sterilize the tumor bed and adjacent lymph nodes postoperatively. Radiation can also be administered prophylactically to those sites that are felt to be at highest risk for harboring metastatic cells. Unfortunately, not all malignant cells are particularly radiosensitive and the radiation dose required to kill most malignant cells frequently will produce profound toxic effects in adjacent normal tissue. This significantly limits the role of radiotherapy in the treatment of many tumors. Even in patients with radiosensitive tumors, large regions of the body cannot realistically tolerate high does of prophylactic or adjuvant radiation therapy due to the accompanying toxicity. This becomes a critical limitation since the concept of cancer as a localized disease has been challenged increasingly in recent years. In many malignancies, it is now felt that by the time the primary tumor reaches a size at which it is clinically detectable it is probably a subclinical systemic disease, that is, some malignant cells have already seeded to other areas of the body. For this reason, future advances in the local treatment of malignancy offer only limited hope for significantly improving cancer survival statistics. Prevention, early detection, and improved systemic therapy appear to offer the best hope for future advances in the control of cancer.

This chapter reviews the development of what, to date, has been the most important step in the control of systemic cancer — antineoplastic chemotherapy. The developing field of immunotherapy is also discussed. Prior to chemotherapy, surgery and radiation cured about one-third of cancer patients. Since the advent of chemotherapy and its widespread use in the last two decades, this figure has climbed steadily, and by 1980 approximately 55% of newly diagnosed cancer patients could be expected to be cured [1,2]. Two critical statistics — (1) survival from the time of diagnosis, and (2) number of patients who achieve complete remission (i.e., no evidence of residual tumor after initial therapy) — have improved markedly. Many of these cures result from the administration of chemotherapy alone and many complete remissions now occur in patients with malignant diseases who had average survival times measured in weeks or months prior to chemotherapy.

II. TUMOR BIOLOGY AND PHARMACOLOGIC PRINCIPLES OF CHEMOTHERAPY

Many of the chemotherapeutic agents described in the chapters of this text are destined to be supplanted by newer compounds of greater efficacy or lesser toxicity. However, whether the next generation of drugs are congeners of existing compounds or work by entirely unique mechanisms of action, the basic pharmacologic principles underlying their biological activity and their clinical application are unlikely to change. Although serendipity and empiricism underlie the discovery and application of many of the major compounds used today [3], in fact there exists a voluminous literature and body of knowledge supporting our current concepts of tumor biology and cancer chemotherapy. These form the basis for therapeutic decisions about drug selection and new drug development and are critical to an understanding of the clinical administration of chemotherapy.

Antineoplastic agents act by interfering with essential molecular processes in the cancer cell. Most of the compounds that are active against neoplastic cells exert their effect by interfering with the cell replication process. However, any chemical or biologic event that is essential to cell function and survival is a potential target for a cytotoxic drug. The essence of the malignant process appears to be an escape from the normal internal or external controls on cell replication and growth. The "transformed" cells found in a malignant tumor proliferate in an unregulated fashion and frequently possess the capacity to invade adjacent normal tissue and metastasize to distant sites. The story of basic cancer research in the modern era is largely the chronicle of thousands of scientists in various disciplines searching for differences between the cancer cell and the normal cell which would account for the process of carcinogenesis. On the molecular level differences have been found in enzyme activity, surface properties, chromosome constitution, and growth kinetics, to name but a few areas of intensive research. However, none of these changes is unique for or common to all malignancies. Furthermore, the cells of a tumor are not necessarily homogenous in composition or activity and therefore may be affected in variable degrees by the administration of an antineoplastic compound. Lacking a "magic bullet" that will selectively kill all tumor cells without damaging the normal cells of the host organism, cancer chemotherapy has been largely nonspecific and empirical: current agents damage malignant cells as well as normal cells, particularly those that proliferate rapidly. When chemotherapy is effective, it is theorized that the malignant cells are more sensitive than normal cells to a given drug dosage (selective toxicity and therapeutic index) and less capable of recovering rapidly. Current principles of drug dose and schedule as well as combination chemotherapy arise from this theory and our understanding of cell growth kinetics.

An understanding of the life cycles of normal and malignant cells and their consequent growth kinetics is essential to appreciate both theoretical and practical aspects of cancer therapy. The cell cycle is defined as the period from one mitosis (cell division) to the next. For cells in a reproductive cycle this interval is divided into four phases (Fig. 1.1). Cells enter a G_1 phase following division. Originally, this phase had been considered a quiescent period and was designated the first "gap" or G_1. However, more recent investigation has shown G_1 to be marked by metabolic activity involving RNA and protein synthesis. G_1 is now recognized as the most variable period of the cell cycle and can be considered as the rate-limiting step in the cell's cycle time. In general, slowly growing cell populations have long G_1 periods [4]. Cells can have quite prolonged G_1 phases to the extent that some cells are said to be in a resting or G_0 dormant stage. Cells in G_0 leave the cell cycle but can reenter and proliferate sometime in the future. Emerging from G_1, the cell enters the S phase, in which DNA is actively synthesized and the chromosomes are replicated. After DNA synthesis is completed the cell enters a phase of apparent rest, G_2, before the initiation of mitosis. Finally, the cell enters mitosis, with its own substages involving the formation of the spindle apparatus and separation of the chromosomes, which results in the formation of two daughter cells.

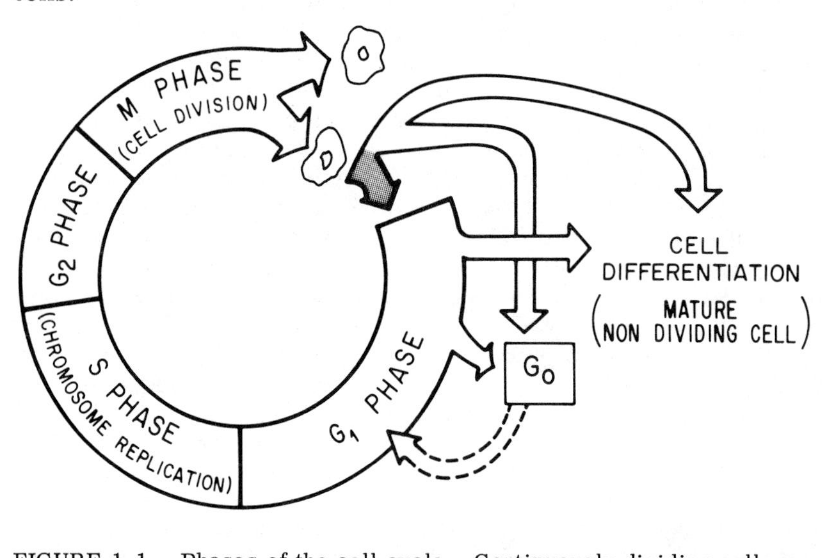

FIGURE 1.1 Phases of the cell cycle. Continuously dividing cells go around the cell cycle from one mitosis (m) to the next. Nondividing cells have left the cycle. Quiescent cells (G_0) are neither cycling nor dying, but may be induced to reenter the cycle. Alternatives for daughter cells resulting from mitosis are shown. In malignant cells with rapid doubling times, most cells either enter a temporary resting state (G_0) or return to the beginning of the mitotic cycle (G_1). The S phase is the period of DNA synthesis. G_2 is a brief postsynthetic resting phase.

This simplified model of the cell life cycle yields a number of important concepts about individual cell growth and cell population kinetics which apply to both normal and neoplastic cells. Any tissue should be considered a mixed cell population [i.e., some cells proliferating (in cycle), some resting (G_0), and some nondividing]. Normal and abnormal tissue growth both depend on cell cycle time, the growth fraction, and the rate of cell loss [3]. Cell cycle time refers to the interval between mitoses; the shorter the interval, the faster new cells are produced. Growth fraction refers to that fraction of cells that are cycling, and the larger the fraction of cycling cells in a population, the faster the increase in cell number. Cell cycle time together with the growth fraction determines the number of cells produced per unit of time. Cell loss determines the number lost in cell death. Taken together, these factors determine the net increase, decrease, or steady state of a tumor or a normal tissue.

At one time it was presumed that tumor cells proliferated faster than normal cells. Malignant tissue was envisioned as a collection of wildly growing cells with short cell cycle times which were not subject to regulatory mechanisms. In fact, those assumptions are frequently invalid. For example, it has been demonstrated that the normal cells which line the intestine of a mouse have a shorter cell cycle time than that of rapidly growing mouse tumors. Similarly, in humans the cell cycle times of normal bone marrow elements and colon epithelium range from 18 to 39 hr, respectively, whereas some human lung cancer cells have a measured cell cycle time of 196-260 hr. Therefore, tumor cells do not necessarily proliferate faster than normal cells [5].

The other determinant of tissue growth, growth fraction, has also been reexamined over the last two decades with profound consequences for chemotherapy strategies. All cancer cells are not in the proliferative cycle. At different times in a tumor's development a variable portion of the cells will be in a growth phase. This means that therapeutic strategies based solely on killing dividing cells will frequently be less than totally effective. Antineoplastic agents vary in terms of where in the cell cycle they exert their effect and can be classified by the selectivity of their mechanism of action.

III. CLASSIFICATION OF ANTINEOPLASTIC DRUGS

Most antineoplastic agents act by interfering with molecular processes in the cancer cell which are essential to the cell replication process. However, any chemical or biological event that is mandatory for normal cell function and survival is a potential target for a cytotoxic drug. Traditionally, these drugs have been categorized as alkylating agents, antimetabolites, antitumor antibiotics, other natural products, miscellaneous drugs, and hormones. This classification scheme distinguishes both the origin of the compounds and their mechanisms of action. The commonly used drugs are listed in Table 1.1 (review in Ref. 6).

TABLE 1.1 Commonly Used Antineoplastic Drugs[a]

Compound	Trade name	Route of Administration	Toxicity			Indications[b]
			BM	GI	Other	
Alkylating agents						
Mechlorethamine	Mustargen (HN_2)	iv, ic	++	+++	Local irritant/vesicant	HD, non-HD lymphoma, MF, lung+
Cyclophosphamide	Cytotoxan	iv, po	++	++	Alopecia, cystitis	HD, non-HD lymphoma, breast ALL+, myeloma, ovary
Chlorambucil	Leukeran	po	++			CLL, HD, non-HD lymphoma, breast+, ovary+
Melphalan (L-PAM)	Alkeran	po	++	+		Myeloma, ovary+, breast+
Triethylenethiophosphoramide	Thiopeta	iv, ic	++			Ovary+, breast+, bladder+
Busulfan	Myleran	po	+		↑ Pigmentation, pulmonary toxicity	CML, polycythemia vera
Imidiazole carboxamide (DTIC)	Dacarbazine	iv	+	+++	Flu-like syndrome, local irritation	Melanoma, sarcoma
Bis-chloroethylnitrosourea (BCNU)	Carmustine	iv	+			Brain, HD, non-HD lymphoma, MF

Chloroethylcyclo-hexylnitrosourea (CCNU)	Lomustine	po	+	+		GI^{+}, brain, HD, non-HD lymphoma, lung^{+}
Chloroethylmethyl-cyclohexylnitroso-urea (MCCNU)	Semustine	po	+	+		Brain, GI^{+}, lung^{+}, melanoma^{+}
Antimetabolites						
Methotrexate (MTX)	Methotrexate	po, iv, im, it	+	+	Stomatitis, renal	AML, ALL, choriocarcinoma, H+N, breast, cervix^{+}, osteosarcoma^{+}, other sarcomas^{+}
5-Fluorouracil (5-FU)	Fluorouracil	iv	+	+	Stomatitis, ataxia ↑ Pigmentation	Breast, GI, ovary, skin (topical)
Cytabrine (ara-C)	Cytosar	iv, it	+	+		AML, ALL, CML (blast crisis)
6-Mercaptopurine (6-MP)	Purinethol	po	+		Alopecia, stomatitis	ALL, AML, CML, choriocarcinoma^{+}
6-Thioguanine (6-TG)	Thioguanine	po	+			AML, CML (blast crisis)
Floxuridine (FUDR)		po				
Antibiotics						
Dactinomycin (ACT-D)	Cosmegen	iv	+	+++	Local irritant, alopecia, stomatitis, dermatitis	Wilms' tumor, choriocarcinoma, testis, neuroblastoma, sarcoma

TABLE 1.1 (Continued)

Compound	Trade name	Route of Administration	Toxicity BM	GI	Other	Indications[b]
Doxorubicin	Adriamycin	iv	++	++	Stomatitis, alopecia, heart failure, arrhythmias, cellulitis	ALL, AML, HD, lymphoma, sarcoma, Wilms' tumor, breast, ovary, lung, bladder$^+$, thyroid, prostate$^+$
Daunomycin		iv	++	++	Stomatitis, alopecia, heart failure, arrhythmias, cellulitis	ALL, AML, CML (blast crisis)
Bleomycin	Blenoxane	im, im	++	+	Dermatitis, fever, pulmonary	HD, lymphoma, H+N, esophagus, cervix, penis, MF, testis
Mitomycin C	Mutamycin	iv	+	++	Cellulitis, alopecia	Ovary$^+$, breast$^+$, H+N$^+$, GI
Other natural products						
Vincristine	Oncovin	iv			Constipation, alopecia, neurotoxicity	ALL, AML, CML (blast crisis), HD, lymphoma, Wilms' tumor, breast, and Ewing's childhood sarcoma

Vinblastine	Velban	iv	+	+	Cellulitis, alopecia, neurotoxicity	HD, lymphoma, breast+, testis, lung+
Miscellaneous drugs						
L-Asparaginase	Elspar	iv, im		+	Anaphylaxis, pancreatitis	ALL, AML
Procarbazine	Matulane	po	+	+	Nervous system, MAO inhibitor	HD, lymphoma+, myeloma+, brain tumors+
Hydroxyurea	Hydrea	po	+	+	Alopecia	CML
Cis-Platinum	Platinol	iv	+	+++	Renal	Testis, H+N, lung, ovary, bladder, prostate

[a]BM, bone marrow; GI, gastrointestinal; iv, intravenous; ic, intracavitary; po, per os; im, intramuscular; it, intrathecal; HD, Hodgkin's disease; MF, mycoses fungosides; ALL, acute lymphoblastic leukemia; CLL, chronic lymphocytic leukemia; CML, chronic myelogenous leukemia; AML, acute myelocytic leukemia; H+N, head + neck.

[b]Check Physicians' Desk Reference for approved indications. This list includes some indications which are a result of investigational studies requiring confirmation, and (+) signifies an indication only as a second line drug or in special circumstances.

Alkylating agents were the earliest compounds recognized to be of widespread clinical usefulness in patients with malignancies, and they remain the most widely utilized class of antineoplastic compounds. Alkylating agents are highly reactive compounds that contain electrophilic alkyl radicals ($R-CH_2-CH_2^+$) and they are particularly active with negatively charged macromolecules. Their cytotoxic activity derives from their high rate of reactivity with nucleic acids, particularly DNA. Alkylation produces breaks in the DNA molecule and cross-linking of the twin DNA strands. This interferes with DNA replication, RNA transcription, and ultimately prevents cell division. As their activity does not depend on DNA synthesis, these agents are considered to affect cells that are in any phase of the cell cycle (phase nonspecific).

Antimetabolites act by interfering with the biosynthesis of nucleic acids, proteins, or other essential cellular constituents (e.g., polyamines). These agents are structural analogs of the normal metabolites or coenzymes required for cell function and replication and they are classified as folate, purine, pyrimidine, or amino acid analogs. Interference with normal cell metabolism occurs either (1) by substituting for a metabolite normally incorporated into a key molecule, rendering such a molecule functionally inoperable; or (2) by inhibiting specific enzymes necessary for cell metabolism. In contrast to the alkylating agents, the antimetabolites are largely dependent on DNA synthesis to be active. They are considered cell cycle phase-specific agents and their activity is often highly schedule dependent.

The antitumor antibiotics form a distinct class of compounds because they are all natural products of various strains of the fungus *Streptomyces* and because their tumoricidal effects share common mechanisms of action. The majority of these antibiotics directly bind and react with DNA and thereby have inhibitory effects on DNA or RNA synthesis. Most of the clinically useful drugs of this class are "intercalators" of DNA. This process can be envisioned as the positioning of a planar molecule between the base pairs of DNA, resulting in steric obstruction and an unwinding of the double-helical DNA structure. This results in inhibition of both RNA transcription and DNA replication. Some of these antibiotics have additional mechanisms of action. For example, the bleomycins act by producing "strand scission" (i.e., breaking and fragmenting of single strands of DNA). Mitomycin C is an antibiotic which is activated in vivo to become a bifunctional or trifunctional alkylating agent, producing DNA cross-links. Although the mechanism of action of those drugs has conventionally been ascribed solely to DNA efforts, other areas now being considered include surface membrane effects and the generation of free-radical oxygen species.

Other natural products include plant derivatives, some of which have formed an important source of anticancer remedies since antiquity. Periwinkle is the source of the *Vinca* alkaloids, while the investigational podophyllotoxin derivatives are extracts from the mayapple. These compounds exert their major antitumor effect by binding the microtubule proteins which form the spindle apparatus during mitosis. The *Vinca* alkaloids arrest cell division at mitosis and are considered cell cycle phase specific. They probably exert additional effects on RNA synthesis. The podophyllotoxin derivatives are semisynthetic plant products which also affect microtubules but appear to exert additional effects by producing DNA strand breaks and inhibiting DNA synthesis.

A. Miscellaneous Drugs

In addition to the classes of drugs described above, a number of agents are utilized commonly which do not fall neatly into these categories. For example, L-asparaginase is an enzyme derived from bacterial cultures of *Escherichia coli* or *Erwinia cartovora*. Some tumor cells appear to be particularly dependent on exogenous asparagine and L-asparaginase depletes the extracellular supplies of this amino acid, thus exploiting the qualitative difference between tumor cells and normal cells in their metabolism of asparagine. Procarbazine is a methyhydrazine derivative which was originally synthesized as a potential monoamine oxidase inhibitor. Its exact mechanism of action is unclear but, among other effects, it causes depolymerization of DNA and suppresses RNA and protein synthesis. Some of its metabolites are highly reactive and their effects resemble those of ionizing radiation. Hydroxurea is a simple chemical compound consisting of a urea molecule with a hydroxyl group replacing a hydrogen atom on one of the two amino groups. It was first synthesized in 1869 but was not used in cancer treatment until the early 1960s. It inhibits ribonucleotide reductase, which impairs DNA synthesis and is S-phase specific in its cytotoxicity. *Cis*-platinum is an inorganic complex composed of a central platinum(II) atom surrounded by chlorine and ammonia atoms in the cis position. This compound acts as a bifunctional alkylating agent, binding to intracellular purines in DNA and causing cross-linking of DNA strands. This drug inhibits DNA synthesis and it is not cell cycle specific.

Hormonal therapy, a unique form of chemotherapy, utilizes natural products or synthetic analogs of the body's endocrine organs. Manipulation of the endocrine system is a strategy which predates the introduction of the chemotherapeutic agents discussed above, and has established efficacy in a number of malignancies. There is now a resurgence of interest in endocrine-related therapies due to two major developments: (1) new laboratory techniques which allow for clear identification and quantification of hormone receptors on tumor cells, and (2) the development and clinical introduction of new agents which block hormone production or hormone receptors much more specifically and effectively than do ablation surgery or the compounds previously available. In addition to estrogens, progestins, and androgens, available hormonal agents now include antiestrogens, adrenal steroid inhibitors, and selective inhibitors of luteinizing hormone (LH) and follicle-stimulating hormone (FSH). Presently, the role of hormonal therapy is exclusively palliative, although there is new interest in the possible synergistic use of these compounds with adjuvant chemotherapy [7].

IV. THERAPEUTIC PRINCIPLES

The clinical use of the drugs described in the preceding section is based on a number of carefully determined therapeutic principles, some of which are common to all pharmaceutical compounds and some which are unique to the antineoplastic agents. Clinically useful chemotherapeutic agents affect processes found in all dividing cells, but they have a greater effect on malignant cells than on nonmalignant cells (i.e., they exhibit "selective toxicity"). However, they also have a low therapeutic index, and their efficacy as well as their toxicity can be dramatically affected by slight changes in their dose, metabolism, or excretion. For these reasons, the dose and schedule of administration of each agent are carefully designed on the basis of theoretical activity and then empirically tested to derive a balance of maximum efficacy and minimum acceptable toxicity. Occasionally, higher than "tolerable" doses may be tested with "rescue" regimens or autologous bone marrow reconstitution (e.g., administration of high-dose methotrexate to block tetrahydrate folate reductase followed by citrovorum factor as a rescue [6]).

The mechanisms of action of the commonly utilized antineoplastic agents were discussed briefly in the preceding section and are explored in detail in subsequent chapters. Factors that affect the serum concentration of the drugs or their active metabolites and the time over which the tumor cells or normal cells are exposed to them are crucial to both efficacy and toxicity. Traditional pharmacologic factors such as route of administration, absorption, distribution, biotransformation, metabolism, and excretion must all be considered. Delivering the drug or its metabolite to the cancer cell in an effective concentration while sparing normal tissues from unacceptable toxicity is difficult and occasionally requires novel therapeutic strategies. A few of these agents may be administered in oral form, but most are given as an intravenous injection. Some are instilled directly into the cerebrospinal fluid or pleural spaces to achieve maximum concentrations and prevent tumor cells from escaping destruction by location in a sanctuary" site. Other drugs have been administered as isolated perfusions in an extremity or an organ (e.g., hepatic artery infusions) to maximize the local drug concentration in the target tissue.

The process of arriving at an optimal dose and schedule of administration for any given drug is described in Chap. 3. A given compound's pharmacologic characteristics (e.g., plasma half-life, tissue distribution, and normal tissue toxicity) as well as the tumor cell kinetics of the malignancy it is being tested against will determine the initial dose, schedule, and method of administration. For example, if a phase-specific drug with a very short half-life is given as a single bolus administration, it may maintain its peak therapeutic level for only a few minutes and affect only the few tumor cells that are dividing during that period. Alternatively, if this drug is administered as a 48- or 72-hr continuous infusion, it can affect all cells dividing over that prolonged period. Similarly, a drug might produce unacceptable toxicity when administered daily, but given in a weekly or monthly schedule it might be quite tolerable and equally efficacious. Failure to test alternative dose schedules may lead to premature dismissal of an antineoplastic agent as being inactive or excessively toxic. In vitro testing and animal tumor models are usually utilized to determine the optimal therapeutic dose and schedule of a drug. Controlled clinical trials in patients are then conducted to determine toxicity in humans [8-10].

In general, the maximally tolerated dose (MTD) is administered and then repeated upon recovery of normal tissues (usually a 3- to 4-week period). This is based on the "log cell kill concept" which theoretically allows for normal tissues to recover while a fixed percentage of tumor cells are killed with each drug administration (Fig. 2). In experimental systems, most antineoplastic agents produce a dose-response curve which is steep and is log-linear; that is, a given dose destroys 90% of tumor cells (1 log);

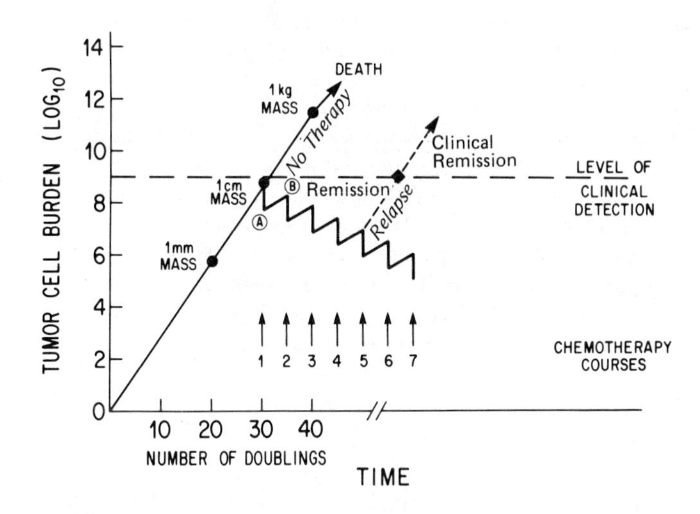

FIGURE 1.2 Theoretical model of cell kinetics during clinical chemotherapy. In animal tumor models, chemotherapeutic agents have been shown to destroy tumor cells by "first-order kinetics"; that is, a given dose of a given drug kills a constant percentage of tumor cells. Effective initial therapy will reduce the tumor cell population by a few logs (point A). One must delay further therapy until the toxic effects of the drug have subsided. However, during this period the tumor cell population will recover to point B. Repeat courses of successful therapy will progressively reduce the remaining tumor burden. During unsuccessful therapy, while the host recovers from toxicity there is a net growth of tumor to a point over and above the starting point, and on successive courses there is a further increase in the number of tumor cells.

twice that dose may destroy 99% (2 logs). Unfortunately, the dose-toxicity curve is also steep and results in a narrow optimal dose range. Clinical data frequently do not support such a close correlation among dose, response, and toxicity. This may be due to competing risks (patients with more advanced disease are more likely to manifest toxicity and less likely to respond) or to idiosyncrasies of drug metabolism. However, recognizing the need to evaluate each agent separately, as an operational policy each cytotoxic agent is usually employed to its maximum but safe and well-tolerated dose.

For most agents, the schedule as well as the dose of drug administration have been empirically determined in animal models and confirmed in clinical trials. Intermittent intensive treatment is usually superior to continuous (i.e., daily) treatment. This advantage is consistent with our current concepts of cytokinetic, pharmacologic, and immunologic factors that are important in controlling malignancy.

Based on the remarkable advances achieved in the treatment of childhood leukemia, lymphoma, and such solid tumors as testicular carcinoma, comprehensive primary treatment regimens frequently employ a long-term treatment strategy. Initially, maximally tolerated agents are given in an "induction" phase in an attempt to produce a complete response (i.e., complete disappearance of the tumor). This is followed by a long-term "maintenance" phase, frequently employing noncross-resistant agents. This phase of therapy may involve 1 to 2 years of chemotherapy administered every 3 to 4 weeks. Some regimens regularly employ a "reinduction" or "consolidation" phase early in the maintenance cycle to achieve further cytoreduction of any residual malignant cells. Recently, some regimens have also incorporated a "late intensification" cycle. Although the results of these concepts have been borne out in some leukemias and lymphomas as well as some of the childhood solid tumors, the value of these strategies in the slower-growing adult tumors remains to be demonstrated.

A. Combination Chemotherapy

The theoretical basis for combination chemotherapy comes from other areas of clinical medicine. For example, in the treatment of hypertension, agents with different mechanisms of action have been combined to achieve better control of blood pressure without additive toxicity. In the treatment of infectious diseases, the use of combination antimicrobial therapy achieves a greater initial effect and delays or prevents the development of drug resistance. In the case of malignant disease there is obviously a need for improved initial treatment. Few anticancer agents produce more than 50% cell kill and the heterogeneity of neoplastic cells within a given tumor and selective pressures favoring the rapid development of drug resistance are felt to account, to a large degree, for the failure to produce cancer cures with single-agent therapy. Therefore, there is a solid biological rationale for the use of combination regimens in antineoplastic therapy.

Moreover, there are separate pharmacologic and cytokinetic rationales for combination chemotherapy's efficacy. Tumor-active agents can be combined which have complementary or subadditive host toxicities. Drugs can also be chosen which exert their effects sequentially, concurrently, or synergistically (e.g., complementary blockade). In some combination regimens, the initial agent is considered to synchronize or recruit cells so that the subsequent phase-specific agent may enhance cell kill. In many cases, the exact drug interactions are unknown. However, it is clear that drug combinations have been very successful empirically in a wide variety of malignancies (reviewed in Ref. 11). In designing a combination regimen, agents are chosen which (1) are individually active against the disease in question in nearly full doses; (2) avoid, if possible, overlapping toxicities; and (3) have differing mechanisms of action. New theoretical principles are also being tested clinically as knowledge of drug action and selectivity increases, and as technology for establishing such principles in vivo has been developed.

Table 2 indicates those theoretical and clinical considerations that favor use of combination over single-drug therapy, and vice versa. In any one specific clinical circumstance, a strategy favoring one or the other might prevail.

V. ADJUVANT CHEMOTHERAPY

The development of active drugs and effective combinations have clearly established the role of chemotherapy as the primary therapy for some malignancies (e.g., leukemia, lymphoma, choriocarcinoma) and as the only reasonable primary or secondary therapy in other malignancies which have spread systemically. However, chemotherapy may also play a critical role in integrated treatment modalities. Local control of malignancy may be

TABLE 1.2 Single-Agent Versus Combination Therapy

Factors favoring single-agent therapy
Less toxic
More predictable and informative
Allows more secondary therapies
Easier to combine with other modalities
Provides "building blocks" for more effective regimens
Factors favoring combination chemotherapy
Greater probability of initial response
Chance for drug synergy
Delays emergence of resistance
Greater curative potential

attempted with radiation or surgery, but this cannot affect the systemic disease, which frequently will become the ultimate cause of death. Therefore, it has become of great interest to determine the role of chemotherapy as an adjuvant to local modalities. In childhood tumors, the administration of chemotherapy following the eradication of the bulk disease has clearly diminished the incidence of recurrence and improved long-term survival rates in such diseases as Wilms' tumor, Ewing's sarcoma, and Burkitt's lymphoma. In adults, this same principle has been applied to a number of solid tumors and in the case of cancers of the testis and breast, statistically significant improvements in survival have been demonstrated. In these diseases, existing chemotherapy combinations are effective enough to recommend that adjuvant chemotherapy be administered. Unfortunately, in many other adult tumors no single drug or combination of drugs exist to which the tumor cells are sufficiently sensitive. Therefore, adjuvant therapy can be recommended in these cases only in the context of an experimental trial. The administration of early systemic adjuvant treatment is an area of active investigation — and controversy. "Preoperative" chemotherapy is also under study in some cancer centers.

VI. TOXICOLOGIC PRINCIPLES

Chemotherapeutic drugs are cytotoxic against a wide variety of cells, with a special predilection against rapidly replicating tissues such as the bone marrow and the gastrointestinal tract. In fact, intermittent regimens have generally gained favor because theoretically they allow full recovery from myelosuppression or gastrointestinal alterations during an interval when the tumor is not able to recover substantially. For most regimens, the induction of tolerable myelosuppression is considered an index for optimal (maximal) dosing; for example, a 3-week interval is considered optimal for full recovery of marrow function following a short burst of alkylating agent or antimetabolite therapy. Some drugs, such as chloroethylnitrosourea, affect bone marrow for longer periods; these and others (e.g., mitomycin C) also lead to cumulative bone marrow stem cell depletions and presumably permanent bone marrow damage with lesser tolerance to subsequent drug administration. The kinetics of recovery from gastrointestinal damage have been less well studied but may be particularly important when one considers combined modality regimens, including radiotherapy or high-dose regimens utilizing rescue techniques for the bone marrow (autologous bone marrow reconstitution).

A major effort is ongoing to avoid common undesirable acute consequences such as nausea and vomiting, and many antiemetic measures are currently being tested. Use of marrow protective or reconstructive measures which allow greater dosages of drugs will undoubtedly uncover many new toxicologic manifestations. Fortunately, other acute consequences are rare with most of the established drugs when administered at conventional doses. Drugs with renal or hepatic toxicities of note will usually be withdrawn at an early stage of testing in favor of others which retain efficacy without these undesirable properties. Conversely, such toxicities are often avoided by stringent patient selection or implementation of organ-specific protective measures such as urine alkalinization for the nephrotoxicity of high doses of methotrexate or hydration for that of *cis*-platinum. For a review of specific acute toxicities and their management, see Ref. 12.

Recently, a number of delayed organ-specific toxicities have become apparent [13]. Each is dose related and in some cases these cumulative consequences of cytotoxic therapy become dose limiting and preclude further treatment. Neurologic toxicity and peripheral neuropathies have long been associated with *Vinca* alkaloid therapy. Recently, irreversible pulmonary toxicity has been associated with a number of agents, most commonly bleomycin. A dose-related cardiac toxicity is associated with prolonged anthracycline administration, primarily adriamycin, and has been the subject of intense investitation.

Renal toxicity can also occur in a predictable manner after repeated exposure to *cis*-platinum. In each of these cases, efforts have been taken or are under way to modify toxicity by the following steps: (1) avoidance of an identified clinical setting (e.g., enhanced cardiac and pulmonary toxicity in a setting or prior or concurrent radiotherapy), (2) development of less toxic dose schedules or analogs (e.g., adriamycin infusions and analog development), (3) prediction of toxicity (animal models or cardiac screening), (4) modification of toxicity (e.g., hydration and diuresis induction with platinum therapy).

Long-term sequelae of chemotherapy have involved a number of additional organ systems and include immune depression, teratogenesis, and oncogenesis. Carcinogenic effects are not unexpected since laboratory models have regularly indicated antineoplastic agent's mutagenic and oncogenic properties. Clinical studies have been helpful in delineating risk factors associated with the development of second malignancies. Prolonged use of alkylating agents combined with radiotherapy in ovarian cancer and in lymphomas have the strongest association with the subsequent development of acute leukemia. Fortunately, less intensive use of these modalities appears to be much less carcinogenic; however, this remains an important consideration in the use of systemic adjuvant chemotherapy in patients who have a high probability for prolonged survival.

VII. IMMUNOTHERAPY AND THE INTERFERON SYSTEM

Chemotherapy involves the administration of agents that are directly cytotoxic to tumor cells. One attractive alternative approach to controlling or eradicating malignancy is the utilization of the body's own immune system to "fight" malignant cells. Immunotherapy or "immune modulation" is a concept with great theoretical appeal and a firm and growing theoretical basis — unfortunately, it has received minimal clinical confirmation to establish its practical utility. In its present application, this modality appears to have only limited potency and it is not a standard therapy for any human malignancy. However, it remains an area of tremendous potential and one of great interest. Its theoretical attractiveness continues to encourage hope that if an effective immune adjuvant therapy could be developed, it might become a major feature of many anticancer regimens.

Whereas most chemotherapeutic agents affect both normal and malignant cells, the basic premise of immunotherapy is that malignant cells possess unique tumor antigens which distinguish them from normal cells. The concept of immune modulation of cancer cells is largely an outgrowth of the "theory of immune surveillance." This theory holds that the body's natural immune system, which protects against infection and rejects "foreign" material, can detect and control the appearance of a spontaneously appearing cancer cell or a small number of such cells [14]. The basic hypotheses of tumor immunotherapy may be stated as follows: (1) tumor cells have antigens that distinguish them from normal cells; (2) an immune response can be developed against these antigens; (3) an appropriate immune response can reduce tumor growth; and (4) modification of the host immune response can increase host resistance to tumor [15]. If these premises could be confirmed in human tumors, immunotherapy would be a nearly ideal therapeutic modality. It would be tumor specific and largely nontoxic, it would be systemic and affect disseminated microscopic sites of disease, and it would act on all tumor cells, whether they were dividing or at rest. Unfortunately, to date the results of immunotherapy trials in patients with cancer have been minimal. However, in some regards this is not surprising. When tested in a standard fashion in patients with large tumors, immunotherapy would not be expected to be very effective. The immune system has finite quantitative limits and immunotherapy's potential, if it is to be realized at all, would be greatest in patients with minimal tumor burdens. Ideally, immunotherapy probably will complement rather than supplant currently available modalities.

Immunotherapy may now be considered to be in its second or perhaps third phase of development [16]. At the turn of the century the first controlled application of immunotherapy was attempted in cancer patients. Prior anecdotal observations had noted that cancer patients sustaining infections occasionally had transient remissions or improved chances for long-term survival. The first clinical attempt to alter the immune system in cancer patients involved the administration of natural or killed bacterial products (e.g., Coley's toxins) which stimulated an antibacterial immune response in patients. In fact, tumor remissions and occasional long-term cures were reported following direct injection of immunostimulants into tumors. This type of immunotherapy is characterized as being "nonspecific"; that is, the immune system is activated against the bacteria or bacterial product and the tumor cells are affected as "innocent bystanders."

The agent most wisely used as a nonspecific immunostimulant is Bacille Calmette-Guerin (BCG), an attenuated bacterial strain which was originally developed at the turn of the century as an antituberculosis vaccine. This compound, its methanol-extracted residue (MER), another killed microorganism, Cornybacterium parvum, and the antihelminthic drug levamisole, are each potent general stimulants of the immune system. Antibody production, macrophage stimulation, and T- and B-cell lymphocyte stimulation may all follow their administration. These agents have each been tested extensively in animals with implanted tumors and have been administered to patients with a wide variety of malignant diseases. Animal studies show that pretreatment of mice and rats with these drugs may afford protection from a subsequent injection of a small number of malignant cells. However, they cannot prevent tumors from forming if large amounts of malignant cells are introduced. In animals with established tumors, administration of the drugs (particularly local injection directly into the tumor) can occasionally produce regression or disappearance of lesions. Unfortunately, immunotherapy trials in humans are not as definitive. They frequently have been poorly controlled and have rarely resulted in convincing data showing that immune manipulation has produced a real beneficial effect [16, 17]. The exceptions are a few studies in which immunostimulants have been injected directly into cutaneous or subcutaneous lesions (particularly in melanoma) and a study by Mathe in 1969 which showed that the administration of chemotherapy and BCG diminished the rate of relapse in children with leukemia. However, these results have not been confirmed by others. Studies of adjuvant immunotherapy in melanoma, lung, breast, and colon cancer have not been consistently successful and in those studies which do suggest that the immunotherapy is beneficial, the improvement in the survival rate has usually been minimal. Results of nonspecific immunotherapy in the setting of disseminated malignant disease have been poor [17].

A second thrust of immune modulation involves the development of "active specific" and "passive" immunotherapy. These modalities became feasible only as advances in cell biology occurred in a variety of related areas and as the tools necessary for readily testing these theories became available. The development of experimental animal tumor systems and the characterization of antigens associated with animal tumors made possible the direct testing of immunization against animal tumor implants described in Chap. 2. The results of immunotherapy in these animal systems have led to a renewed interest in applying immunotherapy in humans.

Active specific immunotherapy involves stimulating the immune system with tumor-specific antigens and this includes the development of antitumor vaccines or direct modification of tumor cells so that their antigens are exposed or presented in a manner that stimulates an enhanced immune response. Allogeneic tumor cell vaccines (derived from attenuated pooled human tumor cells) are under development for lung and breast carcinoma, sarcoma, leukemia, and malignant melanoma. Exposure of tumor cells in vitro to enzymes (e.g., neuraminidase) has been used to increase antigen exposure. These cells are then reintroduced to stimulate an immune response. Unfortunately, no clinical trial has shown conclusive benefit from the use of these techniques.

Passive immunotherapy involves the transfer to the tumor-bearing organism of immunologically active cells, sera, or other biological products which are specifically targeted against malignant cells. The passively transferred agent may be directly operational against the malignant cell or may be "informational" and specifically direct the host organism's immune system against the malignant cells. Transfer of sensitized cells is difficult since the body will reject foreign cells that are not identically matched by histocompatibility antigens. Use of whole antisera is not feasible for the same reason; that is, the antibodies in the sera will not be specifically directed against tumor antigens. The development of monoclonal antibodies may eventually play an important role in this scheme, but for now their potential in this area remains largely theoretical. To date, the avenues furthest pursued have involved the transfer of subcellular fractions of immune cells (e.g., immune RNA and transfer factor). These are felt to be informational and theoretically will induce a specific antitumor response in the host's immune system. Transfer factor is a dialyzed extract derived from the lysate of sensitized lymphocytes. Immune RNA is also extracted from previously sensitized lymphocytes and can confer specific antitumor immunity, at least in animal models. These modalities have a strong theoretical attraction, but serious problems have arisen in their practical application and both have questionable clinical utility at this time [18-20].

A. Interferon

Currently, the most publicized studies in immune modulation concern the use of interferon (IF). However, IF is not new, having been first described in 1957, and it is not a pure immune modulator. It is known to have a variety of mechanisms of action and only some of these involve the immune system.

IF was discovered through studies of "viral interference." This phenomenon represents the recognized capacity of one virus to inhibit or interfere with the replication of a second virus in the same tissue or the same host. In 1957, Issacs and Lindenmann noted that elimination of the viral particles themselves from the allantoic fluid of influenza-infected chick embryos did not inhibit the fluid's capacity to induce interference. They theorized that a soluble mediator was present and named it "interferon" [21]. Subsequently, this substance was identified as a protein and biological assays showed it to be present in most animal species, including chickens, mice, guinea pigs, rats, hamsters, parrots, dogs, sheep, cows, monkeys, and humans. It is now presumed that IF plays a major role in the intrinsic defenses of most organisms against viral infections. Under normal circumstances, therefore, interferon is a cell product formed in virus-infected cells during the course of viral replication. However, IF formation may also occur in cells exposed to incomplete or inactivated virus particles, as well as to some other biological products, as discussed below. No specific organ acts as a site for interferon production. Tissue cultures from the thymus, spleen, liver, lung, kidney, and brain as well as fetal tissues (amnion and chorion) have been shown to produce interferon.

Initial studies showed that IF clearly had antiviral properties, and consideration of potential antitumor activity was raised soon after its discovery. Unfortunately, for a number of reasons the testing of IF's antitumor activity in humans is only now becoming feasible. The greatest problem has been the difficulty of producing a quantity and quality of material suitable for clinical testing in humans. The problems involved include the species specificity of IF, the heterogeneity of IF, and the relative impurity of available material. It is important to emphasize that interferon is not a single substance. As an initial consideration, IF is species specific. The IF produced by different species is not identical; dog IF, for example, will not produce an antiviral effect in humans. For this reason, IF derived from animal material has not been used in human clinical trials. Furthermore, within any one species the nature of IF depends on its cell of origin and the type of agent used to induce its production. In humans, three main types of IF have been identified based on their cell of origin: leukocyte (α), fibroblast (β), and lymphoblastoid IF (γ). How these three differ clinically remains to be determined [22].

The type of IF produced also depends on the inducing agent. Conventionally, viruses or double-stranded RNA inducers, such as polyriboinosinic acid-polyridocytidilic acid (poly I:C), have been used to generate IF. However, immunocompetent cells may also be stimulated to produce IF by unrelated substances such as phytohemagglutinin, concanclavin A, pokeweek mitogen, antilymphocyte sera, and C. parvum. The resulting IF differs both physically and antigenically from virally produced material and appears to be a separate entity. However, the clinical significance of these differences is also unknown. The majority of early clinical cancer trials with IF used leukocyte-derived IF supplied by the Finnish Red Cross Center and prepared from leukocytes harvested from normal blood donors. However, questions have arisen as to the contamination of this material with fibroflast IF as well as with other serum proteins. Recently, the availability of large amounts of homogeneous IF obtained from recombinant DNA introduced into bacteria or cultured cells has allowed the initiation of large-scale clinical testing of high-quality IF.

At this time the potential of interferon as an antitumor agent remains unknown. In vitro studies of IF indicate that its addition to cells growing in culture can have significant biological effects. IF can inhibit the growth of white blood cell precursors in a dose-dependent fashion and it can inhibit the growth of cell lines derived from human malignancies such as various leukemias and lymphomas, osteosarcoma, malignant myeloma, and adenocarcinomas of the colon, breast, and prostate [22]. IF has also shown "activity" in animal tumor models, but these studies warrant careful examination. Because of the known antiviral effects of IF, initial studies were done in animal tumors with a viral etiology. Experimental animal tumors exist in which tumors can be predictably induced by the introduction of oncogenic virus. In this setting, pretreatment of susceptible animals with IF, prior to inoculation with the virus, can prevent tumor formation. However, other studies have shown IF to afford minimal or no improvement in survival when given in similar experimental conditions. Other experimental models also give encouraging but guarded results. Some in-bred strains of animals have a very high incidence of spontaneously developing malignancies, presumably of viral etiology (e.g., AKR mice). Treatment of these animals with IF from the time of birth can result in a diminished incidence of malignancies and prolonged survival rates. When IF is administered to animals after the transplantation of viable tumor cells, it can result in tumor regression, but the antitumor activity is inversely proportional to the number of cells inoculated. The majority of positive anticancer results in animal studies have occurred with IF as "prophylaxis" and few have shown actual regression of established tumors. Furthermore, few studies have looked at the effects of combined IF and cytotoxic drugs.

Clinical anticancer studies utilizing interferon remain limited. The first clinical study in humans was done at Sweden's Karolinska Institute in 1971. Patients with the bone tumor osteosarcoma were given IF as adjuvant therapy following surgical resection. A decreased rate of subsequent relapses was reported for the 33 patients entered into the study [23]. However, this was not a prospectively randomized study (patients' relapse rates were compared only to historical controls and contemporary patients treated at other Swedish hospitals), the numbers were small, and other questions have been raised (e.g., challenges as to the original histological diagnoses) which make these results far from definitive. Recently, a more conventional phase II study of IF was conducted at the M.D. Anderson Hospital [24]. In this study antitumor activity (disease regression) was reported in patients with breast cancer (7/17), multiple myeloma (6/10), and lymphoma (6/11). Only two patients had complete responses (complete disappearance of their measurable tumor); however, these represent the most encouraging clinical results to date. Other studies are ongoing to confirm these results and define the range of clinical settings in which this agent might have real activity. In early reports of phase I and II clinical trials of recombinant DNA-derived interferon, activity has been seen against renal cell carcinoma, Kaposi's sarcoma, multiple myeloma, melanoma, lymphoma, mycosis fungoides, and chronic lymphocytic leukemia [25-31].

Interferon's antitumor activity is believed to arise from three possible mechanisms of action: (1) inhibition of tumor viruses and cell transformation, (2) direct inhibition of tumor growth (i.e., a cytostatic effect), and (3) indirect inhibition of tumor growth via immune mechanisms. The initial rationale for studying IF as an antitumor agent was based on its antiviral action and, indeed, IF can inhibit the multiplication of tumor viruses. However, this theory alone has limited utility as an explanation of interferon's anticancer mechanism. First, in some studies in mice with the Friend leukemia virus, although proliferation of leukemia cells can be reduced, the replication of the Friend virus itself is unaffected. More important, although viruses can induce some experimental animal tumors and although a viral etiology has been suspected in some human tumors, no human tumor has ever been proven to be caused by an oncogenic virus. Other possible explanations of interferon's anticancer activity have recently become more attentive. IF may be directly cytostatic. The addition of IF to tumor cells growing in culture can slow growth and can suppress the incorporation of [^{3}H] thymidine into DNA. Since IF can alter cellular enzymes (e.g., nucleases and phosphorylases), it has been proposed that IF may be a direct inhibitor of DNA synthesis through this mechanism. As a separate property, IF can alter the plasma membrane. Cells treated with IF have been shown to have an altered surface charge and an altered expression of some surface antigens. Perhaps as a direct result of plasma membrane alterations or as a result of effects of cell cycling, there is also some suggestion that IF may module the activity of other chemotherapeutic agents [32, 33]. Finally, IF may exert antitumor effects as an immune modulator. IF has several significant effects on the immune system. IF-treated macrophages show enhanced phagocytosis and IF administration can enhance the cytotoxicity of sensitized lymphocytes as well as augment natural killer (NK) activity. The cell surface changes caused by IF may also increase the immune system's recognition of malignant cells. For these reasons, IF remains an area of major interest. The immediate prospect of generating pure exogenous IF through recombinant DNA technology or stimulating endogenous IF through interferon-inducing drugs holds out the promise that the mechanisms of action and clinical activity of this compound may be much more fully appreciated in the near future.

REFERENCES

1. C.G. Zubrod, Semin. Oncol., 6: 490-505 (1979).
2. V.T. DeVita, V.T. Oliverio, F.M. Muggia, P.W. Wiernik, J. Ziegler, A. Goldin, D. Rubin, J. Henney, and S. Schepartz, Cancer Clin. Trials, 2: 195-216 (1979).
3. C.G. Zubrod, Med. Pediatr. Oncol., 8: 107-114 (1980).
4. R. Baserga, N. Engl. J. Med., 304: 453-459 (1981).
5. R. Baserga, Multiplication and Division in Mammallian Cells, Marcel Dekker, New York, 1976.
6. B.A. Chabner, C.E. Myers, C.N. Coleman, and D.G. Johns, N. Engl. J. Med., 292: 1107-1113, 1159-1168 (1975).
7. S.S. Legha, H. L. Davis, and F. M. Muggia, Ann. Intern. Med., 88: 69-77 (1978).
8. F.M. Muggia, Cancer Clin. Trials, 1: 139-144 (1978).
9. F.M. Muggia, M. Rosencweig, D.F. Chiuten, M.S. Jensen-Akula, L.M. Charles, Jr., T.T. Kubota, V.M Bono, Jr., Cancer Treat. Rep., 64: 1-9 (1980).
10. P.J. Creaven and E. Mihich, Semin. Oncol., 4: 147-163 (1977).

11. R.H. Blum and E. Freti, Methods Cancer Res., 27: 215 (1979).
12. R. Spiegel, Cancer Treat. Rev., 8: 197-207 (1981).
13. W.J. Harrington, Ann. Intern. Med., 24: 141-155 (1979).
14. Y.A. Pilch, G.H. Myers, F.C. Sparks, and S.H. Golub, Curr. Probl. Surg., 1-61 (1975).
15. J.L. Fahey, S. Brosman, R.C. Ossorio, C. O'Toole, and J. Zighelboim, Ann. Intern. Med., 84: 454-465 (1976).
16. F.M. Muggia, Cancer Immunol. Immunother., 3: 5-9 (1977).
17. S.K. Carter, Cancer Immunol. Immunother., 1: 275-281 (1976).
18. A.F. LoBuglio and J.A. Neidhart, Med. Clin. N. Am., 60: 585-590 (1976).
19. Y.A. Pilch and J. B. DeKernion, Semin. Oncol., 1: 387-395 (1978).
20. H. Walters (ed.), Handbook of Cancer Immunology, Garcand, New York, 1978.
21. A. Issacs and J. Lindenmann, Proc. R. Soc., 147: 258-267 (1957).
22. T.J. Priestman, Cancer Treat Rev., 6: 223-237 (1979).
23. H. Strander, Blut, 35: 279-299 (1977).
24. J.V. Gutterman, G.R. Blumenschein, and R. Alexanian, Ann. Intern. Med., 93: 399-406 (1980).
25. S.E. Krown, A.I. Einzig, J.D. Abramson, and H.F. Oettgen, Proc. Am. Soc. Clin. Oncol., 2: 58 (1983).
26. R.D. Leavitt, V. Rantanatharathorn, H. Ozer, S. Rudnick, and R. Ferraresi, Proc. Am. Soc. Clin. Oncol., 2: 54 (1983).
27. J. Costanzi, R. Pollard, M. Ascherl, P. Medellin, J. Bell, J. Gluckian, J. Mokanson, Proc. Am. Soc. Clin. Oncol., 2: 46 (1983).
28. M.S. Ernstoff, M. Reiss, C.A. Davis, S.A. Rudnick, and J.M. Kirkwood, Proc. Am. Soc. Clin. Oncol., 2: 57 (1983).
29. E.T. Creagan, D.L. Ahmann, S.J. Green, A.J. Schutt, J. Rubin, H.J. Long, S. Fein, and J.R. O'Fallon, Proc. Am. Soc. Clin. Oncol., 2: 58 (1983).
30. S. Sherwin, D. Longo, P. Bunn, Jr., S. Fein, P. Abrams, J. Olms, C. Schoenberger, J. Parkis, and R. Oldman, Proc. Am. Soc. Clin. Oncol., 2: 211 (1983).
31. P. Volberding, M. Gottleib, J. Rothman, S. Rudwick, M. Conant, M. Derezin, W. Weinstein, and J. Groopman, Proc. Am. Soc. Clin. Oncol., 2: 53 (1983).
32. C. Welander, J. Gaines, H. Homesley, and S. Rudnick, Proc. Am. Soc. Clin. Oncol., 2: 42 (1983).
33. R.L. Stolfi, D.S. Martin, R.C. Sawyer, and S. Spiegelman, Cancer Res., 43: 561-566 (1983).

2

EVALUATION OF POTENTIAL ANTINEOPLASTIC AGENTS

RUTH I. GERAN*

National Cancer Institute
National Institutes of Health
Bethesda, Maryland

---

*Retired

I. INTRODUCTION

In 1955 the National Cancer Institute (NCI) started a large evaluation program, using rodent cancer models, in an attempt to select systematically the chemicals and natural materials with the best probability of being most beneficial to cancer patients. Since that time over half a million materials have been evaluated in this program.

The NCI anticancer evaluation program has evolved through the years, with the constant awareness of the need to incorporate new ideas into testing techniques and to try different preclinical models in the ideas into testing techniques and to try different preclinical models in the light of new evidence. The models used initially were selected on the basis of a report edited by A. Gellhorn and E. Hirschberg which reviewed the results of a study, organized by the American Cancer Society in 1953, in which 74 assays for evaluating anticancer agents were investigated. The objective of the Gellhorn-Hirschberg report was to provide information for the selection of screening models by the National Cancer Institute, which was about to launch its large systematic anticancer drug development program. Many of the assays reviewed had been developed by earlier in vivo screening programs, including those at the Sloan-Kettering Institute, the National Cancer Institute, the Cancer Institute in Moscow, the Chester Beatty Research Institute, the Children's Cancer Research Foundation, the Southern Research Institute, and the University of Tokyo. The Gellhorn-Hirschberg report concluded that there was not evidence at that time (1955) that any of the 59 microbiological, developmental, or biochemical "non-tumor" systems described in that report could replace a tumor system as a screening tool for carcinostatic agents; that they found no single tumor system that could select all useful anticancer agents; and that there was a need for more extensive studies of antitumor compounds at the clinical level [1]. Because of information derived from the Gellhorn-Hirschberg report, the screen of the Cancer Chemotherapy National Service Center (CCNSC) of the National Cancer Institute consisted in 1955 of three mouse models—sarcoma 180, leukemia L1210, and carcinoma 755—with additional models available for special purposes [2, 3]. These three principal models were chosen because they represented the basic types of malignancies, because all agents considered clinically useful at that time were active in at least one of these models, and because all three of the models were needed to select the clinically active agents of that period. However, the three-model panel was considered an interim screen, and developmental studies to explore better screening systems were also initiated at that time [4].

By 1960 it had been observed that almost all new agents active in the three-model panel had been active in the leukemia L1210 model. L1210 was therefore retained, but sarcoma 180 and carcinoma 755 were replaced in the hope that new assays might detect different chemical types of agents inactive in the previous screen. The emphasis at that time was on finding agents for leukemia (rather than for solid tumors) since in leukemia there is a higher percentage of proliferating cells than in solid tumors and therefore leukemia patients and models were expected to respond more readily to chemotherapy. In 1965 CCNSC was integrated into the overall cancer chemotherapy program of the National Cancer Institute and the screen was reduced to two models: L1210 leukemia and Walker carcinosarcoma 256 in rat. This two-model panel was adopted because a retrospective study had shown that all clinically useful cytotoxic agents at that time except mithramycin were detected by one or both of these models [5]. By 1968 it had been observed that the Walker carcinsarcoma 256 model was too sensitive and, since several agents were in development because of their activity in the Walker carcinosarcoma 256 model, use of this model was curtailed [6]. Synthetic compounds were then tested only in L1210 leukemia, and natural products were tested in L1210 leukemia plus P388 leukemia, which was considered somewhat more sensitive than the L1210 model. Over 120 models (in vivo and in vitro) used by the program by 1972 are described in Appendix II of the 1972 protocols for screening [7].

The present (1981) evaluation system of the Division of Cancer Treatment was initiated in 1975 and has been described in many recent published reports [6-13]. The tumor panel consists of eight cancer models in mice: five transplanted mouse tumors and three human tumors implanted under the kidney capsules of mice. In addition, the mouse P388 leukemia model is used as a prescreen to select new chemical structures for tumor panel evaluation. These nine models are described in detail in Table 2.1. It became possible for this new panel to include human tumors because, while rejected if implanted subcutaneously into normal mice, human-tumor xenografts could be grown in immune-deficient athymic mice implanted either subcutaneously or under the kidney capsule. Athymic mice are often referred to as "nude" mice because the same gene modification responsible for athymia also reduces hair growth. The panel with this increased number of diverse models was chosen because of a new emphasis on developing therapy for solid tumors which are clinically much more prevalent than leukemia and in the hope that broad-spectrum preclinical activity may be more predictive for clinical efficacy than preclinical activity in any one model.

Thus the anticancer evaluation program of the National Cancer Institute has constantly evolved through the years, with each modification based on a rational decision, and it no doubt will continue to develop as additional experience is gained and new opportunities present themselves.

II. EVALUATION OF POTENTIAL ANTINEOPLASTIC AGENTS IN THE DIVISION OF CANCER TREATMENT OF THE NATIONAL CANCER INSTITUTE

Both rationally designed and randomly offered materials are important in the Division of Cancer Treatment (DCT) program. Resources are being devoted to the search for and development of less toxic analogs of clinically

TABLE 2.1 Nine Murine in Vivo Models Currently Being Validated by the U.S.A. National Cancer Institute

---

Colon CX-1 adenocarcinoma (human) originated as a surgical explant from the primary conon tumor of a 44-year-old woman with no previous chemotherapy. The tumor line is carried in athymic mice subcutaneously in the axillary region. Typical test tumor is moderately well differentiated adenocarcinoma consistent with gastrointestinal origin. For testing the tumor fragment is implanted under the kidney capsule of athymic mice [either N:NIH(S)-nu or BALB/cAnN-nu, both of which are the product of backcrossing a heterozygous female with a homozygous male for 10 generations]. The test agent is administered subcutaneously in the nape of the neck every fourth day for four injections starting 24 hr after tumor implant. On day 15 after tumor implant the change in tumor mass is determined. A confirmed test with a mean tumor weight change not more than 20% of that of the control is considered moderately active, and not more than 10% of that of the control is considered to show good activity.

Colon 38 carcinoma (mouse) was originally induced in 1973 by repeated subcutaneous injections of 1,2-dimethylhydrazine. Typical test tumor shows an epithelial/stromal ratio of 80:5 with 15% hemorrhage or necrosis. Epithelium contains immature or rudimentay acini and rosettes. For testing, the tumor fragment is implanted subcutaneously in the axillary region of either B6D2F1 mice (which are products of a cross between female C57B1/6N and male dBA2N) or B6C3F1 mice (products of a cross between female C57BL/6N and male C3H/HeNMTV). The test agent is administered intraperitoneally on day 2 and day 9 after tumor implant. On day 20 tumor weights are determined from caliper measurements. A confirmed test with a median tumor weight not more than 42% of that of the control is considered moderately active, and not more than 10% of that of the control indicates good activity.

Leukemia L1210 (mouse) was originally induced in 1948 in spleen and lymph nodes of a mouse by painting skin with methylcholanthrene. For testing, 10^5 tumor cells are injected intraperitoneally into CD2F1 mice (products of cross between female BALB/cANN and male DBA2N) and the test agent is administered intraperitoneally daily for 9 days starting 24 hr after tumor implant. The median survival time of the test mice is compared to that of the control mice and a confirmed increased life span of at least 25% shows moderate activity, while a confirmed increased life span of at least 50% indicates good activity.

Leukemia P388 (mouse) was originally induced in 1955 in a DBA/2 mouse by painting with methylcholanthrene. For testing, 10^6 P388 leukemia cells are implanted intraperitoneally into CD2F1 mice (the products of a cross

TABLE 2.1 (Continued)

---

between a female BALB/cAnN and a male DBA2N), and the test agents are administered intraperitoneally daily for 5 days. The median survival time of the test mice is compared to that of the control mice and a confirmed increased life span of at least 20% for a synthetic compound or of at least 30% for a natural product is construed as moderate activity, and a confirmed increased life span of at least 75% is required to be regarded as good activity.

Lung Lewis carcinoma (mouse) arose spontaneously in 1951 as carcinoma of the lung in a C57BL/6 mouse. Typical test tumor is composed of sheets of polyhedral cells with little intervening stroma. For testing, 10^6 cells are injected into the tail vein of B6C3F1 mice (the products of a cross between a female C75BL/6N and a male C3H/HeNMTV) and the test agent is administered intraperitoneally daily for 9 days starting 24 hr after tumor implant. The median survival time of the test group is compared to that of the control and a confirmed increased life span of at least 40% indicates moderate activity, while a confirmed increased life span of at least 50% is considered to show good activity.

Lung LX-1 carcinoma (human) originated in April 1975 as a surgical explant from a subcutaneous metastatic tumor of the right arm of a 48-year-old man with oat cell lung carcinoma who had been treated in February 1975 with *C. parvum*, cytoxan, and radiation. The tumor line is carried in athymic mice subcutaneously in the axillary region. Typical test tumor consists of poorly differentiated carcinoma composed of nests of various sizes of tumor cells, with numerous mitotic figures, and with no evidence of mucin production or gland formation. For testing, the tumor fragment is implanted under the kidney capsule of athymic mice [either N:NIH (S)-nu or BALB/cAnN-nu, both of which are the product of backcrossing a heterozygous female with a homozygous male for 10 generations]. The test agents are administered subcutaneously in the nape of the neck every fourth day for three injections starting 24 hr after tumor implant. On day 11 after tumor implant the changein tumor mass is determined. A confirmed test with a mean tumor weight change not more than 20% of that of the control is considered moderately active, and not more than 10% of that of the control is considered to show good activity.

Mammary CD8F1 adenocarcinoma (mouse) tumors arise spontaneously in CD8F1 female mice (which are the product of a cross between a female of an inbred virus-infected colony of BALB/c-CMC and a male of an inbred colony of DBA/8-CMC). First-generation transplants of the excised spontaneous tumors are used for testing. For testing, 0.3 ml of a 1:20 tumor brei (prepared from a minimum of four spontaneous tumors) is implanted

TABLE 2.1 (Continued)

subcutaneously in the axillary region. Staging day is when tumors can be selected within the range 100 to 700 mg. On that day test agents are administered as a single injection intraperitoneally, with no further treatment. Seven days later median tumor weight changes are determined. A confirmed test change to no more than 20% of that of the control is considered to be moderately active while a confirmed test with a change not more than 0% of the control is construed to show good activity. The acceptable control median tumor weight range on final evaluation day is 400-2000 mg.

Mammary MX-1 carcinoma (human) originated in 1974 as a surgical explant from the primary mammary tumor of a 29-year-old woman with no previous chemotherapy. The tumor line is carried in athymic mice subcutaneously in the axillary region. Typical test tumor is poorly differentiated mammary carcinoma, highly cellular with no evidence of gland formation or mucin production. For testing the tumor fragment is implanted under the kidney capsule of athymic mice [either N:NIH(S)-nu or BALB/CANN-nu, both of which are the product of backcrossing a heterozygous female and a homozygous male for 10 generations]. For testing, the agents are administered subcutaneously in the nape of the neck every fourth day for three injections starting 24 hr after tumor implant. On day 11 after tumor implant the change in tumor mass is determined. A confirmed test with a mean tumor weight change of not more than 20% of that of the control is considered moderately active, and not more than 10% of that of the control is considered to show good activity.

Melanoma B16 (mouse) arose spontaneously in 1954 on the skin at the base of the ear in a C57BL/6 mouse. Typical test tumor shows about 70% melanoblasts with indistinct boundaries, about 20% hemorrhage and necrosis, about 10% stromal elements with capillaries, numerous mitotic figures, and pigment granules scattered throughout. In testing, 0.5 ml of a 1:10 tumor brei is implanted intraperitoneally in B6C3F1 mice (products of a cross between female C57BL/6N and male C3H/HeNMTV) and the test agents are administered intraperitoneally daily for 9 days starting 24 hr after tumor implant. The median survival time of the test is compared to that of the control and a test with a confirmed increased life span at least 25% longer than that of its control is considered moderately active, while a test with a confirmed increased life span at least 50% longer than its control is construed to show good activity.

effective agents such as adriamycin and cis-platinum, and these new analogs initially receive special testing in direct comparison with the parent compound. At the same time much effort is also being invested in the evaluation of randomly offered materials representing leads to new chemical types of agents that have the possibility of being effective clinically without concomitant toxicity. It is recognized that some of the current promising leads originally entered into the NCI evaluation program as materials with very little promise as anticancer agents.

A. Acquisition

Materials enter the Division of Cancer Treatment evaluation program from many diverse sources, including industrial, agricultural, and pharmaceutical companies, government agencies, universities, and individual scientists.

Figure 1 shows the number of new materials being acquired annually for anticancer evaluation. Evaluation of the approximately 5000 crude natural products is more complex than the testing of the 13,000 to 14,000 annual new synthetic compounds which is described here; this is because it is necessary to fractionate an active crude material product sample several times in order to isolate the purified active ingredient so that it can be identified.

It was estimated that 353,881 new chemicals were produced, worldwide, during the year 1980 [14]. Since only 300 to 500 materials can be tested annually in the eight-model tumor panel, careful consideration is given to the selection of the materials that are subjected to tumor-panel testing. The usual procedure for NCI selection of the 300 to 500 materials for tumor-panel testing is as follows. First, when a material comes to the attention of the Drug Synthesis and Chemistry Branch of the Division of Cancer Treatment (DCT), NCI staff determines if the compound has not been tested before, and NCI committees determine if the structure is sufficiently different from structures already in the program

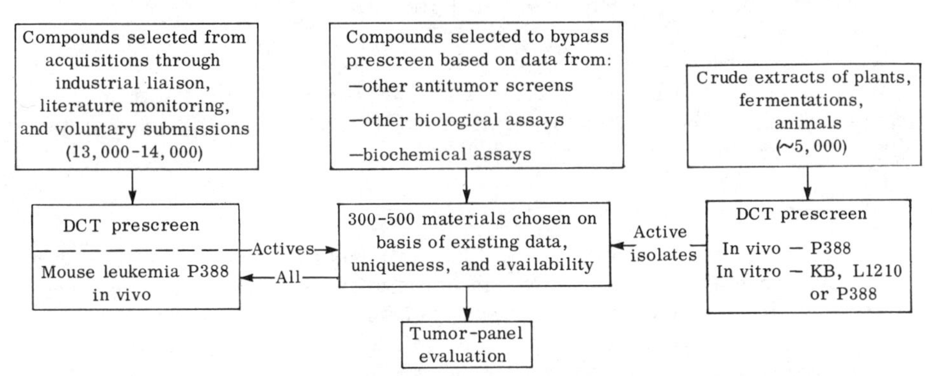

FIGURE 2.1 Number of new materials acquired annually for anticancer evaluation.

and if the biological information available warrants immediate tumor-panel testing without waiting for intervening data from the P388 leukemia prescreen. For example, compounds reported by the offerer to be effective against other human diseases, or compounds reported to have biological activity that could be associated with anticancer capability, can be accepted immediately for tumor-panel testing and for simultaneous testing in the P388 leukemia model if an adequate supply of the compound can be obtained. The approximate amount of material required for testing in all nine models is (in milligrams) 180 times the optimum dose (mg/kg per injection) when given intraperitoneally daily for 5 days. That is, if the optimum dose intraperitoneally for five injections were 50 mg/kg per injection, approximately 9 g would be needed for tumor-panel testing and for the P388 leukemia prescreen.

Second, in an attempt to select rationally additional chemical structures for tumor-panel testing, NCI chemists choose approximately 13,500 synthetic compounds annually to submit to biological testing in the P388 leukemia in vivo prescreen in an effort to find new chemical structures that reproducibly increase the median life span of the treated tumored mice at least 20% longer than that of their untreated control tumored mice. The synthetic compounds that are accepted for P388 prescreening are those that are sufficiently different chemically from compounds previously tested in the DCT evaluation program and that are predicted by the NCI staff with the assistance of mathematical modeling [15, 16] to have a reasonable probability of activity in the P388 prescreen. Approximately 100,000 compounds of known chemical structures have now been tested in the P388 mouse leukemia model: this exceptionally large amount of biological and chemical information affords an unusual opportunity for a computer-aided system to estimate statistically the probability of P388 activity of a candidate compound based on the biological activity of its substructural features as they appeared in previously tested compounds. A sample of 0.6-1.5 g is required for testing in the P388 leukemia prescreen if the optimum dose of the compound has not been established previously.

If a compound is chosen by the DCT selection procedures, the offerer is invited to submit a sample. It is then assigned an identifying NSC number such as those shown in Table 2.2. The "NSC" series originated from the name of the 1955 evaluation program at the NCI, the Cancer Chemotherapy National Service Center.

B. Mouse Leukemia P388 in Vivo Prescreen

The purpose of the prescreen is to find new chemical structures for tumor-panel testing. The P388 leukemia model is used as the prescreen because it is sensitive to many different types of chemical structures, and at the same time it is insensitive to over 90% of the test agents subjected to it. On a year-by-year basis since 1975 the P388 model has indicated moderately active 4.4-7.9% (an average of 5.9%) of the new synthetic agents. These active materials have a diversity of chemical structures.

TABLE 2.2 Selected Clinical Anticancer Agents

Common name	Chemical name	NSC
Adriamycin	L-lyxo-[Hexopyranoside-3-β-glycoloyl-[1, 2, 3, 4, 6, 11]-hexahydro-3, 5, 12-trihydroxy-10-methoxy-6, 11-dioxo-1-α-naphthalacenyl-3-amino-2, 3, 6-trideoxy-α-hydrochloride	123127
Asparaginase	Asparaginase, L-	109229
Bleomycin	Bleomycin sulfate: a mixture of glycopeptide antigiotics iso	125066
Carmustine	Urea, 1, 3-bis(2-chloroethyl)-1-nitroso-	409962
Chlorambucil	Butyric acid, 4-[_-[bis(2-chloroethyl)amino]paenyl]-	3088
cis-platinum	Platinum, diamoninodichloro-, (SP-4-2)-	119875
Cytosar	Cytosine, 1-β-D-arabinofuranosyl-, monohydrochloride	63878
Cytoxan	2H-1, 3, 2-Oxazaphosphorine, 2-[bis(2-chloroethyl)amino]-tetrahydro-,	26271
Dacarbazine	Imidazole-4-carboxamide, 5-(3, 3-dimethyl-]-triazeno)-	45388
Dactinomycin	Actinomycin D. specific stereoisomer of N, N'-[(2-amino-4, 6-dimethyl-3-oxo-3A-phenoxazine-1, 9-diyl)-bis[carbonylimino (2-hydroxypropylidene)carbonyliminoisobutylidene-carbonyl b a [N-methyl-L-valine]dilactone	3053

TABLE 2.2 (Continued)

Common name	Chemical name	NSC
Daunomycin	L-lyxo-hexopyranoside, 3-β-acetyl-[1,2,3,4,6,11]-hexahydro-3,5,12-trihydroxy-10-methoxy-6,11-dioxo-1-α-naphthacenyl-3-amino-2,3,6-trideoxy-α-hydrochloride	82151
Fluorouracil	Uracil, 5-fluoro-	19893
Hydroxyurea	Urea, hydroxy-	32065
Lomustine	Urea, 1-(2-chloroethyl)-3-cyclohexyl-1-nitroso-	79037
Melphalan	Alanine, 3-p-[bis(2-chloroethyl)amino]phenyl-monohydrochloride, L-	8806
Mercaptopurine	Purine-6-thiol, monohydrate	755
Methotrexate	Glutamic acid, N-p-[2,4-diamino-6-pteridinyl)methyl]-amino benzoyl-	740

Mithramycin	Antibiotic produced by Streptomyces	24559
Mitomycin C	Azirino-[2',3':3,4]-pyrroloale[1,2-a]-indole-4,7-dione,6-amino-1, 1a, 2,8,8a,8b-hexahydro-8-(hydroxymethyl)-8a-methoxy-5-methyl-, carbamate (ester)	26980
Mustargen	Diethylamine, 2,2'-dichloro-N-methyl-, hydrochloride	762
Myleran	1,4-Butanediol, dimethanesulfonate	750
Procarbazine	p-Toluamide, N-isopropyl-α-(2-methylhydrazino)-, hydrochloride	77213
Semustine	Urea, 1-(2-chloroethyl)-3-(4-methylcyclohexyl)-1-nitroso-, trans-	95441
Streptozotocin	D-Glucose, 2-deoxy-2-(3-methyl-3-nitrosoureido)-	85998
Thioguanine	Purine-6-thiol, 2-amino-	752
Thiotepa	Phosphine sulfide, tris(1-aziridinyl)-	6396
Vinblastine	Vincaleukoblastine, sulfate, hydrate	49842
Vincristine	Leurocristine, sulfate (1:1)	67574

Unless dose levels are suggested by the supplier, each new synthetic compound in the prescreen is tested initially at 200, 100, and 50 mg/kg per injection intraperitoneally for 5 days. Testing is performed at one of the many laboratories under contract to the National Cancer Institute: examples are Battelle Columbus Laboratories in Ohio, Arthur D. Little in Massachusetts, Southern Research Institute in Alabama, ITT Research Institute in Illinois, and Mason Research Institute in Massachusetts. In an effort to ensure the reproducibility of data from all contract laboratories, since any biological system has inherent biological variations, very careful quality control of all rodent models is required. For example, NCI contract laboratories receive from the NCI frozen tumor bank a replacement of the P388 leukemia every 2 months since, with age, a tumor line carried in vivo may change its drug-sensitivity pattern. Also, in order for each P388 leukemia experiment to be considered satisfactory, its control group (of about 30 mice) must have a median survival time between day 9 and day 13 after tumor implant, it must have a specified number of survivors (approximately 90%) on day 7, it must have a specified number of deaths (approximately 90%) by day 18, and the test group (of six mice) that receives the positive control drug, 5-fluorouracil, in every odd-numbered experiment must have a median life span at least 35% longer than the control group. Computerized scatter diagrams of the responses of all control mice from all contract laboratories are reviewed every 3 months.

Within approximately 4 months a computerized data report is sent to the supplier, evaluating the response of the material in the P388 prescreen. Inactive materials receive no further evaluation; the cost to the NCI of testing an inactive compound in the P388 prescreen in 1981 is approximately $184, and there is no charge to the compound's supplier. A material initially active is retested to confirm the activity in a different experiment. A material with confirmed activity in the P388 prescreen progresses through the NCI systematic committee-review procedure, and if its structure is deemed to be sufficiently different from existing panel compounds, it is accepted for tumor-panel testing.

C. Tumor-Panel Testing

The tumor panel consists of eight cancer models in mice—five transplanted mouse tumors and three human tumors implanted under the kidney capsules of mice. These models are described on Table 2.1, listed in alphabetical order by malignancy site of origin or type. Shown for each model is a description of the tumor, the site of tumor implant for testing, the usual testing host strain, the route and schedule of drug administration, the parameter of evaluation, and the criteria of confirmed responses (percent test compared to control) used by the National Cancer Institute to discern good activity and moderate activity of agents. More detailed protocols for these models may be obtained from the Screening Section, Drug Evaluation Branch, DCT, NCI.

In this tumor panel an attempt has been made to pair a transplanted mouse tumor with a human xenograft tumor for several specific malignancies—colon, breast, and lug, since these are the most common sites of human malignancies. The purpose of pairing models is to determine whether human cancer tissue predicts for clinical therapy better than mouse cancer tissue does.

In addition to the "screening" for activity of previously untested materials, activity-evaluation anticancer rodent models are used for many other purposes: studies, for example, to investigate the best route and schedule for administering a specific compound, to rank structural analogs [17], to rank compounds of diverse chemical structures [18, 19], or to investigate the possibility of enhancing effectiveness by the concomitant use of more than one compound [20].

Examples of tumor-panel evaluations are shown on Table 2.3. The 28 compounds listed on Table 2.2 and evaluated on Table 2.3 were selected (from among the approximately 40 agents now used clinically) to serve as examples of types of agents described in other chapters of this book. The drugs are listed on Table 2.3 according to the chapter in this book to which they are most closely related. That is, natural products have been grouped together as related to Chap. 4, antimetabolites including an antifol as well as compounds similar to purines and pyrimidines have been grouped together as related to Chap. 6, alkylating agents are designated as related to Chap. 7, nitrosoureas and amide-related compounds have been grouped together as related to Chap. 8, and cis-platinum is designated as related to the Chap. 9 metals.

The evaluations on Table 2.3 may change in the future since testing is still in progress. Note that for both ratings A and B, the NCI criteria shown in Table 2.1 were met on the drug regimen indicated, in two separate experiments, and in the first six models, confirmation was at a second laboratory.

Although firm conclusions cannot be stated until the tumor-panel testing is completed, the present Table 2.3 data seems to form patterns. In general (looking at the data for all 28 agents), the leukemia P388 and leukemia L1210 models are the most sensitive, and the colon CX-1 model is the least sensitive of the nine models; and (looking at the data for all nine models), cis-platinum (the Chap. 9 compound) is the most active, with good activity in eight of the nine models, and asparaginase and bleomycin (Chap. 4) and myleran (Chap. 7) are the least active of the 28 compounds, with good activity in none of the nine models so far, as tested with the schedules and drug routes specified. None of the Table 2.3 agents that were active in any model were inactive in P388 leukemia. Some of the Table 2.3 agents related to Chap. 4 (dactinomycin, mithramycin, vincristine, and adriamycin) were more active in the human LX-1 lung model than in the mouse Lewis lung model: however, this pattern is not seen with the other Table 2.3 agents. Twenty-two of the twenty-eight Table 2.3 agents show good confirmed activity in at least two of the nine models.

TABLE 2.3 Preliminary Evaluation[a] of 28 Selected Clinical Anticancer Agents in Nine Murine Cancer Models

	Prescreen	Conventional tumor panel					Xenograft tumor panel					
Model:	Leukemia P388, i.p.	Melanoma B16, i.p.	Mammary CD8F1, s.c.	Colon 38, s.c.	Leukemia L1210, i.p.	Lung Lewis, i.v.	Colon CX-1, src		Lung LX-1, src		Mammary MX-1, src	
Number and site of drug injections:	9 i.p.	9 i.p.	1 i.p.	2 i.p.	9 i.p.	9 i.p.	4 s.c.	10 s.c.	3 s.c.	10 s.c.	3 s.c.	10 s.c.
Agents related to Chap. 4												
Dactinomycin	A	A	A	B	B	-		A		B		A
Mithramycin	B	-		-	-	-	-	-	-	A	+-	A
Mitomycin C	A	A	A	B	A	-						
Vinblastine	A	A		A	B	-		-		-	-	+-
Vincristine	A	A		-	B	-		-		A		A
Daunomycin	A	A		-	A	-		-		-		-
Asparaginase	B	-			-	-						
Adriamycin	A	A	A	+-	A	+-	+-	+-	A	A	-	A
Bleomycin	B	-	B	B	-	B	-	-	-	B	-	B
Agents related to Chap. 6												
Methotrexate	A	-		B	A	+-		-		C		-
Thioguanine	B	-		A	A	-		-		-		-
Mercaptopurine	B	-		A	A	-		-		-		-

Fluorouracil	A	B	A	A	A	+-		-		-		-
Cytosar	A	B	-	B	A	B		-		-		A
Agents related to Chap. 7												
Myleran	-	-			-	-		-		-		-
Mustargen	A	A			A	-		-		-		A
Chlorambucil	B	B		-	B	-		-		-		A
Thiotepa	A	B			A	-		-		-		A
Melphalan	A	A	A	A	A	B		A		A	A	A
Cytotoxan	A	A	A		A			-	-	B	A	A
Agents related to Chap. 8												
Hydroxyurea	B	-		-	A	-	-		-	-		-
Dacarbazine	B	A		B	A	B		-	A	A		B
Procarbazine	B	C			A	B		-	A	A		A
Lomustine	A	A	A	A	A	A	-	-	A	A	-	A
Streptozotocin	B	B		-	A	-						
Semustine	A	A		A	A	A		-	A	A		-
Carmustine	A	A		-	A	A		-	A	A		A
Agents related to Chap. 9												
cis-Platinum	A	A	A	B	A	A	C	A	C	A	A	A

[a] A, good activity that in a tumor-panel model warrants further development of a "unique" structure; B, moderate activity not sufficient to warrant further development; C, active but not yet retested; -, negative as tested; +-, erratic response; blank, not yet tested on the regimen indicated on Table 2.2.

The 1981 approximate cost estimates are: $7000 to $10,000 for the activity evaluation of a compound in the tumor panel; $300,000 for the development of a clinical formulation, the activity evaluation, and the toxicological evaluation of a synthetic compound up to the point of phase I clinical trial (and probably twice as much for a natural product); and $1,000,000 for the clinical evaluation of an agent for 1 year. Because of the large investments involved in formulation, toxicology, and clinical trial, tumor-panel data are obtained and very careful consideration is given to a new compound's biological activity and chemical structure at this point before further NCI funds are committed for development.

Table 2.3 is a sample of the kind of evaluation that results from tumor-panel testing. Table 2.3 testing is a very small portion, however, of a much larger validation study still in progress. At the present time (1981) over 2000 materials have been tested in at least some of these tumor-panel models. This study, designed as a comprehensive prospective project to provide preclinical-clinical correlations, will necessarily include an analysis of data on the clinical trials of each agent. Thus it remains to be determined whether or not any of the current models or any combination of the current models selects new chemical structures that will be less toxic clinically than present therapies and that will be beneficial for human malignancies, especially solid tumors.

The Division of Cancer Treatment evaluation program is still developing. The procedures and the choice of models will probably continue to change in the future, both as a result of the present correlation study and as a result of developmental programs now in progress. These developmental programs are investigating alternative assays, searching for better models to detect agents chemically different from those already known to be relatively ineffective against human solid tumors and known to have undesirable side effects. Attributes desirable in a DCT preclinical model include: predictability for clinical efficacy, quantitative and qualitative reproducibility, specificity that discriminates between desirable and undesirable drug effects, cost and time efficiency, and feasibility for testing many materials.

Examples of some of the alternative assays that are currently being investigated or developed by the DCT include the following. In an "astrocytoma" in vitro assay, immature AC glioma cells (from a rat brain tumor originally induced transplacentally with ethylnitrosourea), which are epithelial-like cells with an abundance of cytoplasm, are transformed by dibutyryl cyclic adenosine monophosphate to the morphology of mature differentiated astrocytes. Treatment with certain anticancer drugs then restores the neuroglial-appearing culture back to the original fibroepithelial estate. In two other alternative assays under study, malignant cells or tissues from human patients are grown under conditions that permit a comparison of responses to a variety of anticancer compounds. In one of these assays, sometimes called a clonogenic assay, cells are incubated with drugs in a two-layer soft-agar system and the assay is terminated on day 21 or as soon as the average control growth is 30 colonies [21-23]. An advantage of the in vitro method is that it eliminates the use of living mice. In the other assay the tissues are grown under the kidney capsules of conventional (not athymic) mice; this in vivo assay is a 6-day test [24, 25]. The advantages of the in vivo method are that it is faster, it eliminates the troublesome problems associated with an artificial medium, and it permits systemic treatment which is necessary to activate compounds such as cytoxan.

Other assays, mostly in vitro, are also being explored by the DCT evaluation program as possible predictors for clinical efficacy. Just as the nine current DCT in vivo models are now undergoing a validation process to determine whether they can selectively distinguish which compounds are beneficial clinically, it would be necessary for any alternative assay for testing unknown materials also to be subjected to a similar validation process after its drug-sensitivity patterns are sufficiently reproducible and its methodology has become sufficiently efficient to permit mass screening. Thus future evaluation procedures will depend on careful study of the relative merits of alternative assays and of the predictability for clinical efficacy of the current models.

D. Formulation and Production

This is a critical step in the drug development process because a compound cannot proceed further in development unless its clinical formulation retains a substantial portion of the biological activity of the bulk compound and unless a supply of the formulation sufficient for both toxicology studies and for therapeutic clinical trials can be produced.

E. Toxicology

These studies are required by the Food and Drug Administration regulations before approval can be granted for initial clinical trials. The purpose of the toxicology studies is to forewarn clinicians of potential toxicities that might be encountered in initial clinical trials, by projecting what major target organs in humans may be affected by the compound and by describing parameters predictive for those organ toxicities.

F. Investigational New Drug Application

The Investigational New Drug application is filed with the Food and Drug Administration for review and approval before the initiation of clinical trials and includes data demonstrating the activity and the safety of the compound.

G. Clinical Trial

Phase I clinical trial with a new agent starts with a few patients at a low dose observing for limiting toxicity. Doses are escalated usually by the Fibonacci series until the maximum tolerated dose is established. The effectiveness of the agent is subsequently investigated in phase II clinical trial in specific representative or "signal" human malignancies: breast, colon, and lung tumors; melanoma, acute leukemia, and Hodgkin's lymphoma. In phase III clinical trial the agent's effect is compared to standard treatment, and in phase IV clinical trial the agent is combined with surgery, radiation, or immune modulators [26].

H. New Drug Application

A New Drug Application is filed with the Food and Drug Administration when the agent is ready to be marketed commercially. There are now 30 cytotoxic anticancer agents commercially available [8].

III. DIFFICULTIES ENCOUNTERED WITH PREDICTING MODELS

There are several difficulties that hamper a model's ability to predict for clinical efficacy.

A. Quantitative Criteria

The sensitivity of an animal model can be adjusted by modifying its various aspects. That is, the "holes" in the screen can be widened or narrowed to control the number of agents selected. It is difficult to adjust for sensitivity adequate to select sufficient potential agents and at the same time have the model mirror clinical experience. The probability of having a successfully predicting cancer model may be reduced because different quantitative criteria are sometimes used for the model and for the human malignancy in which drug effect is being compared. This problem was highlighted by Schabel and his colleagues, who gave the following example. With the human solid tumor under study the criterion for a clinically useful drug was a 50% reduction in objectively measured tumor volume, while with the animal solid tumor under study the criterion for activity was a 50% limit on the growth of the tumor compared to its untreated control. That is, reduction in tumor mass was not required in the animal solid tumor model and therefore a drug called "active" by the experimental chemotherapist failed the clinical criterion [27].

B. Experimental Design

Another problem in cancer chemotherapy is that the ability of an animal model to predict accurately the clinical potential of agents may be reduced by the experimental design adopted to expedite a large screening program.

For rodent anticancer models, transplanted solid-tumor fragments are often implanted subcutaneously in the axillary region, the test material is administered intraperitoneally, and the activity of the agent is judged by the lack of growth of the test fragments compared to the growth of the control fragments. Human solid tumors, however, appear in many anatomical sites, such as breast, colon, lung, skin, esophagus, and bladder. At some of these sites a drug could be administered directly to or into the tumor without entering the circulatory system first. Thus there usually is a tumor-site difference between a patient and a model and also a drug-route difference between possibilities for a patient and the usual route for a model. Tumor-site differences provide different circulation patterns and thus different growth environments for tumors. Agents may be activated or inactivated by the liver or blood [28]; and therefore drug-route differences of the same agent may deliver different chemical products to the tumor if one of the drug routes circumvents the site of the activation-inactivation process. It is thought that the advantages of a systemically administered compound are that it reaches metastasizing cells and also gains intratumoral entrance via the circulatory system. However, it seems possible that the combination of the tumor-site and drug-route differences might in some cases preclude the selection by that model of what might have been the best compound for that patient, particularly if systemic administration happens to inactivate that compound and if the tumor has not metastasized.

C. Side Effects

A considerable problem in cancer chemotherapy is that most clinical anticancer drugs have unpleasant side effects. The benefit from most current clinical anticancer drugs is purported to be due to their ability to kill cancer cells or to keep them from reproducing. This property of being a cytotoxic or a cytostatic agent is also considered to be responsible for the drug's toxic effects that may result from its killing or inhibiting the reproduction of proliferating cells other than tumor cells. Each of the current clinical anticancer drugs may produce toxic reactions that are different in different patients, and chemotherapy for some patients may be devoid of toxic effects. In the same patient the severity of the toxicity of a drug may vary from treatment to treatment [29].

It is very difficult to predict from responses in a cancer activity-evaluation model what clinical toxicities might be expected. From mass-screening activity evaluations, toxicity can be described only grossly at the present time: for example, by lethality, by body weight loss, or by a therapeutic index that shows the margin of safety between an active dose and a toxic dose. A wide margin of safety in mice is often viewed as an indication that the compound may be given in the clinic at a dose low enough to be nontoxic and at the same time beneficial. Detailed studies of mechanisms underlying toxicity and activity are the province of toxicologists, pharmacologists, and molecular biologists.

D. Response Differences

Investigators have questioned whether the problem of selecting useful predicting systems in the area of cancer chemotherapy might be complicated beyond all comprehension [30] and achievability.

Finding quick, inexpensive, dependably predictive models to select drugs for treating human cancer is indeed a challenge. The basis of this difficulty, however, may not be due so much to the preclinical models as to the far more fundamental problem of response differences between patients receiving the chemotherapy. It is the patient-response differences which may be "complicated beyond all comprehension"; for example, different drugs are required for different human malignancies, and different patients with the same malignancy require different therapies. These differences in patients' responses may be due to any of an unlimited number of differences between patients, such as variations in genetics, in physiology (e.g., metabolic rates), in location of the tumors (varying the influence of circulation), in the state of metastasis, in the biochemistry of the tumors, and in the drug resistance of different kinds of cells in the heterogeneous population in the tumor.

In discussing the heterogeneity of a tumor's cell population, Zubrod commented that tumors of a given morphological cell type do not constitute a homogeneous entity that will uniformly respond to a given chemotherapy. He indicated that, after chemotherapy, he has observed differences in the duration of remission in patients in the four subtypes of acute lymphocytic leukemia, defined (by the use of surface antigen markers) as common, T-cell positive, B-cell positive, and null cells [31]. Pratt and Ruddon listed some of the mechanisms of resistance to anticancer drugs (such as increased DNA repair by a cell resistant to alkylating agents) that permit drug-resistant clones of cells to survive and reestablish the tumor mass after the drug-sensitive cells have been killed [32]. Additional factors that may modify the activity (and toxicity) of anticancer agents, suggested by Spreafico and his colleagues, include circadian rhythmicity and the age of the host, which affects the host's capacity to eliminate drugs and to recover from toxicity and additional medication [33]. Thus a drug response of one person does not necessarily predict for the response to the same drug of another person.

The drug sensitivities of the genetically standardized mice used for the Division of Cancer Treatment evaluations are undoubtedly more uniform than the drug sensitivities of our genetically heterogeneous human population. These "complications" are basic biological difficulties inherent in the problem of evaluating potential antineoplastic agents.

IV. ADDITIONAL APPROACHES

"Tumors have been observed in practically all species of multicellular animals," according to Heston in 1975 [34]. He further commented that it is particularly significant that some form of tumor occurs in the most lowly multicellular organisms with little normal cell differentiation because this indicates that the basic neoplastic change involves a very primitive physiological process. Tumor hosts mentioned by Heston included earthworms, planaria, cockroaches, drosophila, goldfish, trout, frogs, parakeets, chickens, and cattle [34]. A 1971 publication of the National Academy of Sciences listed over 1800 species of laboratory animals from aardvarks to zebras (without reference to which are used for cancer research) [35]; thus assays for the evaluation of potential antineoplastic agents at this time appear to be unlimited. Investigators can, of course, use the assay of their choice to evaluate agents for their own purposes. However, to attain its goal, it is necessary for the Division of Cancer Treatment to attempt to identify the model or models best suited for selecting agents most beneficial for human malignancies.

Many methods have been and are being used by investigators in the search for improved cancer therapy. This means attacking the source of cancer from a number of facets [36-41], including genetics, virology, immunology, pain alleviation, metastasis, pathology, physiology, metabolism, endocrinology, pharmacology, molecular biology, carcinogenesis and possible prevention, biological markers, and the effects of hyperthermia, radiation, and nutrition. The activity evaluations of special types of potential antineoplastic therapies require special testing procedures. These therapies include radiation, materials that might affect immunological responses [42], or materials that might affect hormones or endocrine glands [43-45].

In addition to the current endeavors, the author would like to suggest two additional approaches that might be profitable in the future. The first suggestion is a systematic search for the differences discussed above (such as metabolic rate) between responders and nonresponders to the same chemotherapy. Walker showed a 46% response rate for patients with glioblastoma multiforme who received carmustine as a single agent [46]. The differences between such responders and nonresponders should provide new evaluation tools that should lead to improved therapies.

A second suggestion is a systematic look at clinically effective anticancer agents to see what characteristics or properties they might have in common that are not shared with chemicals that have been adequately tested clinically and found to be clinically ineffective including, for example, their effect on erythrocyte deformability [47-49]. Any characteristics that clinically effective agents have in common that are not shared with adequately tested clinically ineffective compounds might be developed into evaluation assays that could lead to improved therapies.

V. CONTACTS FOR ANTINEOPLASTIC EVALUATION

To offer a compound to the Division of Cancer Treatment for possible anticancer evaluation, the proper contact is the Chief, Drug Synthesis and Chemistry Branch, Developmental Therapeutics Program, Division of Cancer Treatment, National Cancer Institute, Bethesda, Maryland. The letter should include the chemical structure, an indication of the size of the sample that could be submitted if invited to do so, and a statement regarding the reason (chemical or biological) the compound might be expected to have potential anticancer activity. There are many advantages to having a new chemical evaluated by the DCT: The evaluation is free of charge to the compound supplier, the quality control of the biological tests is monitored by the DCT staff, and the resulting computerized data which are sent to the supplier also enter automatically into the review procedures of the DCT, which is searching for new types of chemicals with sufficient anticancer potential to warrant development toward eventual clinical use.

An alternative is a commercial evaluation. There are many commercial testing laboratories which the compound supplier can contact directly, and some of the laboratories that conduct testing under NCI contract also conduct testing commercially. An estimate of the cost should be obtained before a compound is submitted for commercial evaluation.

Another possibility is to develop evaluation tests based on the rationale for the synthesis of a compound or series of compounds.

Additional alternatives would be contacts with individual cancer investigators directly: however, many cancer investigators are grantees who have received their grants for specific purposes and are not free to change the scope of their work to evaluate random agents under their grant. Recent journals and books concerned with cancer, such as ones listed in the references, might be a source of ideas for contacts for evaluations. Contacts might be possible through local organizations such as a university, the local unit of the American Cancer Society, or a cancer center. The International Cancer Research Data Bank program, which is a component of the NCI Office of International Affairs, maintains (among others) the CANCER PROJ data base, containing 20,000 descriptions of ongoing research projects. Biomedical libraries around the country which are connected to the National Library of Medicine through the Medlars system are able to access CANCER PROJ data and, upon request, one of these biomedical libraries can arrange for a search of the CANCER PROJ data and provide a listing of cancer research projects within a specified geographical region for a specified activity (such as anticancer drug evaluation).

VI. CONCLUSIONS

Based on statistics from previous years it was estimated that there would be 815,000 new cancer cases in the United States during 1984, and that the site of over half of these human malignancies would be lung, digestive tract, or breast [50]. In 1984 many cancer patients were being treated for their malignancies with a variety of different chemotherapeutic agents, such as the agents listed on Table 2.2. These include carmustine, *cis*-platinum, cytosar, dacarbazine, and lomustine, which are all anticancer drugs in clinical use that were selected by the National Cancer Institute on the basis of their activity in rodent in vivo models. Some success in selecting chemotherapeutic agents has been achieved. However, the search is continuing for new and better anticancer agents that will provide improved clinical therapy. Predicting which of the approximately 350,000 new compounds per year might be most beneficial clinically for cancer patients is indeed a difficult challenge. The current approach of the Division of Cancer Treatment has evolved as a result of 25 years of careful study and planning by the United States National Cancer Institute with the advice and cooperation of scientists from all over the world.

The large study now in progress is to determine the relative value of these NCI in vivo models in selectively distinguishing clinically beneficial agents. The small preliminary evaluation presented in Table 2.3 indicates that 22 of the 28 selected clinical anticancer agents have shown good confirmed activity in at least two of the current nine DCT in vivo models.

So far no other assay has been shown to be superior as a predictor for clinical efficacy to in vivo rodent tumor models. However, the DCT approach to anticancer evaluation is continually evolving and some of the in vitro assays now in DCT development may soon be subjected to a validation study to determine their predictability for clinical efficacy, as soon as the assays are sufficiently reproducible and their methodologies permit mass screening.

REFERENCES

1. A. Gellhorn and E. Hirschberg (eds.), Cancer Res. Suppl., 3: 125 (1955).
2. S. M. Sessoms (ed.), Cancer Chemother. Rep., 1: 10 (1959).
3. K. Endicott, J. Natl. Cancer Inst., 19: 275 (1957).
4. C. G. Zubrod, S. A. Shepartz, J. Leiter, K. M. Endicott, L. M. Carrese, and C. G. Baker, Cancer Chemother. Rep., 50: 349 (1966).
5. A. Goldin, A. A. Serpick, and N. Mantel, Cancer Chemother. Rep., 50: 173 (1966).
6. A. Goldin, S. A. Schepartz, J. M. Venditti, and V. T. DeVita, Methods Cancer Res., 16: 165 (1979).
7. R. I. Geran, N. H. Greenberg, M. M. Macdonald, A. M. Schumacher, and B. A. Abbott, Cancer Chemother. Rep., Part 3, 3: 88 (1972).
8. V. T. DeVita, V. T. Oliverio, F. M. Muggia, P. W. Wiernik, J. Ziegler, A. Goldin, D. Rubin, J. Henney, and S. A. Schepartz, Cancer Clin. Trials, 2: 195 (1979).
9. J. M. Venditti, in Pharmacological Basis of Cancer Chemotherapy, Williams & Wilkins, Baltimore, 1975, p. 245.
10. S. A. Schepartz, Jpn. J. Antibiot., Suppl., 30: 35 (1977).
11. S. A. Schepartz, Recent Results Cancer Res., 63: 30 (1978).
12. J. M. Venditti, A. Goldin, I. Miller, and M. Rozencweig, in Advances in Cancer Chemotherapy (H. Umezawa, ed.), Japanese Scientific Society Press, Baltimore, 1978, p. 201.
13. A. Goldin and J. M. Venditti, Recent Results Cancer Res., 70: 5 (1980).

14. Chemical and Engineering News, April 13, 1981, p. 46.
15. L. Hodes, G. F. Hazard, R. I. Geran, and S. Richman, J. Med. Chem., 20: 469 (1977).
16. L. Hodes, Computer-aided Selection of Novel Antitumor Drugs for Animal Screening, Symposium Series 112 on Computer-Assisted Drug Design, American Chemical Society, Washington, D.C., 1979.
17. J. S. Driscoll, L. Dudeck, G. Congleton, and R. I. Geran, J. Pharm. Sci., 68: 185 (1979).
18. R. I. Geran, G. F. Congleton, L. E. Dudeck, B. J. Abbott, and J. L. Gargus, Cancer Chemother. Rep., Part 2, 4: 53 (1974).
19. T. A. Marks, R. J. Woodman, R. I. Geran, L. H. Billups, and R. M. Madison, Cancer Treat. Rep., 61: 1459 (1977).
20. J. A. Mabel, P. C. Merker, M. L. Sturgeon, I. Wodinsky, and R. I. Geran, Cancer, 42: 1711 (1978).
21. K. L. Rosenthal, W. A. F. Tompkins, G. L. Frank, P. McCulloch, and W. E. Rawls, Cancer Res., 37: 4024 (1977).
22. A. W. Hamburger, S. E. Salmon, M. B. Kim, J. M. Trent, B. J. Soehnlen, D. S. Alberts, and H. J. Schmidt, Cancer Res., 38: 3438 (1978).
23. S. E. Salmon (ed.), Prog. Clin. Biol. Res., 48 (1980).
24. A. E. Bogden, P. M. Haskell, D. J. LePage, D. E. Kelton, W. R. Cobb, and H. J. Esber, Exp. Cell Biol., 47: 281 (1979).
25. T. W. Griffin, A. E. Bogden, R. E. Hunter, A. Ward, D. T. Yu, S. Reich, M. E. Costanza, and H. L. Greene, The subrenal capsule assay as a predictor of response to chemotherapy, submitted for publication to Cancer.
26. V. T. DeVita, Cancer Treatment, Publ. 80-1807, National Institutes of Health, Bethesda, Md., 1979.
27. F. M. Schabel, D. P. Griswold, T. H. Corbett, W. R. Laster, J. G. Mayo, and H. H. Lloyd, Methods Cancer Res., 17: 5 (1979).
28. L. S. Goodman and A. Gilman, The Pharmacological Basis of Therapeutics, Macmillan, New York, 1965, p. 951.
29. National Cancer Institute, Chemotherapy and You, Publ. 80-1136, National Institutes of Health, Bethesda, Md., 1980.
30. H. E. Skipper, Cancer Chemother. Rep., 16: 11 (1962).
31. C. G. Zubrod, Cancer Res., 38: 4377 (1978).
32. W. B. Pratt and R. W. Ruddon, in The Anticancer Drugs, Oxford University Press, New York, 1979.
33. F. Spreafico, M. G. Donelli, A. Vecchi, A. Bossi, and S. Garattini, Recent Results Cancer Res., 49: 88 (1974).
34. W. E. Heston, Cancer, 1: 33 (1975).
35. Institute of Laboratory Resources of the National Research Council, Animals for Research, National Academy of Sciences, Washington, D.C., 1971.
36. H. Busch (ed.), Methods in Cancer Research, 15 vol., Academic Press, New York, 1979.

37. T. A. Connors, Recent Results Cancer Res., 21: 1 (1969).
38. H. M. Dyer, Index of Tumor Chemotherapy, National Institutes of Health, Bethesda, Md., 1949.
39. J. S. Mitchell (ed.), The Treatment of Cancer with Special Reference to Radiotherapy and Chemotherapy, Cambridge University Press, Cambridge, 1965.
40. M. Mizell, in Recent Results in Cancer Research Supplement (M. Mizell, ed.), Springer-Verlag, New York, 1969.
41. A. N. Parshin, in Cancer—A General Guide to Research and Its Treatment, Macmillan, New York, 1962, p. 70.
42. M. A. Chirigos, Cancer Treat. Rep., 62: 1611 (1978).
43. CCNSC Endocrinology Bioassay Program, Cancer Chemother. Rep., 1: 65 (1959).
44. S. Iacobelli, I. Nenci, and F. O. Ranelletti, Cancer Treat. Rep., 63: 1166 (1979).
45. A. B. Russfield, Tumors of Endocrine Glands and Secondary Sex Organs, Publ. 1332, Public Health Service, Washington, D.C., 1966.
46. M. D. Walker, Malignant Brain Tumors—A Synopsis, American Cancer Society, Towson, Md., 1975.
47. R. I. Weed, Am.J. Med., 49: 147 (1970).
48. H. L. Reid, J. Clin. Pathol., 29: 855 (1976).
49. M. H. Cohen, J. Natl. Cancer Inst., 63: 525 (1979).
50. Ca—A Cancer Journal for Clinicians, 31(1): 30, 31 (January-February 1981).

3

PHARMACOLOGICAL EVALUATION OF ANTINEOPLASTIC AGENTS

ROBERT B. DIASIO

Medical College of Virginia
Virginia Commonwealth University
Richmond, Virginia

I. INTRODUCTION

After a new agent has been demonstrated to have antineoplastic activity in a suitable tumor screen (Chap. 2), further studies are needed to clarify its pharmacology before the agent can be thoroughly examined for antineoplastic activity in the clinic. Pharmacology may be defined as the study of the physical and chemical properties of a drug, and the resultant biochemical and physiological effects produced upon interaction with living matter. The pharmacological evaluation of new drugs includes two separate but parallel approaches: evaluation of the disposition of drug following administration in vivo at the level of the whole animal, and evaluation of the biochemical and molecular action of the drug at the cellular level.

It is important to emphasize that antineoplastic drugs comprise a diverse group of compounds with different chemical structures that may produce a variety of biological effects in addition to inhibition of tumor cell growth. Particularly important are the resultant toxic effects produced in normal host cells. Some of these toxic effects may result from inhibition of cell division of normal cells similar to the growth inhibition produced in tumor cells. For example, the inhibition of cell division of a gastrointestinal mucosal cells resulting in mucositis or the inhibition of normal hematopoietic cells resulting in anemia, leukopenia, or thrombocytopenia. Other toxic effects may be unrelated to a direct effect on cell division of the host cells but may result from interference with the normal function of a particular host tissue, resulting in toxicity such as neurologic, cardiovascular, or renal toxicities. For example, the anticancer agents cis-dichlorodiamine platinum not only can interfere with the cell division of tumor cells but also may cause renal and auditory nerve damage by the interaction of platinum with the kidney and cranial nerve VIII [1]. An early understanding of the pharmacology of a new agent should permit better evaluation of the agent in subsequent clinical studies, hopefully enabling more rational use of the agent by maximizing the antitumor effects and minimizing the toxicity to the host.

This chapter reviews the major principles of pharmacology relating to antineoplastic agents. Initially, there is a brief discussion of the chemical and physical factors that determine the interrelationship between drug and biological material. This is followed by a discussion of those factors that determine the disposition of a drug within the whole animal and ultimately determining the amount of the drug that can affect both tumor and host cells in the periphery. The factors that determine the drug disposition at the cellular level, the mechanism of action and possible sites of resistance are also discussed. Finally, there is a brief discussion of the impact of new analytical techniques on the study of the pharmacology of antineoplastic agents.

II. CHEMICAL AND PHYSICAL FACTORS

In evaluating the pharmacology of antineoplastic agents it is useful first to determine the physical and chemical properties of a drug since these properties can markedly influence the disposition of the drug at both the whole animal and cellular level. The solubility of a drug in physiological solutions is the most important factor to consider initially. Since physiological fluids are aqueous solutions, it is usually necessary for the drug to be soluble in aqueous media to be clinically useful. Furthermore, the solubility of the drug may be affected greatly by pH changes that occur in various physiological sites. This is particularly important in the whole animal, for example, orally administered drugs are exposed to large fluctuations in pH in the gastrointestinal tract while renal-excreted drugs are exposed to pH changes in the kidney. These alterations in pH affect solubility, which in turn can affect absorption [2].

The chemical and physical properties of a drug are also important, as they determine the ease with which a drug will pass through membrane barriers encountered at both the whole animal level and at the cellular level. It is the unique physical and chemical characteristics of the cell membrane that determine whether a drug will be able to traverse these barriers. Current concepts in cell biology suggest that the cell membranes are bimolecular lipid layers sandwiched between monomolecular protein layers [3]. Interrupting the integrity of the cell membranes are openings or pores through which some drugs may pass by filtration (Fig. 3.1). The molecular weight and structural complexity of a drug, including whether or not it is bound to protein, affect the passage of drug through these pores, which have been estimated to have a radius of a few angstrom units. The amount of the drug that can pass through these pores is usually determined by hydrostatic pressure, as well as electrostatic, osmotic, and concentration gradients [4].

Some drugs are capable of dissolving in the cell membrane and traversing by simple diffusion. In general, drugs that are nonpolar and lipid soluble are more capable of utilizing this mechanism than are polar and aqueous soluble drugs. A useful index of the relative lipid solubility and polarity of a particular drug is the partition coefficient, calculated by determining the relative distribution of a drug in a two-phase system consisting of a lipid solvent, such as ether, chloroform, or octanol, and an aqueous solvent adjusted to physilogical pH.

$$Cp = \frac{[HA] \text{ in organic solvent}}{[HA] \text{ in aqueous solvent}}$$

This constant can be utilized to predict the ease with which a drug may pass through a cell membrane by simple diffusion; thus a large partition coefficient would suggest a greater lipid solubility in the membrane and hence an increased ease of passage through the cell membrane [4].

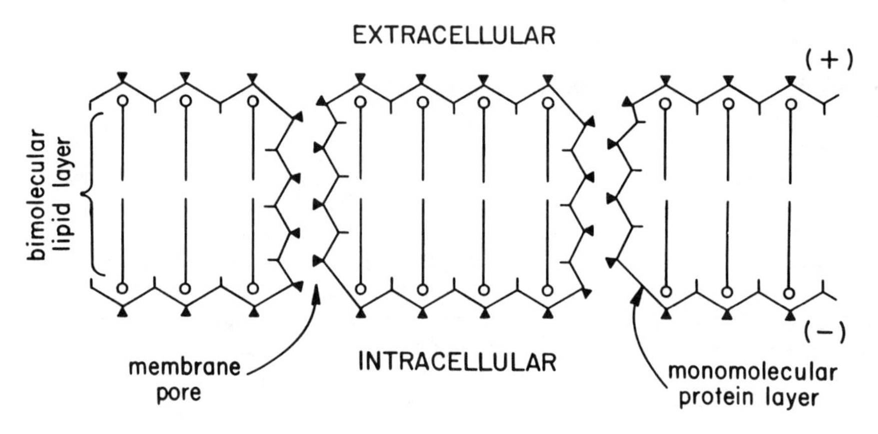

FIGURE 3.1 Schematic diagram of a cell membrane.

As noted above, drugs may be exposed to marked variations in pH, particularly in vivo. The pK_a of a drug will determine whether the drug is in the ionized form at a particular pH. Since nonionized drugs are more likely to pass through the cell membrane by the mechanism of simple diffusion than are ionized drugs [2], it is useful to calculate the pK_a of a drug as defined by the Henderson-Hasselbach equation to predict the amount of the drug that is nonionized at a particular pH that will be able to diffuse through the membrane.

$$pK_a = pH + \log \frac{[HA]}{[H+][A-]}$$

as the pH of a solution decreases, the degree of ionization of basic drugs will increase and less drug will diffuse through the membrane; conversely, as the pH of a solution increases, the degree of ionization of basic drugs will decrease, allowing more drug to diffuse through the membrane. In general, drugs utilizing this mechanism are driven by a concentration gradient. Consequently, the drug will diffuse through the membrane until equilibrium is reached, at which point the concentration of the drug is the same on both sides of the membrane.

A third group of drugs traverse the cell membrane not by simple filtration or diffusion but by specialized transport mechanisms [5]. The physical and chemical properties of these drugs permit complexing with membrane carriers which enable the drugs to traverse the cell membrane, then dissociating from the carrier on the other side, releasing the drug intracellularly. These carrier molecules are characterized by structural specificity. While these carriers are utilized for the transport of naturally occurring metabolites, an exogenous compound such as an antineoplastic drug (e.g., the folate antimetabolite methotrexate) may compete with the natural metabolite for the carrier mechanism. In general, carrier-mediated transport systems can be demonstrated to saturate at high concentrations of substrate. When the compound is carried across a concentration gradient, energy must be expended and the process is referred to as "active transport." In this situation, rather than obtaining equal concentrations of the drug inside and outside the cell membrane, as is observed with filtration and simple diffusion, the drug concentration inside the membrane can be greater than that outside the membrane. Active transport can be demonstrated by utilizing metabolic inhibitors which inhibit the production of cellular energy and result in decreased drug uptake into the cells. Thus an initial examination of physical and chemical properties of the drug is valuable in predicting the disposition of the drug both at the whole animal and cellular level.

III. DISPOSITION OF DRUG IN THE WHOLE ANIMAL

This section reviews those factors that determine drug (and drug metabolite) concentrations that ultimately reach the tumor (or host cells) in the periphery following administration of the drug to a whole animal. While antineoplastic activity in an in vitro tumor model may identify a potentially effective drug, to be potentially clinically useful, the drug must have antineoplastic activity following administration to a whole animal harboring a tumor. Among the factors that contribute to drug effectiveness in vivo are the route of drug administration; the metabolism at sites other than the target site (e.g., the liver, where the drug may be activated or inactivated); the distribution of the drug (including the amount bound to protein) and the amount of drug sequestered in tissue depots (e.g., fat); and the excretion of the drug. The interrelationship of these factors is shown in Fig. 3.2. Several other factors may also affect drug disposition, particularly in the cancer patient. These include the effect of neoplasm and associated medical conditions, and the possible interaction of the antineoplastic drugs with each other as well as with nonneoplastic drugs. By measuring the concentration of the drug or drug metabolites in plasma at various times after drug administration, it is possible to develop an understanding of the pharmacokinetics, such as the change in concentration of drug (or drug metabolite) over time. This information, together with data on toxicity and antitumor activity, can then be used to develop a schedule for drug administration in the clinic.

A. Route of Administration

The route by which an antineoplastic agent is administered can markedly affect the amount and rate of the drug reaching the tumor cells within the

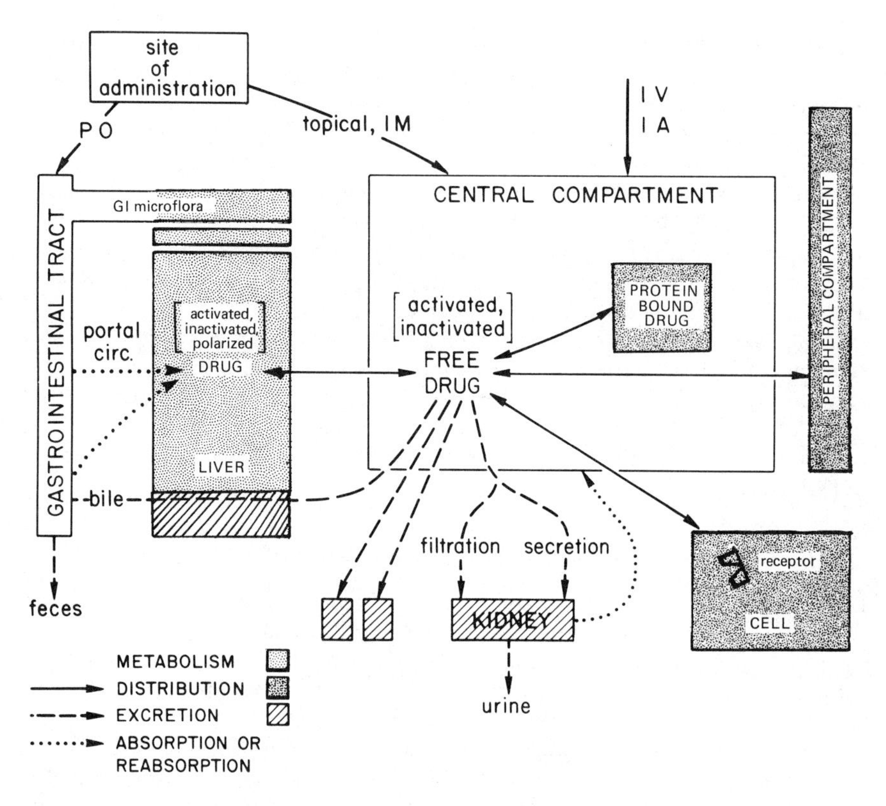

FIGURE 3.2 Factors influencing the disposition of an antineoplastic agent in the whole animal.

whole animal. This is important not only in large animal and clinical studies, but also in early tumor screening studies with small animals. In certain rodent tumor lines mechlorethamine was shown to be ineffective when administered by the intraperitoneal route, the usual route of administration in tumor screening studies in mice and rats. This might have led to the premature conclusion that the drug was ineffective in this particular tumor line; however, the drug was demonstrated in other studies to have activity when administered intravenously or intraarterially [16].

In evaluating a potential route of drug administration, it is helpful to compare pharmacokinetic data obtained by a particular route with that obtained following intravenous administration. This permits an assessment of the amount of drug absorbed via this route into the circulation (over time) since comparatively speaking, the intravenous route assures direct delivery of essentially all of the drug into the circulation. The pharmacokinetic parameters examined most often are the peak plasma or serum concentration (the highest concentration of the drug obtained over a period of time following drug administration), the peak time (the time at which the peak concentration occurs), and the AUC (the total area under the curve generated by plotting the changing drug concentrations in the plasma or serum over time). Thus, if the values obtained for the peak concentration, peak time, and AUC are similar to those obtained with the intravenous route, it is probable that the drug is absorbed well from this particular route of administration. The peak concentration and peak time can also be used to identify drug concentrations in the plasma at which toxicity is observed as well as determining a potential minimally effective concentration for antitumor activity [7].

In choosing a route of administration, one must also be aware of the possible increased toxicity with drug administered via a particular route. For example, certain alkylating agents, such as mechlorethamine, are very reactive chemicals, capable of alkylating biological tissues exposed to these drugs. For this reason, this type of drug cannot be administered orally, subcutaneously, or intramuscularly but must be administered either intravenously or intraarterially to avoid local toxicity [8].

Systemic delivery of a drug is not always the optimal route since intensive local treatment may be more desirable. Local or regional administration of a drug permits delivery of relatively high concentration of the drug to the tumor area. Furthermore, drugs administered in this way are potentially unaffected by degradation or inactivation that may occur in the circulation. A further potential benefit may be achieved with drugs that are activated on delivery to the tumor bed but are inactivated before reaching other host tissues.

Intravenous Route

The intravenous route is the most frequently utilized route of administration for antineoplastic agents. For some drugs, particularly those that are not well absorbed through cell membrane barriers, this may be the only means by which the drug may be administered. For other drugs, the intravenous route may offer pharmacological advantages [4]. For example, some drugs administered orally can undergo biotransformation, such as chemical or metabolic degradation in the gastrointestinal tract or metabolism in the liver. Furthermore, the intravenous route offers the advantage of achieving higher and more predictable plasma concentrations of drug. It is usually easier to achieve a rapid peak concentration of the drug, if this is desirable. For those patients who are unconscious, unable to swallow, or unable to retain gastric contents, the intravenous route is specifically advantageous. An additional benefit of intravenous administration is that if potentially dangerous side effects develop, further administration of the drug may be stopped immediately, unlike many of the other routes. The intravenous route also offers the possibility for more control of the dose administered; it permits bolus injection or sustained continuous infusion if necessary. The capability to deliver the drug predictably is particularly advantageous with antineoplastic drugs that are known to have a steep dose-response curve. One should be cognizant that usually there is little difference between the dose that produces toxicity and that which is needed to produce an antitumor response. Also, local toxicity caused by many drugs, such as the alkylating agents or anthracyclene drugs, necessitates that they be administered into a free-flowing intravenous line.

The disadvantages of the intravenous route with antineoplastic drugs are essentially the same as those associated with other drugs. These include the risk of infection, anaphylaxis, emboli, hypotension, cardiar arrhythmia, and local irritation. It should be emphasized that the intravenous route of administration may be particularly unappealing to the cancer patient needing treatment. Patients often relate that the most noxious aspect of cancer treatment is the frequency of "needle sticks." Intravenous administration is also more expensive since an office or clinic visit is required, with the possibility of hospitalization each time the drug is administered. These required hospitalizations are often more disturbing to the patient than are the side effects of the drugs. A potential solution to this problem has been the development of chronically indwelling catheters through which blood may be drawn for routine laboratory tests and through which drug may be administered each time the patient requires therapy [9]. Furthermore, several new devices attached to chronically indwelling catheters permit continuous infusion of drugs, which frees the patient from spending much of his or her limited life span in a physician's office or in the hospital [10].

Oral Route

Oral administration is attractive for both physicians and patients because of the convenience and because less time and money are required. This is particularly beneficial when the drug schedule necessitates frequent administration to maintain an effective concentration of the drug.

One must first be assured, however, that the drug is well tolerated and not unduly toxic when administered by this route, and second, that it is predictably and sufficiently absorbed to assure attaining the plasma concentration required. An obvious prerequisite is that the drug is able to be absorbed through the gastrointestinal mucosa. Characteristically, drugs that can be administered by the oral route are low-molecular-weight water-soluble compounds that are minimally ionized at the pH level found in the gastrointensintal tract (particularly in the small intestine) with a high lipid/water partition coefficient [2]. Furthermore, within the gastrointestinal tract, the agent should not be degradable to any great extent by hydrolysis or by enzymes [4]. One must also be aware of potential metabolism in the liver. Since drugs are absorbed via the portal circulation, they may be sufficiently catagolized during the "first pass" through the liver, rendering most of the drug inactive by the time it reaches the tumor cells [3]. Finally, oral absorption may also be affected by coexisting disease. The presence of some types of cancer may cause variations in transit time through the gastrointestinal tract, changes in pH, and alteration in the digestion of food such that the absorption of drug may be erratic.

Other Routes for Systemic Delivery of Drugs

Other routes of administration have been utilized for systemic delivery of drugs, but these have not been widely used with antineoplastic agents. This is largely due to the profound local toxicity observed with many of these agents. Another problem is the difficulty in obtaining precise control of systemic drug levels, particularly because antineoplastic drugs characteristically have steep dose-response profiles. A notable exception is the occasional clinical intramuscular administration of methotrexate [11]. Other routes of administration, such as by rectal suppository, have been attempted with the antimetabolite prodrug ftorafur [12]. The bioavailability information on this route of administration is limited, however, and further studies are needed before this could be recommended.

Local or Regional Administration

Local administration of antineoplastic drugs has been utilized with accessible tumors such as dermatological malignancies. Topical cytotoxic agents have been used for basal cell carcinoma, squamous cell carcinoma, and in the treatment of the premalignant condition actinic keratoses. 5-Fluorouracil mixed with a vehicle such as polyethylene glycol has been demonstrated to be an effective treatment in some of these disorders, particularly actinic keratoses. Administered in this manner, the drug can achieve a high local concentration with little evidence of absorption into the systemic circulation [13]. Other antineoplastic agents have been utilized topically, although none have been as widely used as 5-fluorouracil.

A unique approach has been used in treatment of early cancer of the urinary bladder in which high concentrations of _tris_-triethylenephosphoramide (TEPA) are administered by intravesicular delivery to achieve relatively high concentrations of the drug locally in the bladder with relatively little absorption into the systemic circulation [14].

Regional therapy has been shown to be particularly clinically useful in the treatment. In contrast to local therapy, which refers to the administration of a drug on an "outside" surface, regional therapy usually refers to the administration of drug into the circulation directly (e.g., selective intraarterial catheterization of a specific organ or region) or into certain sequestered regions (e.g., the intraperitoneal or intrathecal regions). With both the local approach and the regional approach the goal is to achieve relatively maximal concentration of drug in a particular area with minimal concentrations systematically. Regional therapy has been shown to be clinically useful in the treatment of primary and secondary central nervous system (CNS) maglignancies, particularly carcinomatous meningitis, where it is often difficult to achieve adequate drug levels by systemic drug administration. This is thought to be secondary to a postulated blood-brain barrier which restricts the passage of drug into the central nervous system. This membrane barrier, similar to other membrane barriers discussed earlier, is traversed most easily by nonionized lipid-soluble drugs [15]. Most antineoplastic drugs, particularly those used in malignancies that can metastasize to the CNS, are relatively polar nonlipid-soluble drugs. The nitrosourea drugs, which have antitumor activity against several primary and secondary CNS maglignancies [16], are the exception, being relatively nonpolar lipid-soluble drugs capable of achieving effective concentrations in the cerebrospinal fluid by systemic delivery. In the setting of carcinomatous meningitis, as in the case of acute lymphocytic leukemia, the CNS can function as a therapeutic sanctuary for the tumor; consequently, tumor cells sequestered in the CNS can escape the effect of antineoplastic agents that are often capable of eradicating the disease elsewhere within the systemic circulation [17]. For this reason it is desirable to deliver chemotherapy directly into the cerebrospinal fluid space. As with all regional therapy and particularly in the CNS, it is most important that the agents be relatively noninflammatory. At the present time, there are only two agents, methotrexate [18] and cytosine arabinoside [19], which have been demonstrated to be clinically tolerable and effective in this setting. Either of these drugs can be administered via repeated lumbar puncture, through surgically formed reservoirs placed either in the lumbar region [20] or adjacent to the ventricles in the brain [21].

Interarterial infusion is another regional approach for delivery of a relatively high concentration of drug directly into the tumor bed. This method is often used together with a radiological technique in order that drug delivery can beaassessed arteriographically. This approach has been attempted with treatment of malignancy localized to a limb [22], primary and secondary tumors in the liver [23], as well as certain other malignancies that can be demonstrated to be accessible by a vascular route. The disadvantages of this approach are similar to those observed with intravenous therapy, with infection and emboli being potential problems. These frequent sequelae limit the use of chronically indwelling catheters and often limit this approach to a "one-time" administration or with the requirement that the catheter be replaced arteriographically at frequent intervals. This necessitates increased hospitalization time, with concomitant increased expense. At present, the lack of significant cures and a most questionable palliation by this method have limited the use of this procedure.

A relatively new regional approach that delivers high concentrations of drug to the tumor bed while limiting the delivery of drug into the systemic circulation is intraperitoneal infusion [24]. This method involves the placement of a chronically indwelling peritoneal catheter which allows for delivery of a relatively high dose of drug into the intraperitoneal space. The drug is subsequently absorbed into the portal circulation draining into the liver, where it is metabolized before reaching the systemic circulation; consequently, the systemic concentration is low and resultant host toxicity is minimized. This procedure has recently been evaluated for treatment of ovarian carcinoma metastatic to the peritoneal cavity [25]. The potential benefit of this approach with other malignancies remains to be demonstrated.

B. In Vivo Metabolism

Following administration of an antineoplastic agent to an animal or person harboring a tumor, biotransformation or metabolism may occur prior to entry into the tumor cells (Fig. 3.2). Metabolism may result in either activation or inactivation of the administered drug. Certain agents such as cyclophosphamide (cytoxan) are metabolically activated prior to entering the tumor cell [26]. This is particularly important following oral administration in which case the drug is absorbed into the portal circulation and subsequently delivered to the liver, where it is activated by microsomal enzymes [27]. The active metabolites of cyclophosphamide released into the circulation can then be taken up by tumor or host cells. Most drugs, however, undergo biotransformation or metabolism, which results in inactivation following administration. This is particularly true with orally administered drugs that may be hydrolyzed, degraded by digestive enzymes, or metabolized within the gastrointestinal tract. Methotrexate, for example, has been shown to be metabolized within the intestinal microflora [28]. Drugs absorbed into the portal circulation may be further degraded by the microsomal enzymes during the "first pass" through the liver, resulting in a much lower effective concentration of drug in the systemic circulation. For certain drugs, such as 5-fluorouracil, which are catabolized mainly in the liver, oral administration may result in potentially ineffective drug levels [29]. For this reason oral administration of 5-fluorouracil is not recommended. The fact that drug catabolism occurs in the liver may be utilized for therapeutic benefit with interperitoneal administration of drug as in ovarian cancer. In this setting, high concentrations of drug may be delivered to the tumor bed (within the peritoneal cavity) with subsequent catabolism of the absorbed drug in the liver resulting in lower concentrations of drug being released into the systemic circulation such that host tissue (e.g., bone marrow) are protected.

Several additional factors may influence the metabolism of an antineoplastic agent. These include interaction with other antineoplastic drugs as well as nonantineoplastic drugs, particularly those commonly used in supportative therapy. The presence of neoplastic as well as nonneoplastic disease in organs where drugmetabolism normally occurs may result in altered metabolism, often resulting in less inactivation of drug. This results in increased levels of drug in the circulation, which can in turn result in increased cytotoxicity. These factors are discussed in greater detail below.

C. Distribution

Once a drug is in the systemic circulation it may be further distributed through the host (Fig. 3.2). The physical and chemical properties of the free drug will determine whether the drug can bind to protein within the circulation. The binding of drug to protein (most often albumin) is reversible and is controlled by hydrogen, ionic, or van der Waal bonds [30]. These properties, together with the rate of circulation and the availability of binding sites, will determine the drug distribution as well as influence the length of time that the drug remains in the body [31]. Protein-bound drug is limited with regard to movement out of the "central compartment." In contrast, free (unbound) drug may be taken into tumor, or host cells, as well as into various peripheral compartments such as fatty tissue (depending on the lipid solubility of the drug). Lipid-soluble drugs that distribute into fatty tissue may result in a decrease in concentration of drug in the central compartment; since less drug is available for uptake into tumor cells there is less therapeutic effect. This can also result in an increase in the length of time the drug remains in the animal. Metabolism at sites such as the liver and the removal from the circulation by various excretory mechanisms affect the length of time that a drug can stay within the central compartment. As implied in Fig. 3.2, the central compartment is "central" in the disposition of drug in the whole animal. For the pharmacologist the central compartment is relatively accessible and is often the only site within the whole animal, particularly in humans, that can be examined in studies of drug disposition over time. Knowledge of the concentration of drug and metabolites in the plasma or serum at specific times can provide an insight into the disposition of drug in the whole animal. These pharmacokinetic data are useful in designing drug schedules.

Pharmacokinetic Measurements

The assessment of drug disposition in the whole animal usually includes measurements of the concentration of drug (and possibly drug metabolites) in serum or plasma at specific times following drug administration. In the most simplistic situation a drug can be assumed to be uniformly and rapidly distributed throughout the body. The "volume of distribution," a pharmacokinetic term used to approximate the concentration of drug in the nonexchangeable compartments of the body, can be calculated by dividing the total amount of drug into the body (in milligrams per kilogram) by the concentration that one finds in the plasma (in milligrams per liter) after sufficient time is allowed for the drug to fully distribute and equilibrate following drug administration [32].

$$V_D = \frac{\text{total amount of drug in body (mg/kg)}}{\text{concentration in plasma (mg/liter)}}$$

When the volume of distribution V_D is relatively large, the drug is slowly eliminated from the body with a relatively low concentration of free drug being observed. The volume of distribution provides an excellent means by which the physical-chemical properties of drug can be correlated with the length of time the drug remains within the animal. This information can be useful in developing a dose schedule (see below).

In evaluating the distribution of a drug, it is also useful to determine the rate of disappearance of drug from the central compartment. The removal of drug is usually a first-order kinetic process with a constant fraction of drug being removed per unit of time. The pharmacokinetic term that is used to describe the rate at which a drug is eliminated from the body is the half-life (t1/2). This is defined as the time required for a drug in the body to decrease to one-half of its initial value [33]. This value provides an overall measurement of the efficiency with which the drug is eliminated. Knowledge of the half-life can be used to adjust drug schedules to achieve optimal drug concentrations with hopefully increased therapeutic effectiveness.

D. Excretion

Drugs are excreted from the whole animal either unchanged or as metabolites. Virtually all excretory organs (with the possible exception of the lung, which does not have a major role in the excretion of antineoplastic drugs) excrete polar compounds more efficiently than do nonpolar lipid-soluble compounds. Usually, lipid-soluble drugs must first be metabolized to more polar compounds before they can be excreted [34].

The major route of excretion of antineoplastic agents is via the kidney with release of drug or drug metabolites into the urine (Fig. 3.2). Similar to excretion of endogenous substances, excretion of drugs (or their metabolites) into the urine is determined by essentially three processes: glomerular filtration, tubular secretion, and tubular reabsorption. Glomerular filtration of a drug is restricted by molecular weight and the concentration of free drug [35]. Tubular secretion of both acidic and basic drugs is via an active carrier-mediated transport process which usually necessitates movement of a drug across a large concentration gradient.

In certain clinical situations, the excretion of the drug must be carefully monitored to avoid major toxicity. For example, the administration of high doses of methotrexate, a weak organic acid, can cause acid-related toxicities. Consequently, use of this drug requires alkalinization of the urine and avoidance of other acidic drugs, such as aspirin, which may compete for the same tubular secretory carriers [36]. In the proximal and distal tubules of the kidney nonionized weak acids and bases may also undergo passive reabsorption back into the circulation. A concentration gradient can develop for back diffusion secondary to reabsorption of water and certain inorganic ions. By alkalinizing the urine it is possible to increase the excretion of weakly acidic drugs since they are more likely to be dissociated, thereby decreasing the possibility of passive reabsorption. Alkalization of urine has the opposite effect on the excretion of weak basic drugs, decreasing the ionization and hence the excretion of weakly basic drugs.

Although the renal route is the major means for excretion of antineoplastic drugs, many drugs after metabolism in the liver are excreted into the intestinal tract via the bile (Fig. 3.2). Here also, reabsorption of drug may occur, with drug being absorbed from the intestine back into the circulation. This enterohepatic circulation can result in the persistence of drug in the body. It is particularly important to identify which antineoplastic agents utilize this route of excretion since the presence of hepatobilialy disease, which can occur with metatases, may markedly affect the excretion of the drug, leading to significant toxicity. This has been shown to be important with the widely used anthracyclene antibiotic adriamycin [37].

It should be noted that some drugs may also be excreted into sweat, saliva, tears, and breast milk. Although not important in a quantitative sense, this can have important toxic implications.

E. Other Factors Affecting Drug Disposition

There are several other factors that may have a major impact on the disposition of drug in the whole animal and one of these is the presence of neoplasia itself. It has been well documented in experimental animals harboring transplantable tumors that impairment of drug metabolism can occur in these animals compared to control animals without tumor [38]. Although direct evidence does not exist for this phenomenon in humans, there is a suggestion that drug metabolism may be altered in the human patient with cancer as well [39]. One must also keep in mind that the patient with cancer may have markedly altered organ function. For example, patients with liver metastates may have altered hepatic metabolism of a drug and patients with gastrointestinal malignancies may have altered gastrointestinal function, with changes in intraluminal pH or transit time, resulting in altered absorption of a drug [40].

Another important factor is the potential drug interaction. Most patients receiving chemotherapy are no longer treated with one antineoplastic agent but with combinations of agents. Therefore, the possibility for interaction of the various drugs must be considered. Interaction may occur at several levels. There is evidence in experimental animals that one antineoplastic drug may affect the uptake and retention of other drugs. L-Aspariginase has been demonstrated to affect the in vivo uptake and retention of methotrexate, 6-mercaptopurine, cytosine arabinoside, and 5-fluorouracil in mice bearing the L5178 tumor [41]. Also important on the disposition of antineoplastic drugs are the effects of supportive drugs.

Patients with neoplasia often are on multiple drugs, including sedatives, analgesics, tranquilizers, and other supportive agents. It is well known that agents such as the barbituates can markedly increase microsomal enzyme activity, resulting in an increased rate of metabolism. For example, the $t_{1/2}$ value of cyclophosphamide can be decreased by prior administration of barbiturate [42]. Drugs can also compete for catabolic pathways, resulting in increased toxicity. Thymidine administered with 5-fluorouracil can markedly increase toxicity by competing for the same catabolizing enzymes as 5-fluorouracil, resulting in increased effective concentrations of 5-fluorouracil, and thereby increased toxicity [43]. Similarly, the use of allopurinol (given to decrease uric acid, which often is increased because allopurinol inhibits xanthine oxidase, the enzyme responsible for 6-mercaptopurine degradation [44]. Other drugs may compete for excretory mechanisms; for example, aspirin competes with methotrexate for the same tubular secretory carriers in the kidney. This causes tubular secretion of methotrexate to decrease, resulting in increased plasma levels and possible increased toxicity [45]. Other drugs may compete for binding sites on protein (e.g., albumin), leading to altered distribution of the antineoplastic agent [46].

F. Developing a Dose Schedule

Understanding the drug disposition parameters discussed above provides a basis for the development of a drug schedule, including the dose to be used and the interval of drug administration. Bioavailability data should aid in the selection of a route of administration. Pharmacokinetic data such as the V_D and t1/2 values should provide an estimate of how quickly the drug is eliminated.

Two other very important factors particularly relevant to antineoplastic drugs that must be considered in developing a dosing schedule are (1) the potential high toxic side effects, and (2) the very steep dose-response profiles of these agents. Thus the effective dose of antineoplastic agents and the toxic dose are frequently very similar. As a consequence, antineoplastic drug schedules are most often dictated primarily by toxicity data rather than pharmacokinetic data. For example, nitrosourea drugs which are rapidly metabolized and released from the circulation are administered only every 6-8 weeks because of late-occurring thrombocytopenia that may occur 4-7 weeks following drug administration [47]. Small increases in drug dose may also be accompanied by large increases in host toxicity. Thus the frequency of readministration of drug as well as the drug dose can be determined by host toxicity.

It should be noted that another factor complicating development of a dosing schedule for antineoplastic drugs is the fact that drug effect is not easily assessed in the whole animal. In contrast to antibacterial chemotherapy, where the response to the dose and frequency of drug administration can be assessed within hours or days with marked clinical improvement and significant changes in laboratory tests (e.g., increased white blood count returning to normal limits, or bacterial culture studies demonstrating a response to therapy), the response with antineoplastic therapy is much more difficult to quantitate; often there is no measurable tumor mass or marker available for follow-up.

The actual selection of the dose and schedule to be used in humans is usually based on studies done in animals, not only small animals (e.g., mice and rats) but also larger animals (e.g., dogs, cats, and Ederly monkeys). Doses based on surface areas have been shown to have relevance in the selection of a comparable dose in other animals as well as humans [48]. Thus a relatively nontoxic dose (expressed per square meter) from large-animal studies can be used to select a relatively nontoxic dose (expressed per square meter) in humans. This dose is used for the initial phase I studies with gradual escalation of dose in subsequent patient studies until toxicity is noted. Following the determination of the maximally tolerable dose, phase II studies can be undertaken in patients with measurable tumors to determine drug effectiveness. Later studies can be undertaken to compare the maximally effective (but tolerable) dose with other standard therapies used for a particular tumor type.

IV. DISPOSITION OF DRUG IN CELLS

Section III reviewed those factors that determine disposition of antineoplastic drugs in the whole animal, thereby defining the concentration of a drug and/or drug metabolites that ultimately reach cells in the periphery. Other factors, primarily at the cellular level, determine the further disposition of antineoplastic drugs into and within these cells. The subject area of cellular or biochemical pharmacology includes the study of uptake of the drug into the cell, metabolic activation or inactivation of the drug within the cell, the interaction of drug or drug metabolite with intracellular targets, and the mechanism of drug cytotoxicity. Particularly important is understanding why the growth of certain tumor cells is inhibited by a drug while the growth of other cells is unaffected, and why the growth of still other cells that were initially responsive subsequently become resistant to the drug. Understanding the mechanism of resistance can provide an insight into the biochemical means by which the resistance can be circumvented. Depicted in Fig. 3.3 are the factors important in understanding the cellular pharmacology of antineoplastic drugs and the possible sites of drug resistance. This approach applies to the study of the cellular pharmacology of antineoplastic drugs in host cells as well. The awareness of a potential difference in the cellular pharmacology of the drug in tumor and host cells may enable possible biochemical modulations of drug action to enhance the therapeutic effect by increasing the toxicity in tumor cells while decreasing the toxicity in host cells.

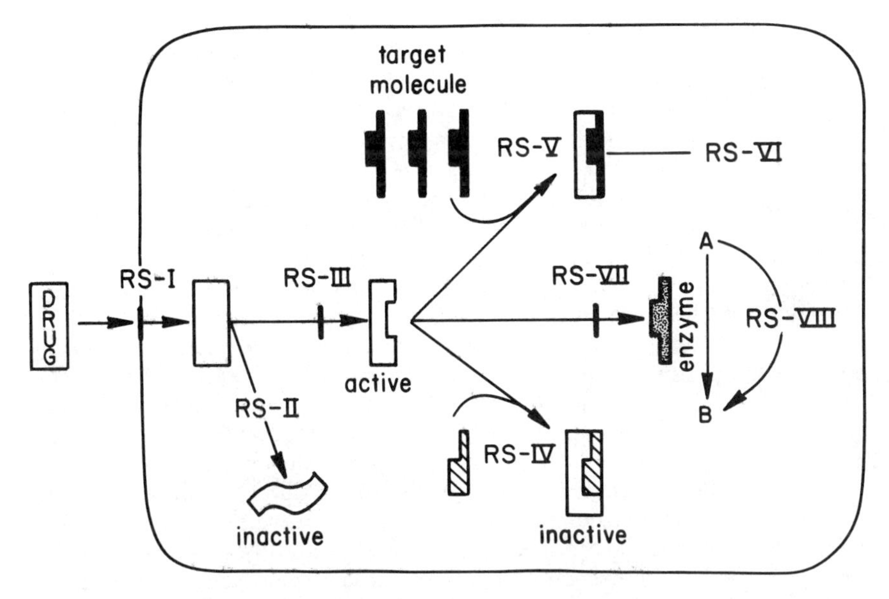

FIGURE 3.3 Disposition of antineoplastic agent in the cell with emphasis on the possible sites of drug resistance; RS-I, inhibition of uptake or transport of drug into cell; RS-II, increased inactivation of drug (or acute metabolite); RS-III, inhibition of activation step; RS-IV, increased reaction with a nonessential molecule; RS-V, increased synthesis of target molecules; RS-VI, repair of cytotoxic damage; RS-VII, decreased interaction of drug with critical enzyme; RS-VIII, bypass of inhibition of critical enzymatic step by alternative pathway. (Adapted from Ref. 86.)

A. Drug Entry into Cells

With most antineoplastic drugs it is necessary for the drug to traverse the cell membrane before antitumor activity can result. This should be accomplished sufficiently fast to achieve the intracellular concentrations needed either for direct interaction with a critical intracellular target or for initial conversion to an active metabolite which can subsequently react with the target. One notable exception is illustrated by the natural product L-asparaginase, an enzyme "drug", isolated from Escherichia coli which catabolizes extracellular asparagine. This results in a decreased amount of extracellular asparagine. Since certain tumor cells, such as lymphocytic leukemic cells (unlike natural host cells) require exogenous asparagine, use of L-asparaginase can theoretically result in selective toxicity inhibiting the growth of these luekemic cells [49].

The synthetic chemist should have an awareness of the potential for uptake of a drug into cells when designing new antineoplastic agents. For example, a drug may be a very potent inhibitor of an intracellular target, therefore suggesting that it is a potentially useful antineoplastic drug, when in fact the drug may be unable to be transported across the cell membrane, thus rendering it completely useless as a therapeutic agent.

The same principles that apply to passage of drugs though cell membranes in whole animals (absorption from the gastrointestinal tract and reabsorption from the renal tubule) are relevant in determining whether a drug may pass through the cell membrane of tumor or host cells. This is particularly important for drugs that traverse by passive or facilitated diffusion. Drugs that are analogs of normally occurring metabolites such as the purine and pyrimidine antimetabolite drugs and the antifolate drugs utilize the same transport routes as do their natural counterparts. Their transport is governed by essentially the same factors that influence the transport of the endogenous compounds across cell membranes [50].

The transport of several antineoplastic drugs into tumor cells in vivo has been well characterized. These include many of the antimetabolite drugs, such as the antifolate methotrexate [51], as well as several alkylating agents [52]. An understanding of the transport of many of the other antineoplastic drugs is less clear. Cellular transport of a drug into tumor cells can be the critical determinant of whether a particular antineoplastic agent shows activity in vivo. Furthermore, it has been demonstrated that tumor cells can develop resistance (see RS-I in Fig. 3-3) to an antineoplastic drug due to an acquired defect in transport leading to diminished intracellular levels of drug [53], actinomycin D [54], daunomycin [55], and the *Vinca* alkaloids [56].

B. Intracellular Metabolism

Antineoplastic agents differ as to the need to be activated. Agents such as methotrexate do not require metabolism within the whole animal or within the tumor. Although methotrexate and other agents may be polyglutamated [57] within both areas these may also have a role in the antitumor effect. Other drugs, such as cyclophosphamide, must be metabolically activated within the host prior to entry of the active metabolite into tumor cells. Cyclophosphamide is activated by the mixed-function oxidase enzymes located primarily within the hepatic microsomes [26,27]. Other drugs, such as the pyrimidine and purine antimetabolites, require metabolic activation after entry of the drug into the tumor cells before reaction with intracellular targets occurs. Thus the pyrimidine base 5-fluorouracil and its nucleoside derivatives have antitumor activity following conversion to specific nucleotide forms within the tumor cell [58, 59]. Similarly, the pyrimidine nucleoside cytosine arabinoside [60] and the purine nucleosides 6-thioguanine and 6-mercaptopurine [61] must first be converted to nucleotides before these drugs can react with critical intracellular targets to produce antitumor activity. Since nucleotides traverse the cell membrane poorly [62], these drugs should not be nucleotides themselves but should be capable of being activated to the nucleotides within the tumor cells. The inability of a drug such as the pyrimidine or purine antimetabolites to be converted to its nucleotide may be a source of primary or secondary resistance to the drug (see RS-III in Fig. 3.3).

The inactivation of a drug or drug metabolite may also occur within the tumor cell, resulting in decreased activity of the antineoplastic agent. For example, cytosine arabinoside may be converted within leukemic cells not only to the active form by conversion to the nucleotide cytosine arabinoside triphosphate but also to inactive forms by deamination of either cytosine arabinoside or its nucleotides to inactive uracil arabinoside metabolites [63]. Understanding the cellular pharmacology of cytosine arabinoside has led to the design of other drugs (e.g., tetrahydrouridine) that can inhibit the inactivating enzymes (e.g., cytidine deaminase) within the tumor cells [64]. Tetrahydrouridine is a hypothetical transition-state compound interacting with cytidine deaminase that is currently in clinical evaluation [65]. Studies are also being conducted to develop agents which may directly or indirectly inactivate the deaminating step at the nucleotide level of deoxycytosine monophosphate deaminase. Hopefully, in this way, primary or acquired resistance to cytosine arabinoside may be overcome.

A comprehensive understanding of the cellular metabolism of antimetabolites and their natural counterparts has led to attempts to modulate the metabolism of these drugs biochemically. Since many of the pyrimidine or purine base and nucleoside drugs utilize "salvage" metabolic pathways that differ from the "de novo pathways," it may be possible to increase the relative proportion of nucleotides formed from salvage pathways by using agents that block steps in the endogenous pathways [66]. PALA [67] and pyrazofuran [68] are two modulators of the de novo pathway of uracil that have been demonstrated to increase the relative proportion of 5-fluouracil nucleotide metabolites, leading to increased tumor cell toxicity. Similar approaches have been used with the purine nucleoside 6-mercaptopurine [69]. Another modulation approach to increase the production of an active metabolite is to increase the availability of necessary substrate (e.g., ribose or deoxyribose) [70], or cofactor [e.g., phosphoribosylpyrophosphate [71].

C. Intracellular Targets

The intracellular target is the location of a critical interaction between the drug (or its activated metabolite) and a specific cellular receptor. With antineoplastic drugs this is usually the site that results in cytotoxicity which is manifested by the inhibition of further cell division. The target or receptor may be a critical enzyme reaction. Thus the drug or drug metabolite may be a substitute for a naturally occurring metabolite, thereby interfering with an important enzyme reaction most often needed in nucleic acid biosynthesis. For example, the antifolate methotrexate after intracellular accumulation may bind to all available dihydrofolate reductase sites, preventing further formation of 5,10-methylene tetrahydrofolate, a cofactor needed for thymidylate and purine biosynthesis, resulting in inhibition of further nucleic acid synthesis [72]. Similarly, the deoxyribonucleotide of 5-fluorouracil may directly inhibit the enzyme thymidylate synthetase, thereby inhibiting synthesis of thymidylate [73].

The importance of acquiring a thorough understanding of the intracellular target is highlighted further by the interaction of methotrexate and 5-fluorouracil since these two drugs may both affect (indirectly and directly) the same target site, the enzyme thymidylate synthetase. It has been shown that the timing of administration of these two drugs determines whether the combination is antagonistic [74] or synergistic [75].

Not all intracellular targets affected by antineoplastic agents are enzyme reactions. For example, a number of drugs have been identified that interact directly with nucleic acids. Alkylating agents such as the nitrogen mustards may alkylate the number 7 nitrogen of guanine, forming bridges across nucleic acid chains which can result in disruption of nucleic acid function [76]. The antibiotics actinomycin D [77] and adriamycin [78] and the inorganic coordinate complex *cis*-dichlorodiamine platinum (*cis*-platinum) [79] may intercalate into the nucleic acid, resulting in alteration of normal nucleic acid function, which in turn results in cytotoxicity with inhibition of growth. Still other drugs, such as the *Vinca* alkaloids, may react with critical proteins (tubulin in microtubules) necessary for metaphase, which can result in disruption of cell division [80]. The hormonal antineoplastic agents, such as the antiestrogen tamoxifen, may react with specific estrogen receptors present in the cytoplasm of tumor cells, blocking further growth of these, which requires hormone for growth cells [81].

Understanding the biochemical and molecular characteristics of the intracellular targets or receptors is also important in determining the mechanisms of cell resistance to anticancer drugs. This can provide insight into potential biochemical manipulations that can be used to regain activity in resistant cells. Several mechanisms of resistance at the intracellular target have been identified (see Fig. 3.3). For example, cells in which thymidylate synthetase activity has been inhibited by methotrexate or 5-fluorouracil, resulting in depletion of thymidylate needed for nucleic acid synthesis, can recover from inhibition of thymidylate synthetase activity by synthesis of thymidylate by an alternative pathway (see RS-VIII in Fig. 3.3) to form thymidylate from thymidine [82]. Similarly, the affinity of the drug or drug metabolites for a critical enzyme reaction (see RS-VII in Fig. 3.3) may become altered. This has been suggested as a mechanism of resistance to 5-fluorouracil [83]. With a critical enzyme reaction, competition from a naturally occurring substrate may lead to resistance to the drug (or drug metabolite). This also occurs with 5-fluorouracil where its deoxyribosylnucleotide competes with the endogenous uracil deoxyribosyl nucleotide for binding sites on thymidylate synthetase [84]. Increased reduction of a critical target may also result in increased resistance (see RS-V in Fig. 3.3). Thus increased production of dihydrofolate reductase has been suggested as a mechanism of resistance to methotrexate [85]. The activated drug may also be inactivated prior to reaction with a target by interacting with a noncritical molecule (see RS-IV in Fig. 3.3). This has been suggested as a mechanism of resistance to alkylating agents which are chemically very active and may react with many other molecules besides the critical target [86]. Finally, resistance may result from repair of damage caused by the drug (see RS-VI in Fig. 3.3). For example, resistance to alkylating agents has been attributed to cellular repair enzymes, which can repair damage caused by alkylation within nucleic acid by excising and replacing abnormal bases and abnormal bridges across the nucleic acid chains [87].

D. Cytotoxicity

When initially evaluating the cytotoxicity of a new drug in cellular pharmacologic studies, the target site may not be apparent, particularly if the drug is novel and dissimilar to any of the known antineoplastic drugs. Consequently, following demonstrated antineoplastic activity in screening studies, one should first assess cytotoxicity by determining the effect of the drug on the synthesis and function of nucleic acid, a common target or site of cytotoxicity with diverse types of antineoplastic agents. Determining the effect of a range of drug concentrations on the synthesis of new DNA, RNA, and protein in tumor cells is often the initial approach. Cellular kinetic studies can be useful in identifying the phase of the cell cycle in which inhibition of cell division occurs. These biochemical and cell kinetic observations can then be further correlated with the effect of a range of drug concentrations on growth of various host and other tumor cells in cell culture.

V. MEASUREMENT OF DRUG AND METABOLITES

The development of new analytic methods with improved sensitivity, specificity, and reproducibility has had a major impact on recent studies of antineoplastic agents at both the whole animal and cellular levels. At the whole animal level, measurement of serum or plasma drug concentrations for bioavailability and pharmacokinetic studies has been used to determine the proper route and schedule of administration. Earlier studies with antineoplastic agents often used radiolabeled drugs to measure drug concentration in plasma or serum. These studies were often limited by the inability to separate drug from drug metabolites with thin-layer and low-pressure column chromatography; both of these techniques lack sensitivity, resolution, and reproducibility. Use of gas chromatography and gas chromatography-mass spectrometry has enabled more precise identification of drug and metabolites with increased sensitivity. These methods have been demonstrated to be valuable in studies of many antineoplastic drugs [88]. More recently, high-pressure liquid chromatography (HPLC) and, in particular, reversed-phase HPLC have been demonstrated to be valuable in simultaneously assessing drug and drug metabolites [89].

Although these methods are now being used during the initial pharmacological evaluation of a new drug, they have not been used extensively with approved antineoplastic drugs in a general oncological setting. One exception is methotrexate (particularly when used in "high-dose regimens"), which must be measured in serum or plasma to determine when to start "rescue" therapy with leukovorin in order to avoid toxicity [90]. Consequently, several different analytical methods have been developed for assaying methotrexate in the clinical setting. The most widely used method is the radiobinding assay [91], which can be carried out in most hospitals having a clinical chemistry laboratory.

Analytical methods currently have a major role in cellular pharmacological studies of antineoplastic agents. High-pressure liquid chromatography combined with the use of radiolabeled drugs has been valuable in studies of drug transport [92] and intracellular metabolism [93]; reversed-phase HPLC being particularly valuable in simultaneously resolving drug and metabolites. These analytical methods have made it possible to coordinate studies at the cellular level with studies at the in vivo or clinical level. Thus it is possible to estimate the dose of drug needed in vivo to obtain a concentration of drug in the tumor cells in the periphery from cellular studies with verification by monitoring drug levels in vivo.

VI. CONCLUSIONS

This chapter has examined an approach to the study of antineoplastic drugs in pharmacological studies at the whole animal level and at the cellular level (including studies in tumor cells and host cells). An attempt has been made to identify those factors in the whole animal that control delivery of a drug or its active metabolite to the tumor or host cell in the periphery. This was followed by a review of the factors controlling disposition of drug or active metabolite at the cellular level. These pharmacological data should enable more rational use of the drug, maximizing antitumor effectiveness while minimizing host cell toxicity. This, in turn, may lead to the design of more effective combination chemotherapy regimens and may suggest biochemical means by which cellular resistance may be overcome.

REFERENCES

1. P. J. Creavan and E. Mihich, Semin. Oncol., 4: 147 (1977).
2. S. E. Mayer, K. L. Melman, and A. G. Gilman, in Pharmacological Basis of Therapeutics (A. G. Gilman, L. S. Goodman, and A. Gilman, eds.), Macmillan, New York, 1980, pp. 1-27.

3. F. S. Sjostrand, in Ultrastructure and Functions of Cellular Membranes in the Membranes (A. S. Dalton and F. Gagenan, eds.), Academic Press, New York, 1968, pp. 151-210.
4. V. T. Oliverio, in Absorption, Distribution, and Excretion of Antineoplastic and Immunosuppressive Agents II (A. C. Sartorelli and D. G. Johns, eds.), Springer-Verlag, New York, 1975, pp. 229-239.
5. I. D. Goldman, in Pharmacologic Principles of Cancer Treatment (B. Chabner, ed.), W. B. Saunders, Philadelphia, 1982, pp. 15-44.
6. L. M. Cobb, Int. J. Cancer, 1: 324 (1966).
7. L. B. Sheiner and T. N. Tozer, in Clinical Pharmacokinetics: The Use of Plasma Concentrations of Drugs in Clinical Pharmacology (K. L. Melman and H. F. Marrelli, eds.), Macmillan, New York, 1978, pp. 71-109.
8. P. Calabresi and R. E. Parks, in Pharmacological Basis of Therapeutics (A. G. Gilman, L. S. Goodman, and A. Gilman, eds.), Macmillan, New York, 1980, p. 1263.
9. D. A. Priebat, P. P. Bradley, and E. W. Nelson, Proc. Amer. Soc. Clin. Oncol., 22: 415 (1981).
10. A. M. Shah, W. C. MacDonald, J. H. Goldie, G. A. Gudaskae, and B. Sullivan, Proc. Am. Soc. Clin. Oncol., 22: 536 (1981).
11. P. Calabresi and R. E. Parks, in Pharmacological Basis of Therapeutics (A. G. Gilman, L. S. Goodman, and A. Gilman, eds.), Macmillan, New York, 1980, p. 1275.
12. H. Handelsman and M. Slavik, Ftorafur (FT-207) NSC-148959. Clinical brochure, Division of Cancer Treatment, National Cancer Institute, Bethesda, Md., 1974.
13. E. Klein, H. Milgrom, H. L. Stall, F. Helm, H. J. Walker, and O. A. Haltermann, in Cancer Chemotherapy II (I. Brodsky and S. B. Kahn, eds.), Grune & Stratton, New York, 1972, pp. 147-166.
14. T. Anderson, Semin. Oncol., 6: 240 (1979).
15. D. P. Rall, in Drug Entry into Brain and Cerebrospinal Fluid in Fundamentals of Drug Metabolism and Drug Disposition (B. N. LaDu, H G. Mandel, and E. L. Way, eds.), Williams & Wilkins, Baltimore, 1971, pp. 76-87.
16. C. B. Wilson, P. Gutin, E. B. Baldrey, D. Crafts, V. A. Levin, and K. J. Enat, Arch. Neurol., 33: 739 (1976).
17. E. W. Moore, L. B. Thomas, R. K. Shaw, and E. J. Freireich, Arch. Intern. Med., 105: 451 (1960).
18. R. A. Bender, Oncology, 30: 328 (1974).
19. P. R. Band, J. F. Holland, J. Bernard, M. Weil, M. Walker, and D. Mand Rall, Cancer, 32: 744 (1973).
20. W. A. Bleyer, D. G. Poplack, and R. M. Simon, Blood, 51: 835 (1978).
21. J. H. Galicich and L. J. Gaido, Symp. Surg. Oncol., 54: 915 (1974).

22. E. T. Krementz, R. D. Carter, C. M. Sutherland, and I. Hulton, Am. Surg., 185: 555 (1977).
23. J. A. Petrek and J. P. Minton, Cancer, 43: 2182 (1979).
24. J. L. Speyer, J. M. Collins, R. L. Dedrick, M. F. Bresman, H. Londer, V. T. DeVita, and C. E. Myers, Cancer Res., 40: 567 (1980).
25. R. L. Dedrick, C. E. Myers, P. N. Bungay, and V. T. DeVita, Cancer Treat Rep., 62: 1 (1978).
26. N. Brock and D. J. Hohorst, Arzneim. Forsch., 13: 1021 (1963).
27. J. L. Cohen and J. Y. Joo, J. Pharmacol. Exp. Ther., 174: 206 (1970).
28. D. M. Valerino, D. G. Johns, D. S. Azharko, and V. T. Oliverio, Biochem. Pharmacol., 21: 821 (1972).
29. R. E. Finch, M. R. Bending, and A. F. Lont, Br. J. Clin. Pharmacol., 7: 613 (1979).
30. C. Davison, in Fundamentals of Drug Metabolism and Drug Disposition (B. N LaDu, H. G. Mandel, and E. L. Way, eds.), Williams & Wilkins, Baltimore, 1971, pp. 63-75.
31. T. Butler, in Fundamentals of Drug Metabolism and Drug Disposition (B. N. LaDu, H. G. Mandel, and E. L. Way, eds.), Williams & Wilkins, Baltimore, 1971, pp. 44-62.
32. A. J. Alkinson and W. Kushner, Am. Rev. Pharmacol. Toxicol., 19: 105 (1979).
33. M. Gilbaldi and D. Perrier, Pharmacokinetics, Marcel Dekker, New York, 1975.
34. G. H. Mudge, Am. Rev. Pharmacol., 7: 163 (1967).
35. I. M. Weiner, in Concepts in Biochemical Pharmacology (B. B. Broddie and J. R. Gillette, eds.), Springer-Verlag, Berlin, 1971, pp. 328-353.
36. J. L. Romalo, N. H. Goldberg, K. R. Hande, et al., Cancer Treat. Rep., 61: 1393 (1977).
37. R. S. Benjamin, P. H. Wiernik, and N. R. Bachur, Cancer, 33: 19 (1974).
38. R. Rosso, M. G. Donelli, G. Franchi, and S. Garatlini, Eur. J. Cancer, 7: 565 (1971).
39. T. L. Loo, D. H. W. Ho, and D. Farquhar, in Cancer Chemotherapy—Fundamental Concepts and Recent Advances (M. D. Anderson Staff, eds.), Year Book Medical Publishers, Chicago, 1975, pp. 57-58.
40. G. Brule, S. J. Elkhardt, T. C. Hall, and A. Winkler, in Drug Therapy in Cancer, WHO, Geneva, 1973, p. 23.
41. A. Nahos and R. L. Capizzi, Cancer Res., 34: 2689 (1974).
42. J. Y. Jao, W. J. Jusko, and J. L. Cohen, Cancer Res., 32: 2761 (1972).
43. T. M. Woodcock, D. S. Martin, L. E. M. Damin, et al., Cancer, 45: 1135 (1980).

44. J. J. Caffey, C. A. White, A. B. Lesk, et al., Cancer Res., 32: 1283 (1972).
45. D. G. Liegler, E. S. Henderson, M. A. Hahn, et al., Clin. Pharmacol. Ther., 10: 849 (1969).
46. W. Settle, S. Hegeman, and R. M. Featherstone, in Concepts in Biochemical Pharmacology (B. B. Brodie and J. R. Gillette, eds.), Springer-Verlag, Berlin, 1971, pp. 175-186.
47. M. Calvin, in Pharmacologic Principles of Cancer Treatment (B. Chabner, ed.), W. B. Saunders, Philadelphia, 1982, pp. 276-308.
48. E. J. Freireich, E. A. Gehan, D. P. Rall, et al., Cancer Chemother. Rep., 50: 219 (1966).
49. R. L. Capizzi, J. R. Bertino, and R. E. Handschumacker, Amer. Rev. Med., 21: 433 (1970).
50. R. M. Wahlhueter, R. S. McIvar, and P. G. W. Plagemann, J. Cell. Physiol., 104: 209 (1980).
51. I. D. Goldman, N. S. Lichtenstein, and V. T. Oliverio, J. Biol. Chem., 243: 5007 (1968).
52. G. J. Goldenberg, C. L. Vanstone, L. G. Israels, D. Ilse, and I. Bihler, Cancer Res., 30: 2285 (1970).
53. G. A. Fischer, Biochem. Pharmacol., 11: 1233 (1962).
54. M. N. Goldstein, K. Hamm, and E. Amrod, Science, 151: 1555 (1966).
55. K. Dano, Biochem. Biphys. Acta, 323: 466 (1973).
56. K. Dano, Cancer Chemother. Rep., 56: 701 (1972).
57. R. L. Schulsky, B. D. Borley, and B. A. Chabner, Proc. Natl. Acad. Sci. USA, 77: 2919 (1980).
58. D. Kessel, T. C. Hall, and I. Wodinsky, Science, 154: 911 (1966).
59. R. D. Armstrong and R. B. Diasio, Cancer Res., 40: 3333 (1980).
60. Y. M. Rustum and H. Preisler, Cancer Res., 38: 543 (1978).
61. J. J. McCormack and D. G. Johns, in Pharmacologic Principles of Cancer Treatment (B. Chabner, ed.), W. B. Saunders, Philadelphia, 1982, pp. 213-228.
62. A. R. P. Patterson, in Molecular Actions and Targets for Cancer Chemotherapeutic Agents (A. C. Sarotrelli, J. S. Lazo, and J. R. Bertino, eds.), Academic Press, New York, 1981, p. 214.
63. C. D. Stewart and P. J Burke, Nature New Biol., 233: 109 (1971).
64. R. G. Stoller, C. E. Myers, and B. A. Chabner, Biochem. Pharmacol., 27: 53 (1978).
65. W. Kreis, T. M. Woodcock, and C. S. Gordon, Cancer Treat. Rep., 61: 1347 (1977).
66. D. S. Martin, R. L. Stolfi, R. C. Sawyer, R. Nayak, S. Spiegelman, F. Schmid, R. Heiner, and E. Cadman, in Nucleosides and Cancer Treatment (M. H. N. Tattersall and R. M. F. Ox, eds.), Academic Press, New York, 1981, pp. 339-382.

67. T. W. Kensler and D. A. Cooney, Adv. Pharmacol. Chemother., 18: 273 (1979).
68. E. C. Cadman, D. E. Dix, and R. E. Handschumacher, Cancer Res., 38: 682 (1978).
69. M. C. Wang, A. I. Simpson, and A. R. F. Patterson, Cancer Chemother. Rep., 51: 101 (1967).
70. D. Kessel and T. C. Hall, Cancer Res., 29: 1749 (1969).
71. E. Cadman, R. Heimer, and C. Benz, J. Biol. Chem., 256: 1695 (1981).
72. W. C. Werkheiser, Cancer Res., 23: 1277 (1963).
73. P. Reyes and C. Heidelberger, Mol. Pharmac., 1: 14 (1965).
74. D. Bowen, J. C. White, and I. D. Goldman, Cancer Res., 38: 219 (1978).
75. J. R. Bertino, W. L. Sawicki, C. A. Lindquist, and V. S. Gopta, Cancer Res., 37: 327 (1977).
76. C. C. Price, in Antineoplastic and Immunosuppressive Agents, Part II (A. C. Sartorelli and D. G. Johns, eds.), Springer-Verlag, Berlin, 1975, pp. 1-5.
77. J. Kamowata and M. Imanishi, Nature, 187: 1112 (1960).
78. H. Walder and M. S. Center, Biochem. Biophys. Res. Commun., 98: 95 (1981).
79. L. A. Zivellig and K. W. Kohn, Cancer Treat. Rep., 63: 1439 (1979).
80. R. J. Owellen, C. A. Hartke, and R. M. Dickerson, Cancer Res., 36: 1499 (1976).
81. R. C. Heel, R. N. Erogden, and T. M. Speight, Drugs, 16: 1 (1978).
82. B. A. Chabner, in Pharmacological Principles in Cancer Treatment (B. A. Chabner, ed.), W. B. Saunders, Philadelphia, 1982, pp. 183-212.
83. C. E. Myers, R. Diasio, H. Eliot, and B. A. Chabner, Cancer Treat. Rep., 3: 155 (1976).
84. C. E. Myers, R. C. Young, and B. A. Chabner, J. Clin. Invest., 56: 1231 (1975).
85. F. W. Alt, R. E. Kellems, and R. T. Schimke, J. Biol. Chem., 251: 3063 (1976).
86. C. R. Ball, in Scientific Basis of Cancer Chemotherapy (G. Mathe, ed.), Springer-Verlag, New York, 1969, pp. 26-40.
87. K. W. Kohn, N. H. Steighigel, and C. L. Spears, Proc. Natl. Acad. Sci. USA, 53: 1154 (1965).
88. W. Sacke, C. Finn, and J. Staroscik, Adv. Mass Spectrom. Biochem. Med., 1: 509 (1976).
89. J. A. Benvenuto, S. W. Hall, D. Farquhar, K. Lu, and T. L. Loo, in Biological/Biomedical Applications of Liquid Chromatography (G. L. Hawk, ed.), Marcel Dekker, New York, 1979, pp. 377-395.
90. R. G. Stoller, K. R. Hande, and S. A. Jacobs, N. Engl. J. Med., 297: 630 (1977).

91. C. E. Myers, M. E. Lippman, H. Eliot, and B. A. Chabner, Proc. Natl. Acad. Sci. USA, 72: 3683 (1975).
92. D. Bowen, R. B. Diasio, and I. D. Goldman, J. Biol. Chem., 254: 5333 (1979).
93. J. P. Sommadossi, D. A. Gewirtz, R. B. Diasio, C. Aubert, J. P. Cano, and I. D. Goldman, J. Biol. Chem., 257: 8171 (1982).

4

NOVEL ANTITUMOR AGENTS FROM PLANTS

ALBERT T. SNEDEN

Department of Chemistry
Virginia Commonwealth University
Richmond, Virginia

I. INTRODUCTION

A. Background

Plants have long been recognized as a valuable source of many different types of potential chemotherapeutic agents. The folklore and phytochemical literature of virtually every country is filled with references to the medicinal use of local plants, including the use of selected species in the treatment of tumors [1].

Research dedicated to the isolation and identification of antineoplastic plant principles began in a rational manner in the late 1940s with the isolation of podophyllotoxin [1] and related lignans from the common mayapple root (Podophyllum peltatum) [2, 3]. However, many of the early plant-derived antitumor agents were fortuitous discoveries resulting from the investigation of plants for compounds with other medicinal uses.

Most of the early research on the development of plant principles as potential cancer chemotherapeutic agents was carried out independently in industrial and academic laboratories. Then in 1955, the Cancer Chemotherapy National Service Center (now called the Developmental Therapeutics Program) was established within the National Cancer Institute (NCI) to coordinate the development and to facilitate the screening of compounds with potential antitumor activity. Subsequently, an extensive program was developed for the collection and screening of plants for antitumor activity [4].

B. Acquisition of Plant Material [5]

Each investigator may use a variety of sources to provide plant material, including local and foreign botanists as well as plant and seed importing companies. The NCI program has relied on the Medicinal Plant Resources Laboratory (MPRL) of the U.S. Department of Agriculture (USDA) since 1960 to supervise the acquisition and identification of plants for screening through a network of collectors and botanists in various countries throughout the world.

Initially, a small sample of plant material (approximately 3 lb) is provided for identification and screening for antileukemic activity. Collection of plant samples may be guided by folklore or a random sampling of plants in a particular area may be carried out [5, 6]. Documentation by the botanist in the field and voucher specimens which are deposited with the MPRL are used to classify each plant sample. The identified samples are sent to a contract screener, where an extract is prepared and tested for anticancer activity against the P388 lymphocytic leukemia in the mouse and the KB cell culture screen [7]. If the plant extract demonstrates activity in one or both of these screens, a large recollection of 100 lb or more is made to be used in the isolation work.

Since the active compound(s) may be concentrated in any part of the plant, each part may be collected and screened individually. Thus the collector may divide each plant into separate samples of leaves, fruits, seeds, roots, stems, twigs, bark, or some reasonable combination. One survey has shown that for woody plants in Kenya, stem bark seems to contain the majority of the active constituents, while the leaves are the poorest source [5]. However, each plant is different, and herbaceous plants, in particular, often have the active compound(s) distributed throughout the plant.

The collected plant material is generally chopped into small pieces in the field and allowed to dry before shipment. After inspection at the port of entry by the Animal and Plant Health Inspection Service of the USDA, large recollections are sent directly to investigators for isolation and identification of the active principle(s).

C. Isolation Procedures

During the last 25 years, there has been a tremendous increase in research directed toward the specific isolation and structural elucidation of antineoplastic plant principles. As would be expected, the isolation procedures employed vary a great deal from researcher to researcher. However, one particular protocol has been used extensively with great success. In this procedure [8-10], the dried ground plant material is first exhaustively extracted with 95% ethanol. The concentrated extract is partitioned between chloroform and water, and the chloroform soluble material is then partitioned successively between petroleum ether and 90% methanol. Each tetrachloride and 80% methanol, and chloroform and 60% methanol. Each fraction is concentrated and tested for antitumor activity against the P388 lymphocytic leukemia in the mouse and against a cell culture derived from a human epidermoid carcinoma of the nasopharynx (KB) [7]. The active fraction(s) is then subjected to a variety of separation techniques, such as countercurrent distribution, column chromatography, preparative thin-layer chromatography, and high-pressure liquid chromatography at the discretion of the researcher in order to isolate the active principles.

Obviously, the isolation techniques used may vary to a considerable extent depending on the type of natural product(s) being isolated. However, any method(s) employed for the isolation of the active principles must not alter or destroy the principle being sought. Consequently, chemical reactions and harsh conditions are usually avoided in the initial isolation procedure. Once the structure or type of the active principle is known, a modified isolation procedure may then involve a mild reaction designed to facilitate the isolation or to remove undesired constituents of the extract. For example, if the active principle is known to be an alkaloid (a plant-derived compound containing one or more amine moieties), the active principle might be isolated by initial treatment of the extract with acid to form a water-soluble amine salt followed by regeneration of the free alkaloid with a mild inorganic base. This procedure has been used successfully to isolate active alkaloids such as solapalmitine [11]. In another case, treatment of an intermediate active fraction with acetic anhydride-pyridine facilitated the isolation of the potent antileukemic ansa macrolide maytansine [12].

The particular methods employed for the isolation of the active plant principles are the prerogative of the individual investigator, but one procedure is used by all. Each fraction generated in the isolation procedure is screened for antitumor activity and only those fractions that show significant activity are pursued. The bioassay systems generally employed are the P388 lymphocytic leukemia in the mouse and the Eagle's carcinoma of the nasopharynx in cell culture (KB) [7, 13]. The P388 in vivo and KB cell culture screens are used because they have proven to be the most sensitive of the currently available screening systems, particularly in the early phases of the isolation procedure, where complex mixtures of compounds are common. Once a natural product has been isolated, identified, and demonstrated to have significant antileukemic activity against the P388 leukemia system [i.e., a T/C > 130, where T/C is the ratio, expressed as a percent, of the median survival time of the treated group (T) of mice divided by the median survival time of the control group (C)], it is eligible for testing against other animal cancer systems described in Chap. 3, such as the L1210 leukemia, B16 melanocarcinoma, and Lewis lung tumors [14]. Advancement into clinical trials depend on the results of these and other animal screens.

D. Types of Active Compounds

Antineoplastic plant principles encompass a wide variety of structural classes. Two excellent reviews by Hartwell [2] and by Cordell and Farnsworth [15] have covered much of the literature through 1976. However, a few examples will serve to illustrate the diversity of naturally occurring antitumor compounds.

Podophyllotoxin (1), as noted previously, was the focus of much of the early research in this area, together with related lignans [3]. Since the original work on podophyllotoxin (1), a large number of lignans have been isolated, but like (1), they exhibit a higher degree of toxicity than therapeutic value. However, two semisynthetic lignans in the epipodophyllotoxin series, VP 16-213 (2) and VM 26 (3), have been found to be less toxic and

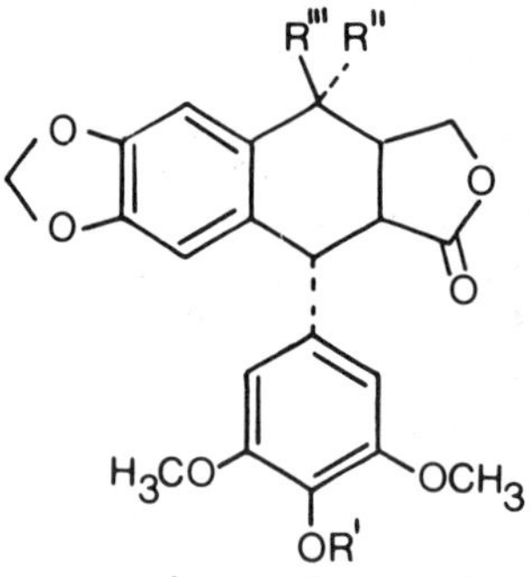

	R'	R''	R'''
(1)	CH_3	OH	H
(2)	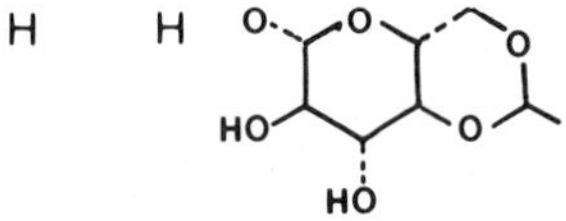 H	H	(glycoside)
(3)	H	H	(thenylidene glycoside)

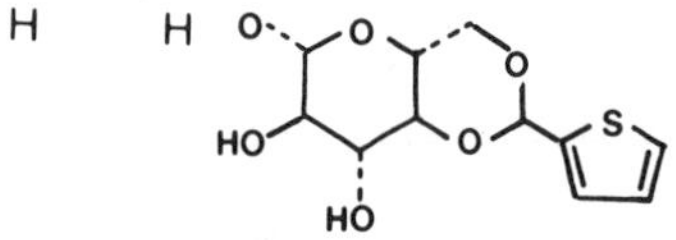

very active in animal test systems [16, 17]. Clinical trials of these latter two lignans appear quite promising [18-20].

Four major classes of terpenes are also represented by active principles. In the monoterpene class, only a few iridoid lactones such as allamandin (4) have shown cytotoxic and, occasionally, in vivo activity [21]. Sesquiterpenes, on the other hand, have yielded a large number of compounds that are both cytotoxic and active in vivo. Many of these compounds are sesquiterpene lactones, such as vernolepin (5) [22] and helenalin (6)

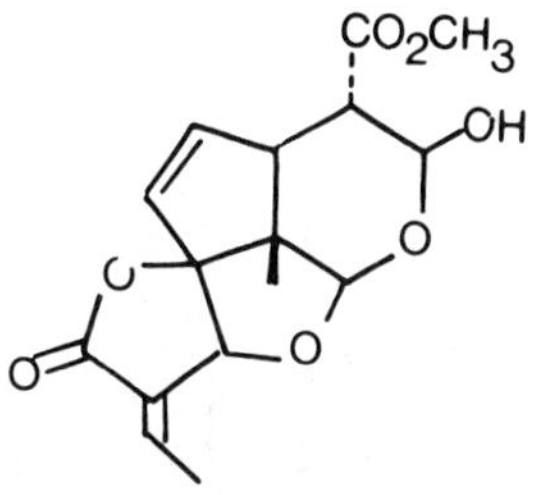

(4) 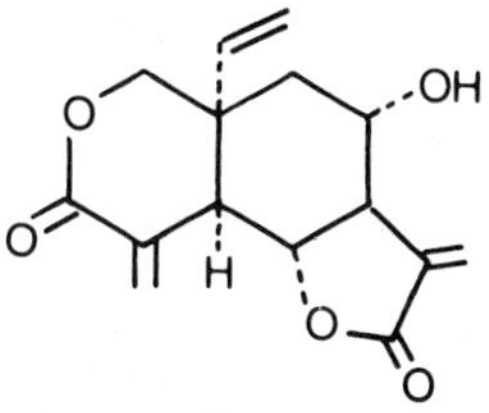 (5) 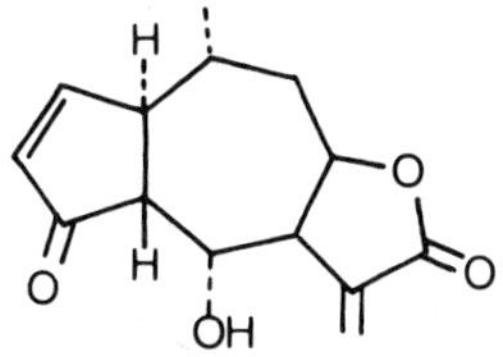 (6)

[23]. None of the sesquiterpene lactones have yet developed any clinical interest due primarily to toxicity and lack of activity in the slow-growing animal tumor systems [2]. Several of the active diterpenes, however, do show significant activity against solid tumor systems, and two diterpenes, taxol (7) from *Taxus brevifolia* [24] and tripdiolide (8) from *Tripterygium*

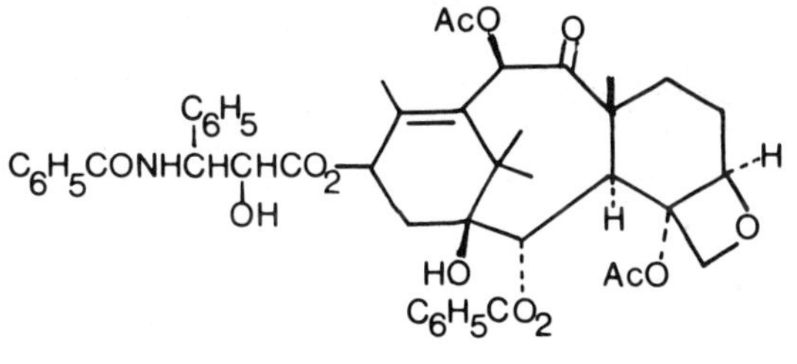

(7) 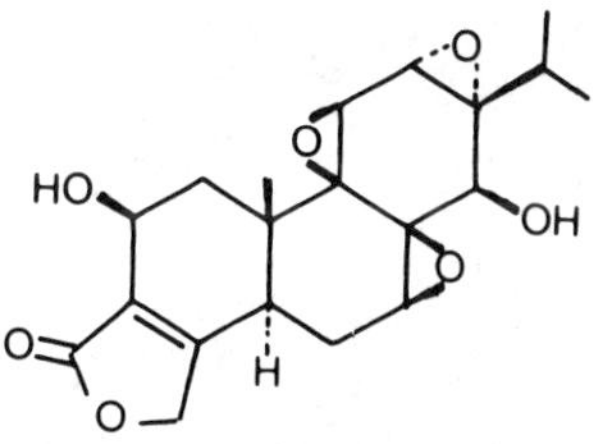 (8)

wilfordii [25], are currently of high interest to the NCI program [14, 26]. Triterpenes have largely been disappointing in the search for antitumor agents. Most of the active compounds found to date have been cucurbitacins such as datiscoside (9) [27] which have minimal activity, or relatively toxic compounds such as pristimerin (10) [28]. The quassinoids are a class of degraded triterpenes related to quassin (11) [29], many of which have exhibited significant antileukemic activity [2, 30]. One family of these compounds will be discussed in more detail later.

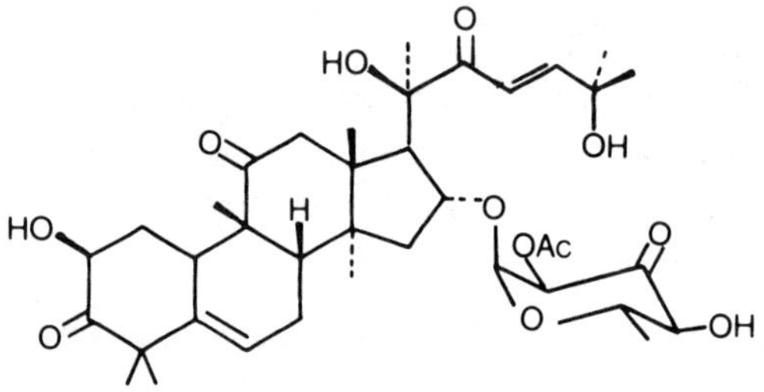

(9)

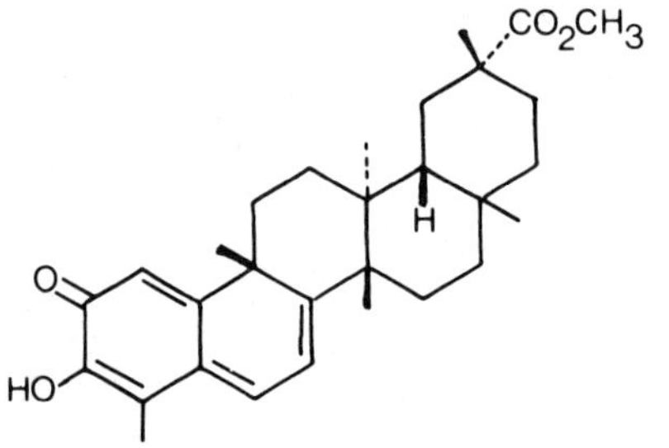

(10)

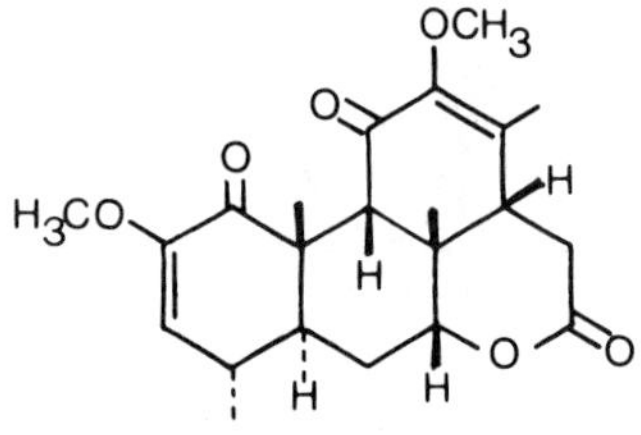

(11)

The class of plant principles that contains the greatest number of antineoplastic compounds is the alkaloids. Several alkaloids besides the Vinca alkaloids have been evaluated in clinical trials. Thalicarpine (12),

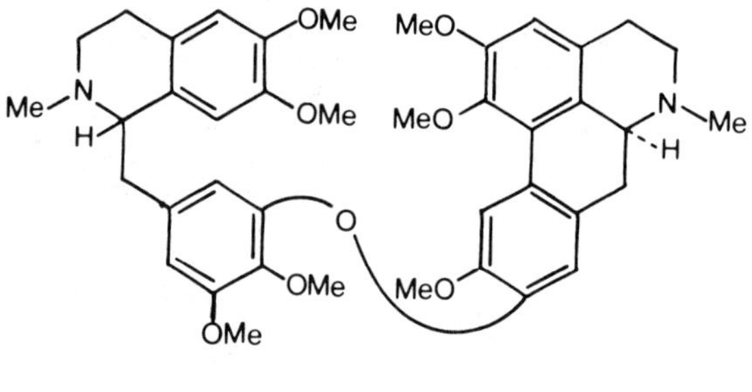

(12)

a dimeric benzylisoquinoline alkaloid isolated from Thalictrum dasycarpum as a hypotensive agent [31], showed minimal toxicity in phase I clinical trials [32]. However, phase II studies of (12) showed no objective responses among 14 patients and further trials have been discontinued [33]. Camptothecin (13), which was isolated from Camptotheca accuminata [34], also exhibited promising activity in animal tumors. It was originally

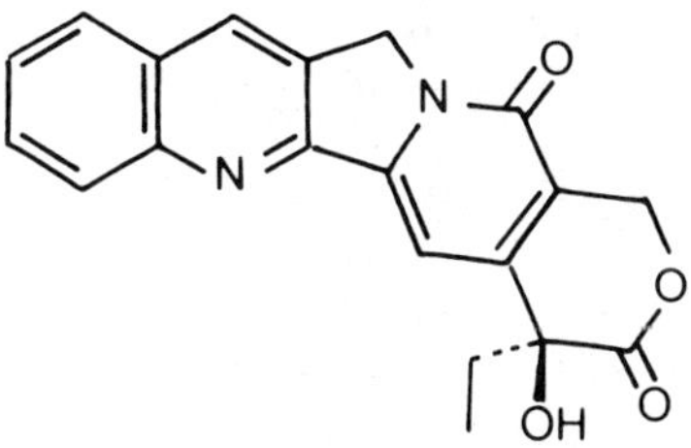

(13)

entered into clinical trials as the sodium salt for increased solubility in water, but toxicity problems have diminished interest in this agent [82]. Other alkaloids of current interest in the NCI program include ellipticine (14) [35] and homoharringtonine (15) [36], which are at various stages of development [14, 26].

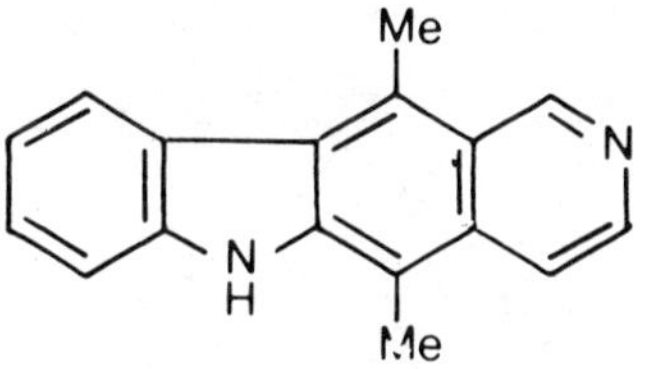

(14)

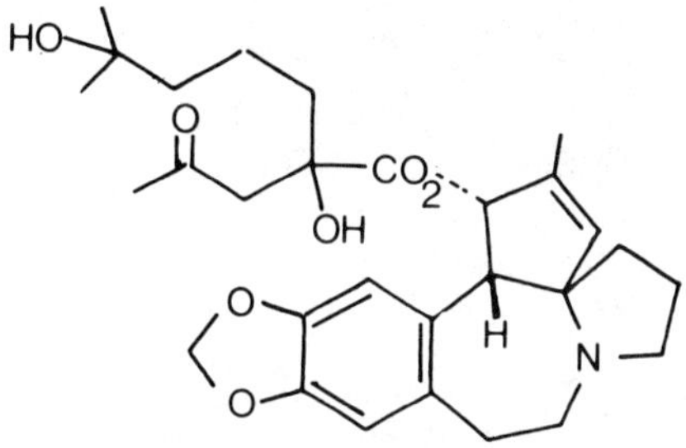

(15)

Other plant-derived compounds, such as sterioid lactones, saponins, ansa macrolides (which will be discussed in more detail later), and a variety of miscellaneous structural types, have also provided active agents [2]. The major characteristic of most of the compounds that show significant activity is that they are highly functionalized molecules. Those compounds that are chosen for further development are generally active in more than one tumor system. Other than these two criteria, however, there are no obvious characteristics which make one class of compounds more likely to produce an antitumor agent than any other.

E. Mechanisms of Action

One of the most important aspects of any study of plant-derived antitumor agents is to determine, where possible, the mechanism by which they exhibit their antitumor activity. A more complete understanding of the mechanisms of action of antineoplastic agents will lead to the synthesis of new tumor-inhibitory compounds as well as rational modifications of existing ones. In examining the existing knowledge of the modes of action of various compounds, it is apparent that several different mechanisms may occur.

Many of the tumor-inhibitory compounds derived from plants contain one or more potential alkylating sites. Consequently, one possible mechanism of action is the alkylation of a nucleophilic moiety on biological macromolecules involved in control of cell division or DNA replication. One such biological nucleophile is a free sulfhydryl (thiol) on a protein, and the alkylation of such sulfhydryls by certain types of tumor inhibitory natural products has been proposed to be the major mechanism of action in several cases [37, 38].

Studies with vernolepin (5) and elephantopin (17) showed that both cytotoxic principles readily alkylated the sulfhydryl of cysteine via Michael addition to the α-methylene-γ-lactone to yield (18) and (19), respectively [39].

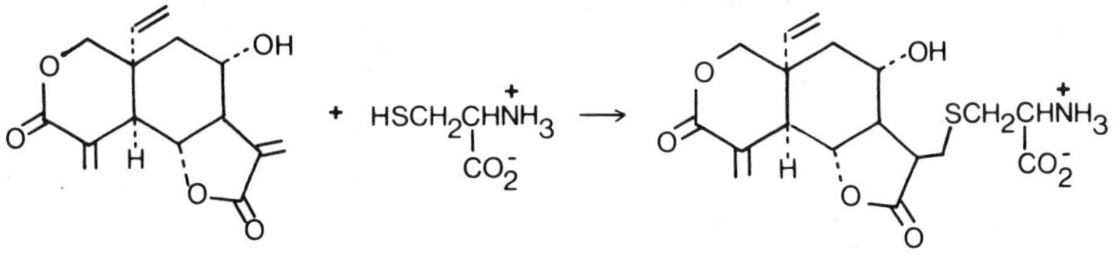

(5) + $HSCH_2CH(CO_2^-)NH_3^+$ (16) ⟶ (18)

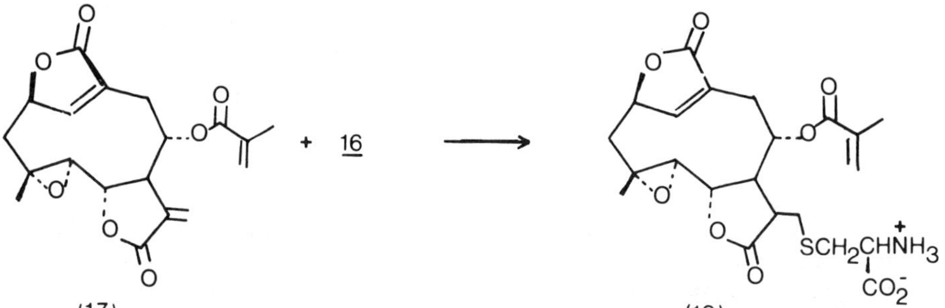

(17) + 16 ⟶ (19)

Subsequent addition of a second molecule of cysteine to the α-methylene-δ-lactone of (5) and the methacrylate ester of (17) also occurred, resulting in adducts that were inactive as antitumor agents. Vernolepin (5) was also found to inactivate glycogen synthetase, evidently reacting with at least three out of the six available free sulfhydryls on the enzyme [40]. In order to delineate the reactivity of the α-methylene-γ-lactone more clearly, (5) and (17) were treated with both lysine and guanine, amino acids with free amine groups. In each case, no reaction occurred, thus indicating that both (5) and (17) were selectively alkylating the thiols [39].

Other tumor-inhibitory plant principles show similar reactivity toward sulfhydryl-containing enzymes. The quinone methide diterpene taxodione (20) was originally isolated from Taxodium distichum and found to have tumor-inhibitory activity against the Walker 256 carcinosarcoma in the rat [41]. Since quinone methides were known to be susceptible to nucleophilic

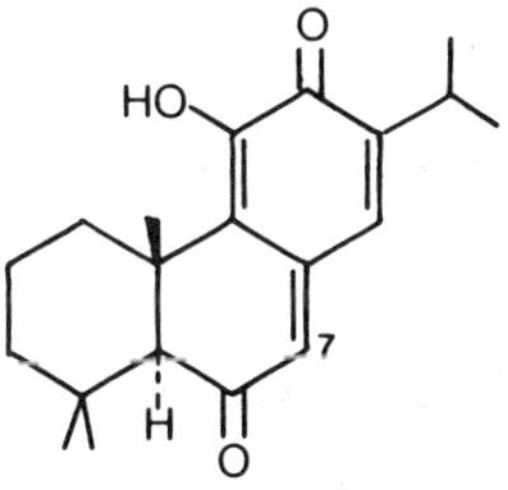

(20)

addition, it was thought that taxodione (20) might exhibit its antitumor activity by alkylating free sulfhydryls in a manner similar to (5) and (17). To examine this possibility, phosphofructokinase, an enzyme that contains 16-18 sulfhydryl groups per protomer, was treated with (20). The activity of the phosphofructokinase was reduced by 50% at a concentration of 1.6 mol of (20) per protomer [42]. This reduction in activity is presumably due to the reaction of (20) with the free sulfhydryls of phosphofructokinase, via addition at C(7).

Obviously, sulfhydryls are not the only biological nucleophiles that might react with a tumor-inhibitory natural product. Another readily available nucleophile is an amine moiety on a nucleic acid or protein. Several studies with model nucleophiles suggest, however, that the reaction of an alkylating site with a sulfhydryl group is more likely to occur. This has been noted in the case of vernolepin (5) and elephantopin (17), and was also suggested by the reactions undergone by oridonin (21), a tumor-inhibitory

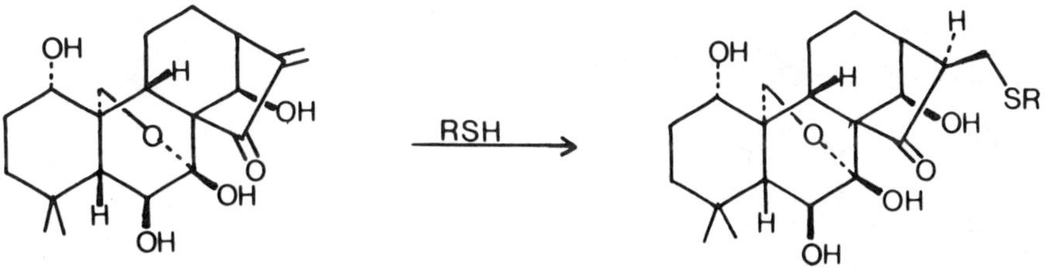

(21) RSH → (22)

diterpene isolated from *Isodon japonicus* [43, 44]. Oridonin (21) was found to react quite readily with a variety of model thiols, including cysteine, via Michael addition to the C(16) methylene to yield adducts such as (22). On the other hand, oridonin (21) did not react with adenosine or cytidine, which are models for the amine-bearing constituents of nucleic acids. Similarly, no reaction was observed between (21) and amino acids such as L-lysine and L-serine.

Other sesquiterpene lactones show similar reactivity. For example, helenalin (6) and tenulin (23) were found to react readily with thiols on L-cysteine and glutathione [45]. In the case of tenulin (23), an adduct with

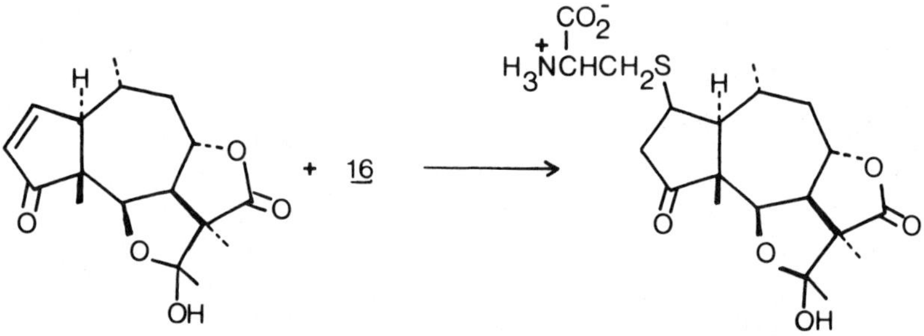

(23) + 16 → (24)

L-cysteine results from Michael addition to the cyclopentenone ring to yield (24). However, neither compound reacted with DNA, d-guanosine 5'-monophosphate (GMP), or d-guanosine 5'-triphosphate (GTP).

Many plant-derived antitumor compounds, however, do react with DNA or RNA, and this reactivity does appear to be related to their antitumor activity. For example, although camptothecin (13) binds extensively to plasma proteins in both humans and mice, its main action appears to be on RNA and DNA synthesis [32, 46]. The maximum interaction of derivatives of (13) with DNA occurs when all the rings other than the lactone are the same as is found in (13). This suggests that the mode of the initial interaction is intercalation into the DNA rather than alkylation. Intercalation followed by alkylation has also been suggested as the mechanism by which nitidine chloride (25) and related alkaloids exert their antitumor effects [47, 48].

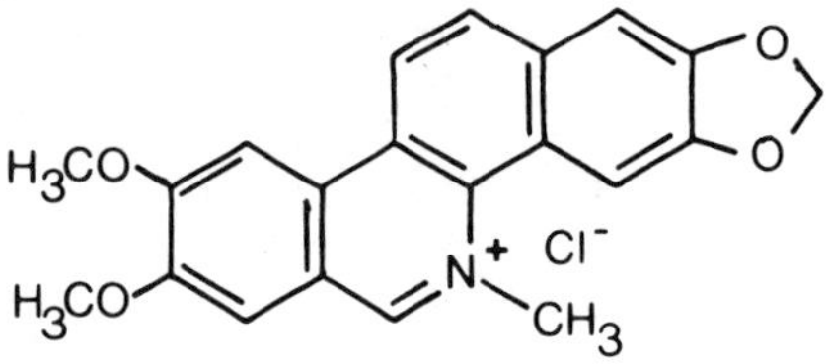

(25)

Thus it seems likely that tumor-inhibitory plant principles may exhibit several different mechanisms of action, with selective alkylation being one of the more important ones. However, further research is required to elucidate which, if any, of the known mechanisms is primarily responsible for inhibition of tumor growth.

F. The *Vinca* Alkaloids

The *Vinca* or *Catharantus* alkaloids vinblastine (26) and vincristine (27) are the most successful of the plant-derived antitumor agents. They are "dimeric" indole-dihydroindole alkaloids isolated from *Catharanthus roseus*

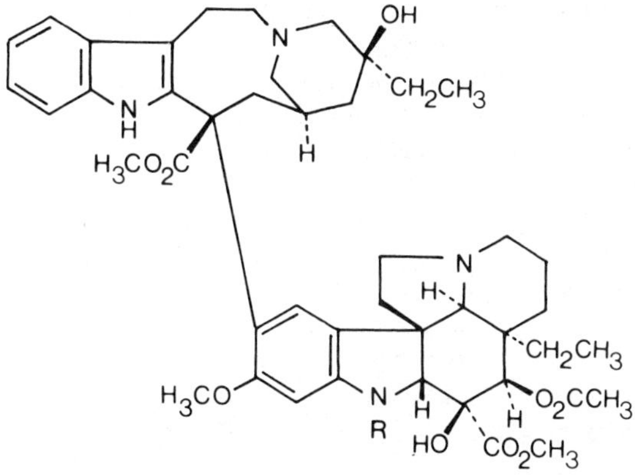

(26) R = CH_3
(27) R = CHO

(also called Vinca rosea), commonly known as periwinkle. Vinblastine (26) was isolated independently by two separate groups of investigators at the University of Western Ontario [49] and at the Lilly Research Laboratories [50] who were investigating the plant for potential hypoglycemic agents. Although (26) did not show any hypoglycemic activity, it did have significant antileukemic activity [51, 52]. This activity prompted further work on the isolation of additional antitumor alkaloids from C. roseus, and vincristine (27) was subsequently isolated by the Lilly group [53]. Vincristine (27) was also found to have significant antileukemic activity. The structures of (26) and (27) were established by chemical and spectral methods [54] and confirmed by x-ray diffraction studies [55]. The only difference in the structures of (26) and (27) is that vinblastine (26) bears a methyl group on the indole nitrogen of the vindoline half of the molecule while vincristine (27) has an N-formyl moiety.

The biological activity, mode of action, and structure-activity relationships of (26) and (27) have been reviewed by Johnson et al. [56] and by Creasey [57]. Briefly, both alkaloids are active against several animal tumor systems, including the P1534 leukemia, the P388 leukemia, the Freund ascites tumor, and the Ridgeway osteogenic sarcoma [32, 56]. Cross-resistance of (26) and (27) was observed in a vinblastine-resistant P815 leukemia [56]. Vinblastine (26) and vincristine (27) act as mitotic inhibitors, inhibiting mitosis in the metaphase [32, 57, 58]. They bind to tubulin, a protein involved in forming the mitotic apparatus in the cell, and this has been suggested as the principal mode of action [32, 57, 58]. Both compounds also exhibit an effect on DNA and RNA synthesis [57, 58].

The clinical use (as the sulfate salts) and toxicity of (26) and (27) has been reviewed by Creasey [57] and by Carter and Livingston [18], among others. Vinblastine (26) is useful primarily in the treatment of Hodgkin's disease and the major toxic effect is hematologic toxicity [18]. Vincristine (27) is useful against childhood leukemia, Wilm's tumor, and non-Hodgkin's lymphomas [18]. The major toxicity found with (27) is neurotoxicity [18]. Both alkaloids have become clinically useful drugs in the treatment of certain cancers, and most of the clinical investigation of (26) and (27) is now directed toward the development of new combination chemotherapeutical regimens using these drugs.

To illustrate the development of plant principles as antineoplastic agents through isolation and clinical trials (a process that may take more than 7 years), two examples from the laboratories of the late S. Morris Kupchan will be examined. These two compounds clearly demonstrate the benefits of activity-guided fractionation procedures.

II. MAYTANSINE

A. Isolation and Structure Elucidation

Maytansine (28) was first isolated in 1971 from an ethanolic extract of the Ethiopian shrub *Maytenus serrata*, a member of the Celastraceae family [58]. Extensive fractionation of the extract using column chromatography and preparative thin-layer chromatography guided by biological activity against the P388 lymphocytic leukemia and KB cell culture eventually yielded maytansine (28) in amounts of less than 1 mg/kg of plant material. Because of the low yield, routine methods of structural determination were impractical and the structure was determined by x-ray crystallographic analysis of the C(9) bromopropyl ether [12, 58].

Maytansine (28) is a highly functionalized ansa macrolide (an aromatic ring joined to a macrocyclic ring at two nonadjacent positions) with an amino acid ester at C(3), an epoxide at C(4, 5), and a carbinol-amide moiety at C(9). Maytansine (28) was found to be active (T/C 125-220) against the P388 leukemia over a dose range of 0.4-50 μg/kg and to exhibit an ED_{50} value of 10^{-4}-10^{-5} against the KB cell culture [59]. Subsequent animal tests showed that (28) was highly active at μg/kg doses against a variety of tumor systems, including the L1210 lymphoid leukemia, the B16 melanoma, the Lewis lung tumor, mast cell P815 tumor, the plasma cell YPC-1 tumor, and W256 carcinosarcoma tumor [14, 60].

The low yield and high activity of the maytansine (28) prompted a search for closely related plants which might be a better source of maytansine (28). The Kenyan species *Maytenus buchananii* was found to contain (28) in higher yield (1.5 mg/kg) as well as the related active maytansinoids maytanprine (29), maytanbutine (30), maytanvaline (31), and normaytansine (32) and the inactive maytansinoids maysine (33), normaysine (34), and maysenine (35) [12, 61]. Because of the higher yield and greater availability, *M. buchananii* was chosen as the source to be used for large-scale isolation of (28). *Putterlickia verrucosa* from South Africa was found to be the

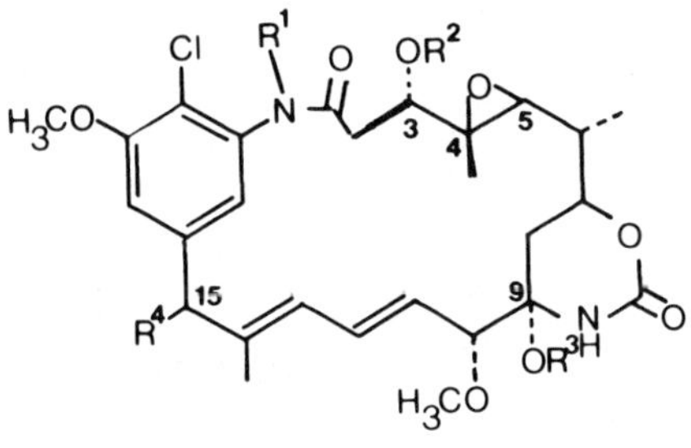

	R^1	R^2	R^3	R^4
(28)	CH_3	$COCH(CH_3)N(CH_3)COCH_3$	H	H
(29)	CH_3	$COCH(CH_3)N(CH_3)COCH_2CH_3$	H	H
(30)	CH_3	$COCH(CH_3)N(CH_3)COCH(CH_3)_2$	H	H
(31)	CH_3	$COCH(CH_3)N(CH_3)COCH_2CH(CH_3)_2$	H	H
(32)	H	$COCH(CH_3)N(CH_3)COCH_3$	H	H
(36)	CH_3	$COCH_3$	H	H
(37)	CH_3	H	H	H
(38)	CH_3	$COCH(CH_3)N(CH_3)COCH(CH_3)_2$	H	OH
(39)	CH_3	$COCH(CH_3)N(CH_3)COCH(CH_3)_2$	H	O_2CCH_3
(42)	CH_3	$COCH(CH_3)_2$	H	H
(43)	CH_3	$COCH(CH_3)_2$	H	O_2CCH_3
(49)	CH_3	OH	CH_3	H
(50)	CH_3	$COCH(CH_3)N(CH_3)COCH_3$	CH_3	H

best source of maytansine (28), consistently yielding 8-9 mg/kg, but had limited availability in large quantities [12]. P. verrucosa was also found to contain (29), (30), and three new maytansinoids, maytanacine (36), maytansinol (37), and normaytansine [12, 129].

Maytansinoids have also been isolated from sources other than the Celastraceae plant family. Maytanbutine (30), colubrinol (38), and colubrinol acetate (39) have been isolated from Colubrina texensis, a member of the Rhamnaceae family [62], and more recently, maytansinoids with a C(15) methoxyl group have been isolated from a Euphorbiaceae plant, Trewia nudiflora [63]. T. nudiflora has also yielded three additional novel antitumor maytansinoids in which the C(3) N-acyl amino acid side-chain ester is linked through the N-acyl group to the aromatic amide nitrogen at C(18) to form a second macrocyclic ring [130]. The structural similiarity of maytansine (28) to antibiotics such as geldanomycin and rifamycin prompted investigation of microbial sources and in 1978, maytansinoids with aliphatic C(3) esters (called ansamitocins) were isolated from a Nocardia sp. [64]. The isolation of 16 new ansamitocins has been recently reported [65].

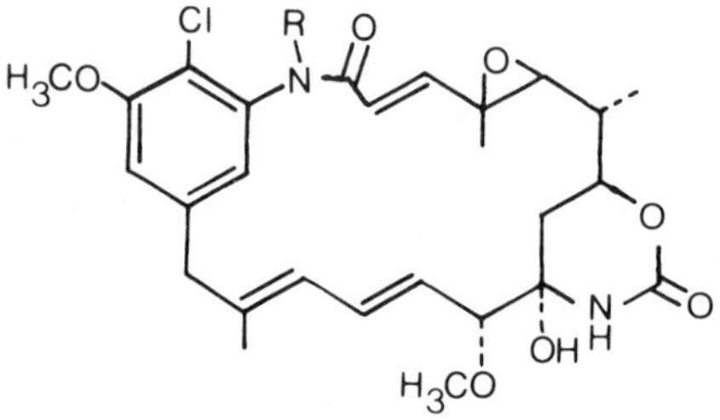

	R
(33)	CH_3
(34)	H

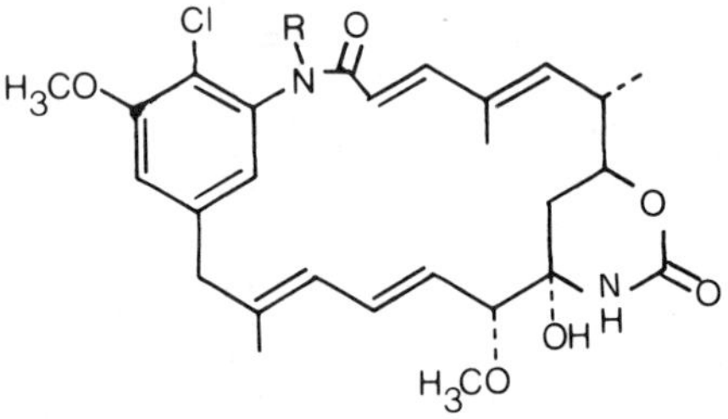

	R
(35)	H
(44)	CH_3

B. Mode of Action and Structure-Activity Studies

Like vincristine (27), maytansine (28) inhibits mitosis in clam and sea urchin eggs by preventing formation of a mitotic apparatus [59, 66]. Maytansine (28), however, is a more potent inhibitor of mitosis than is vincristine (27). The antimitotic activity of (28) has been suggested to result from interference with tubulin polymerization in the cell [66], and (28) does inhibit the polymerization of brain tubulin in vitro [59, 66, 67]. Maytansine (28) has also been shown to bind to tubulins at the same site as vincristine (27) [66, 68, 69], and it has been suggested that this binding may be due to the C(9) carbinolamide acting to alkylate free sulfhydryls in tubulin [52]. This hypothesis is supported by the ease with which (28) and (30) alkylate *n*-propane thiol to give the corresponding C(9) thioethers [59, 66]. Maytansine has also been shown to inhibit mitosis at metaphase in L1210 leukemia cells [60, 70, 71], HeLa cells [72], and P388 leukemia cells [70, 73].

In L1210 and P388 leukemia cells, both RNA and DNA synthesis were inhibited by maytansine (28), but DNA synthesis was affected to a greater extent [70, 71]. This inhibition of DNA synthesis was proposed to occur via the alkylation of a nucleophilic site on a nucleic acid by the C(9) carbinolamide moiety of (28) [74]. Support for this proposal was provided by the demonstration that (28) and synthetic carbinolamides (40) and (41) did indeed alkylate covalently closed circular DNA in vitro [74]. However, later work with (28) and ansamitocin P-3 (47) showed that the inhibition of DNA synthesis was more likely a secondary effect of the mitotic inhibition rather than a direct reaction with the nucleic acid [72, 75].

Structure-activity studies of maytansine (28) and its homologs have been somewhat limited by insufficient material for extensive chemical modification work. Of the several functional groups that might be involved as reactive sites and thus contribute to the antileukemic activity, two have been shown to be required for optimal activity [59]. These are the C(3) ester and the C(9) carbinolamide. Comparison of the testing results for (28) to (31), all of which have amino acid esters at C(3), with the data for (33) to (35) and (37) showed that only those maytansinoids with C(3) esters

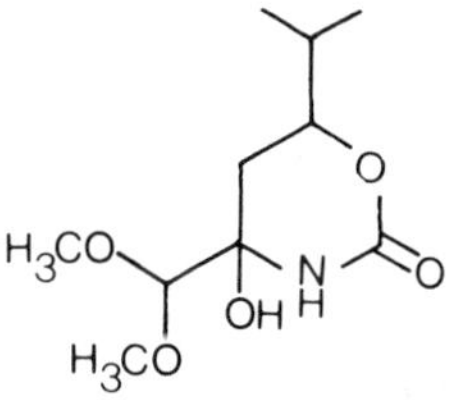

(40)

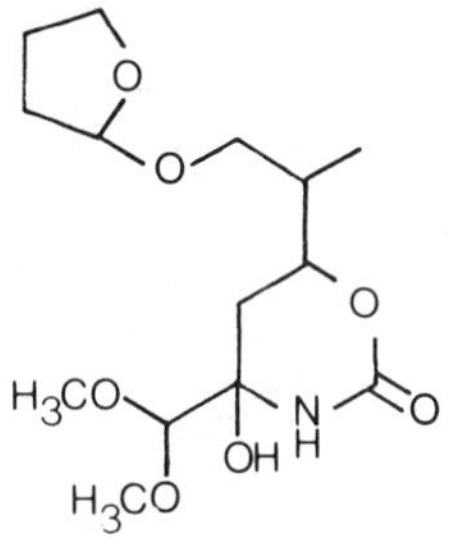

(41)

were significantly active against the P388 leukemia in vivo, the KB cell culture, the sea urchin egg mitosis, and the tubulin polymerization assays [59]. It was evident from these data that differences in the structure of the amino acid ester did not change the antileukemic activity significantly, and comparisons with the data obtained for aliphatic C(3) esters prepared from maytansinol (37) indicated that any ester was sufficient for activity [59]. This was further demonstrated by the testing data for the ansamitocins, all of which are C(3) aliphatic esters [76].

The C(9) carbinolamide was also demonstrated to be required for antileukemic activity. When the C(9) carbinol of (28) or (30) was blocked by conversion into the corresponding methyl or ethyl ether, antileukemic activity against the P388 leukemia in vivo assay was significantly reduced. Inhibition of tubulin polymerization and cytotoxicity against the KB cell culture were also decreased, but antimitotic activity in sea urchin eggs was not affected. In the latter assay hydrolysis of the C(9) ether may be taking place [59].

Very little is known about the roles of the remaining functional groups in the antileukemic activity of the maytansinoids. It has been suggested that the C(4, 5) epoxide may not be required for optimum antileukemic activity [59, 77]. The presence of a C(15) acetate or methoxyl group does not particularly affect antileukemic activity [59, 62, 63], but a C(15) hydroxyl moiety may inhibit this activity [77]. Demethylation of the C(18) nitrogen does not diminish antileukemic activity [61, 77, 129]. However, demethylation of C(20) has been achieved by microbial conversion of ansamitocin P-3, and the 20-O-demethylated derivative exhibited greater activity against the P388 leukemia than ansamitocin P-3 [78].

C. Synthesis

The potent antitumor activity of maytansine (28) and the low yield from plant sources made it an attractive and challenging target for total synthesis. The eight chiral centers and highly functionalized macrocyclic structure of (28) are major problems in synthesis design which have been addressed by at least 10 groups of researchers [79-87, 131-135]. Two of these groups have succeeded in overcoming the problems and have recently published syntheses of (28) [79, 80].

Optically active maytansine (28) was synthesized by E. J. Corey and his co-workers at Harvard University [79a]. Previously, syntheses for racemic and optically active N-methylmaysenine (44) had also been reported by this group [79b, c]. This approach to the synthesis of (28) involved the synthesis of dienal (45) [79d] and ketal thioacetal (46) [79b].

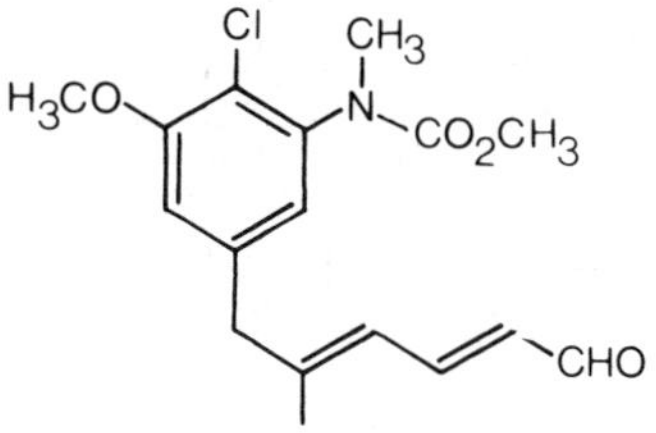

(45)

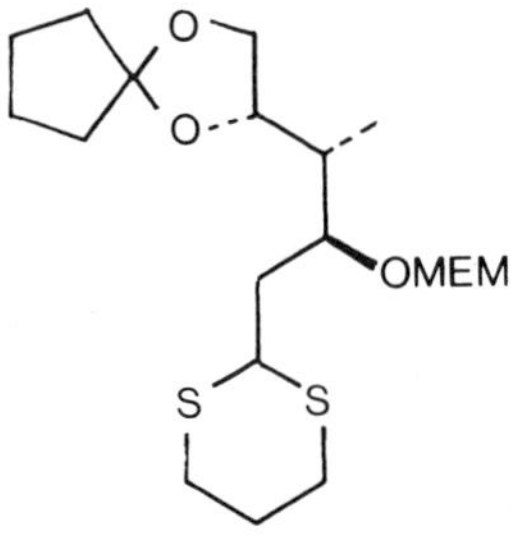

(46)

Cyclization of (47) to yield (48) was followed by the conversion, again in several steps, of (48) into maytansinol 9-O-methyl ether (49). In the final steps, (49) was acylated with the imidazolide of N-acetyl-N-methyl-L-alanine to give maytansine 9-O-methyl ether (50). The ether was then

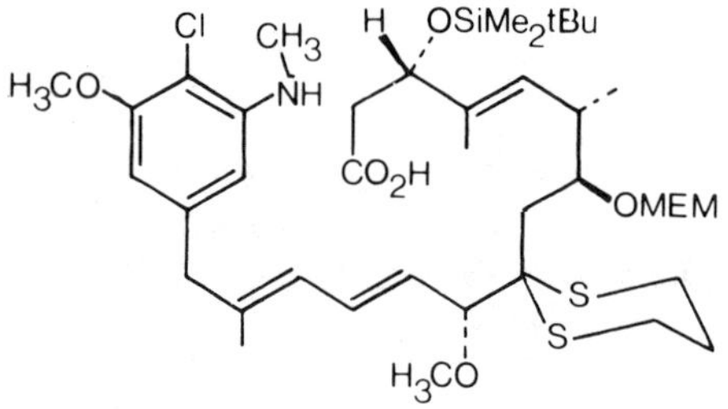

(47)

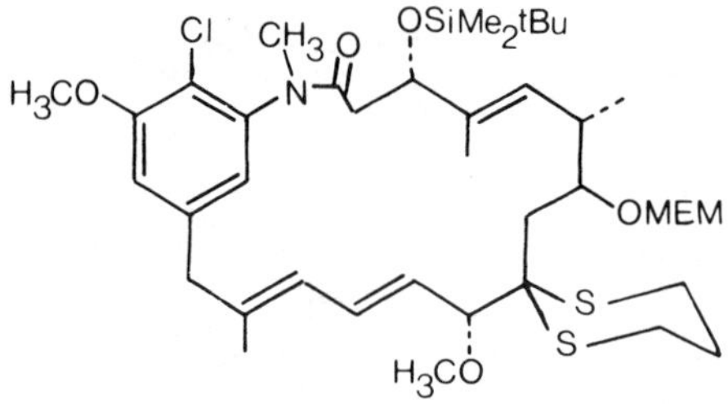

(48)

removed by mild hydrolysis to provide optically active maytansine (28). This synthesis of over 30 steps was a product of over 5 years of effort and resulted not only in the total synthesis of (28) but also in the addition of several new reactions and methods of controlling stereochemistry to the chemical literature.

Approximately 1 month earlier than the work noted above was published, Meyers and co-workers reported the total synthesis of racemic maytanisol (37) [80a]. Since (37) had previously been converted into maytansine (28) [88], this work constitutes a formal synthesis of racemic (28). Previously, these same workers had achieved syntheses of racemic maysine (34) [80b] and racemic N-methylmaysenine (44) [80c]. In this synthesis of (28), key intermediates (51) and (52) were converted into (53), which then served as the precursor for both racemic maysine (33) and

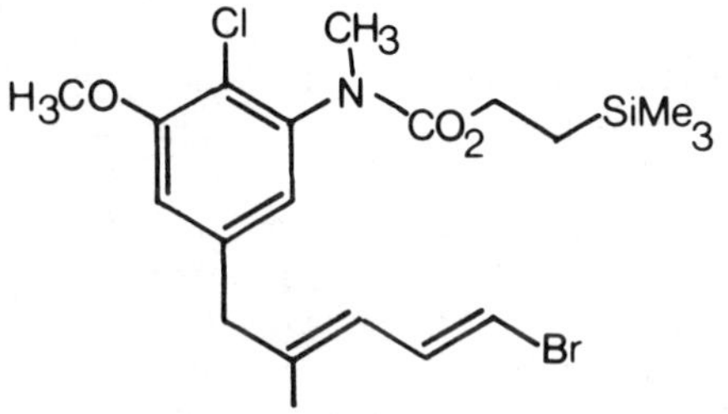

(51)

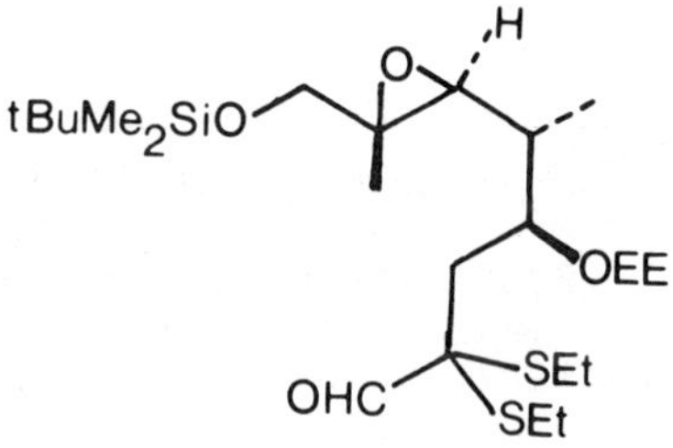

(52)

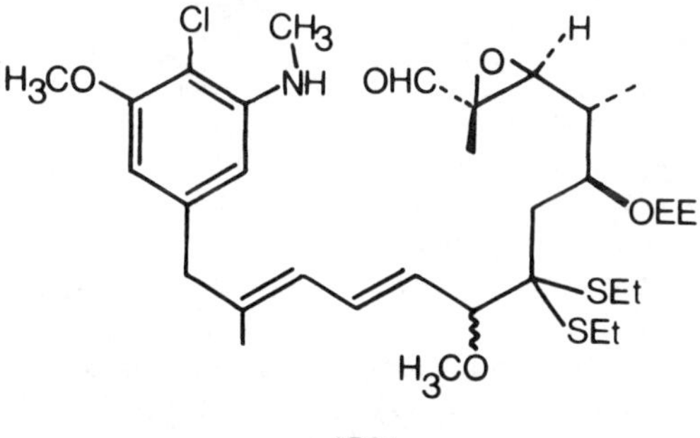

(53)

racemic maytansinol (37). This work was the product of over 8 years of research, and, like that of the Harvard group, resulted in the development of a variety of reactions for forming and protecting various functional groups with control of stereochemistry.

The benefits of both synthetic efforts include the availability of key intermediates with different stereochemistry or only selected functional groups. These intermediates may now be used to elaborate further the key structure-activity relationships among the maytansinoids and to generate "unnatural" maytansinoids which may prove to have very different biological activity from the "natural" compounds.

D. Clinical Trials

Phase I clinical trials of maytansine (28) have been conducted under the auspices of the National Cancer Institute, and several toxic effects have been noted in humans. The major dose-limiting toxic effects were gastrointestinal [89-93] and neurological [92,93]. In initial clinical trials, (28) was administered on days 1, 3, and 5 repeated in 4-week cycles. Nausea, vomiting, stomach cramps, and diarrhea were first evident at dose levels of 1.8 mg/m^2 and became severe at 2.7 mg/m^2 beginning on days 4-5 [89]. Severe diarrhea was also a major problem in trials with doses of 0.6-0.9 mg/m^2 administered on a 3-day schedule repeated every 2-3 weeks [90] and with doses of 1.6-2.0 mg/m^2 administered as a single intravenous infusion every 3 weeks [91]. In a trial with doses administered weekly by intravenous bolus or 24-hr infusion, similar gastrointestinal toxicity was severe at doses $\geq$1.1 mg/m^2 per week [93].

Severe central and peripheral neurological toxicity, similar to the toxicity exhibited by vincristine (27), also presents a major problem with maytansine (28) [92,93]. In the phase I clinical study using weekly doses, severe neurological toxicity was prevalent at a cumulative dose >6.0 mg/m^2 [93]. Myelotoxicity, however, was found to be minimal in several studies [91-93], and maytansine (28) was found to lack cross-resistance with vincristine (27) [91,93].

A few partial responses were seen in phase I clinical trials in patients with melanoma [90], breast carcinoma [90], acute lymphocytic leukemia [91], ovarian carcinoma [91], non-Hodgkin's lymphoma [91,93], and thymoma [93], but no spectacular results occurred.

The toxicity results from phase I trials were not discouraging enough to halt further study, and maytansine (28) was entered into phase II clinical trials at several institutions [94-101]. These phase II studies have, however, been disappointing. Maytansine has failed to demonstrate any significant tumor-inhibitory activity in patients with advanced colorectal carcinoma [94], advanced head and neck cancer [97], melanoma [96,100], breast cancer [96], refractory non-Hodgkin's lymphoma [136], or small-cell lung carcinoma [137] at doses which resulted in severe neurological and gastrointestinal toxicity. Some minimal responses have been observed in patients with lung cancer [95], malignant thymoma [98], and advanced lymphomas [101]. Any further clinical trials of maytansine (28) will probably occur only after the pharmacology and the mode of action of this agent is more thoroughly understood. Potentially, (28) might prove useful in combination with drugs which exhibit severe myelotoxicity, since this effect is minimal with maytansine (28).

III. BRUCEANTIN

A. Isolation and Structure Elucidation

Several compounds related to quassin (11) which had been isolated from plants in the Simaroubaceae family were used as antiamebic agents for many years before several of these principles were found to have antileukemic activity [29]. Holacanthone (54) was the first quassinoid isolated on the basis of its antileukemic activity [102], but bruceantin (55) has generated the most interest as a potential anticancer agent. Bruceantin (55) was isolated in 1972 from a 95% ethanol extract of the stem bark of the Ethiopian tree Brucea antidysenterica [103]. The isolation using solvent partition and column chromatography techniques was guided by bioassay against the P388 lymphocytic leukemia in vivo and the KB cell culture. The structure of (55) was determined by spectroscopic and chemical methods and by comparisons to the previously known bruceine B (56). Bruceantin (55) was evidently the second quassinoid to show significant antineoplastic activity against the P388 leukemia (e.g., T/C 220 at 0.5 mg/kg), and exhibited its effect over a dose range of 0.3-1.0 mg/kg [104,105]. Bruceantin (55) has subsequently

(54)

	R
(55)	CO–CH=C(CH$_3$)–CH(CH$_3$)$_2$
(56)	$COCH_3$
(57)	COC_6H_5
(58)	CO–CH=C(CH$_3$)–C(CH$_3$)$_2$–OAc
(64)	$COCH_2CH(CH_3)_2$
(65)	CO–CH=C(CH$_3$)–C(CH$_3$)$_2$–OH
(71)	$COCH{=}C(CH_3)_2$
(72)	$COCH_2CH(CH_3)CH(CH_3)_2$
(73)	H

exhibited significant activity against several other animal tumor systems, including the L1210 lymphoid leukemia, an adriamycin-resistant P388 leukemia, a cytoxan-resistant P388 leukemia, the B16 melanocarcinoma, and the Lewis lung carcinoma [104].

Eight additional quassinoids closely related to (55) were also isolated from *B. antidysenterica*: bruceantarin (57), bruceantinol (58), dehydrobruceantin (59), dehydrobruceantarin (60), dehydrobruceine (61), dehydrobruceantol (62), and isobruceine B (63). Bruceantin (55), bruceantarin (57),

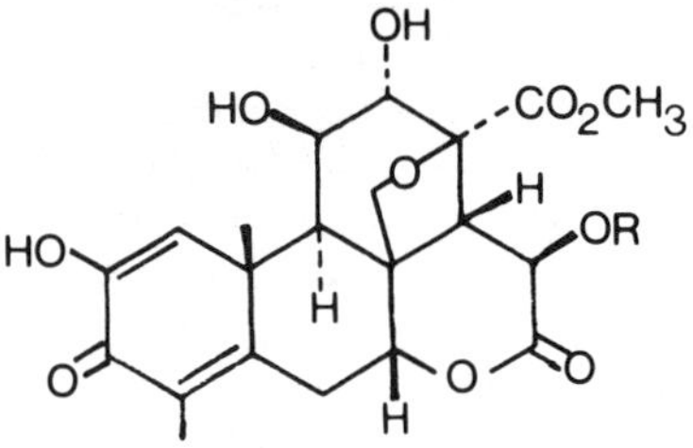

(59) 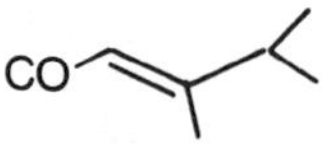 CO
(60) COC_6H_5
(61) $COCH_3$
(62) 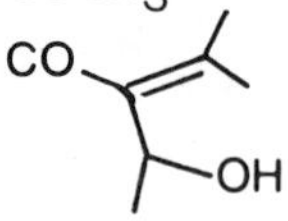 CO

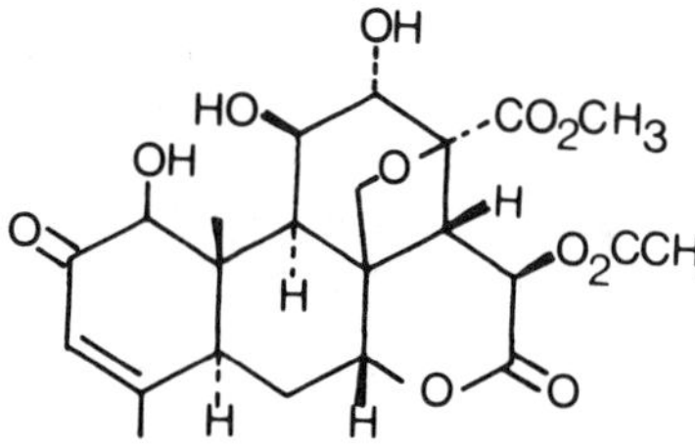

(63)

bruceantinol (58), and bruceine B (56) were later isolated from the Ghanian species *B. guineensis* [103]. The structure of bruceantinol (58) has recently been revised [105]. Three of these related quassinoids, (57), (58), and (63), also showed significant antileukemic activity against the P388 in vivo system.

The significant antitumor activity of (55) in the animal tumor systems cited above and the interest shown by the NCI in (55) has resulted in a continued search for additional related quassinoids. Of particular interest are various collections of *B. javanica*. *B. javanica* from Fiji has yielded bruceines A (64) and C (65) in addition to (55) to (58) [106]. Taiwanese *B. javanica* hielded two antileukemic quassinoid glucosides, bruceoside-A (66) and bruceoside-B (67), as well as brucein-D (68), which exhibits activity against the Walker 256 carcinosarcoma in vivo [107]. The inactive brucein-E (69) was also isolated from this species. A related glucoside, bruceine-E-2-β-D-glucoside (70), has been isolated from *B. javanica* collected in China [108].

B. Mode of Action and Structure-Activity Studies

Bruceantin (55) was found to inhibit protein synthesis in HeLa cells, rabbit reticulocytes, reticulocyte lysates, and cultured P388 leukemia cells [109,

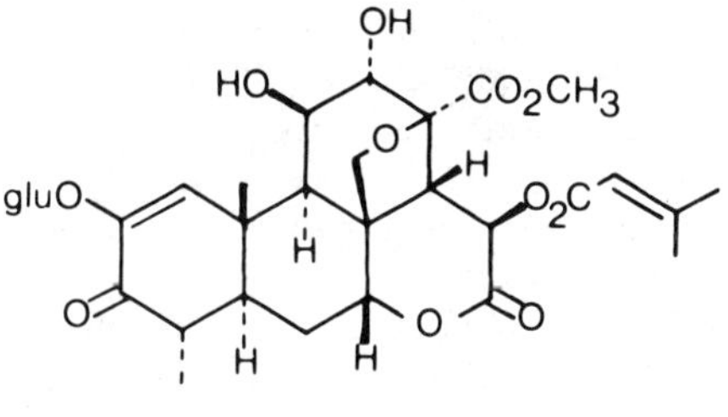

(66)

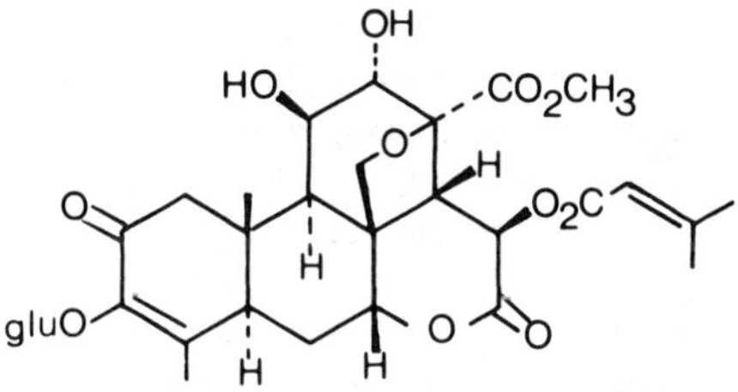

(67)

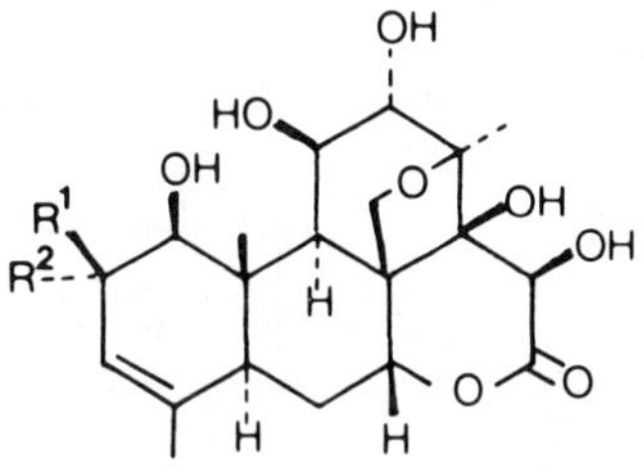

(68) R^1, R^2 =O

(69) R^1 = H
R^2 = OH

(70) R^1 = H
R^2 = Oglu

110]. In HeLa cells, bruceantin (55) partially inhibited DNA synthesis but had no effect on RNA synthesis [109]. In P388 cells, however, bruceantin (55) did reduce RNA synthesis as well as DNA synthesis [110]. More recently, bruceantin (55) has been found to specifically block peptide bond formation on eukaryotic ribosomes and to exhibit poly(U)-directed polyphenylalanine synthesis [111]. In these systems, (55) apparently binds to a site on the peptidyltransferase that is very similar to the binding site for trichodermin, since the subsequent binding of trichodermin is inhibited. However, bruceantin (55) did not inhibit the initiation of protein synthesis in yeast ribosomes. Therefore, it was proposed that the different effects on reticulocytes and reticulocyte lysates observed previously [109] might be due to (55) having a different affinity for each [111]. A recent study of bruceantin (55) and related quassinoids in P388 leukemia cells found that protein synthesis was inhibited only after previously initiated polypeptide synthesis was completed and the free 80S ribosome was released [138]. Bruceantin (55) acted as an elongation inhibitor of protein synthesis, possibly by interfering with the peptidyl transferase reaction and binding to the free 80S ribosome.

There are evidently two major structural features of bruceantin (55) and related quassinoids which affect the antileukemic activity, the C(15) ester and the A-ring diosphenol moiety. Antileukemic activity is greatly changed by variations in the C(15) ester [102, 104, 112]. Bruceantin (55), bruceantinol (58), and brusatol (71), obtained by hydrolysis of bruceoside-A (66) [108] are the most active compounds against the P388 in vivo system. Those bruceolides with saturated esters at C(15) such as bruceantarin (57), dihydrobruceantin (72), and bruceine-B (56) all exhibit marginal activity in this system, while those without any ester at C(15) such as bruceolide (73), brucein-D (68), and brucein-E (69) are inactive.

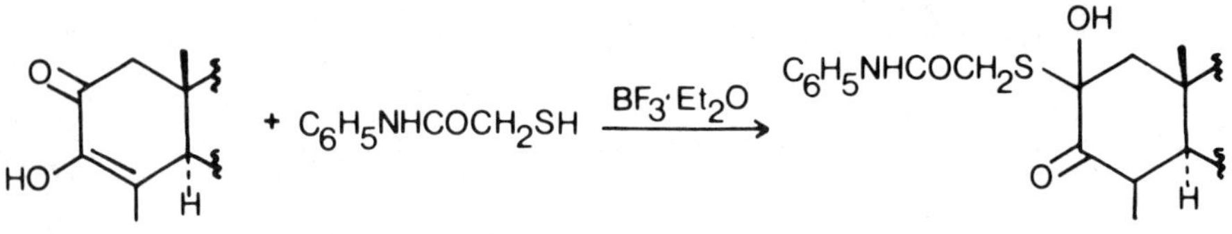

$$(57) \text{ or } (72) + C_6H_5NHCOCH_2SH \xrightarrow{BF_3 \cdot Et_2O} (75)$$

The C(15) ester was thought to be involved in enhancing transport of the compound across cell membranes [103, 104]. This was supported by the results of studies in HeLa cells and rabbit reticulocytes, where (55) and (72) were most active in inhibiting protein synthesis [109]. Bruceantarin (57) and bruceine-B (56) were approximately 10 times less active, and bruceolide (73), which lacks the C(15) ester, was 100 times less active. In reticulocyte lysates, however, all five compounds were approximately equal in inhibiting protein synthesis. In the studies with P388 leukemia cells, both (68) and (69), neither of which contain an ester at C(15), were approximately equivalent to (55) in their ability to inhibit protein synthesis [110]. It was also found that transport of (55) and (71) through the cell membrane in P388 cells was somewhat retarded, suggesting that the ester does not enhance transport, at least in P388 cells.

The A-ring diosphenol moiety has also been shown to be involved in and required for significant antileukemic activity [104]. Those compounds in which the diosphenol moiety has been altered, such as (59) and (60), show no activity against the P388 in vivo system. Tetrahydrobruceantin (74),

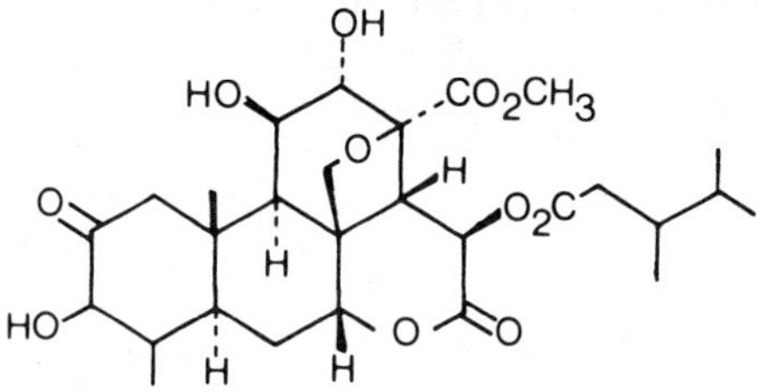

(74)

which has a reduced A ring is also inactive. Thus it would seem that an intact A-ring diosphenol is required for activity. However, bruceoside-A (66) is also active against the P388 leukemia in vivo but has an altered A ring [108]. Since brusatol (71), which is obtained by hydrolysis of (66), is much more active than (66) in vivo and contains a "normal" diosphenol A ring, it is possible that in vivo hydrolysis of (66) may occur and lead to activity against the P388 leukemia.

In light of the ability of bruceantin (55) to inhibit protein synthesis, the A-ring diosphenol was proposed to be involved in alkylation of biological sulfhydryl moieties on macromolecules. In studies of the reaction of thioglycolic acid anilide with (55), (72), and (74), it was found that (55) and (72) formed C(2) hemithioketal adducts [e.g., (75)], while (74) formed a substitution product at either C(2) (76) or C(3) (77) [113]. This difference

(74) + $C_6H_5NHCOCH_2SH$ $\xrightarrow{BF_3 \cdot Et_2O}$ (76) or (77)

in chemical reactivity toward a model sulfhydryl suggested that the difference in biological activity of the three compounds might result from a similar difference in activity in vivo. It also served to reinforce the requirement for an intact A-ring diosphenol as a reactive site. Additional evidence for this came from the studies with HeLa cells, rabbit reticulocytes, and reticulocyte lysates [109]. In HeLa cells and rabbit reticulocytes, (74) was approximately 200 times less potent than (55) and (72) in inhibiting protein synthesis. In the reticulocyte lysates, (74) was 100 times less potent than (55) and (72).

Although there has not been any further investigation of the role of other functional groups in bruceantin (55) in antileukemic activity, information has been obtained regarding similar antileukemic quassinoids. The ring-D lactone with adjacent ester is required in several cases [30], and the epoxymethano bridge between C(8) and C(11) or C(8) and C(13) has also been shown to be required for significant activity [114].

C. Synthetic Approaches

The potent antileukemic activity of bruceantin (55) makes it an attractive target for synthetic chemists. Recently, the conversion of bruceoside-A (66) into bruceantin (55) via bruceolide (73) has been reported [115]. Although there are several groups of researchers pursuing approaches to (55), no total synthesis has yet been achieved. The highly functionalized ring system and 10 contiguous chiral centers pose special problems in designing an efficient synthesis.

The synthesis of the quassinoid ring system has been investigated by several groups using a Diels-Alder reaction to establish several chiral centers at one time [116-119, 139, 140]. Valenta and co-workers have synthesized (77) by elaborating the Diels-Alder product of (78) and (79) [116].

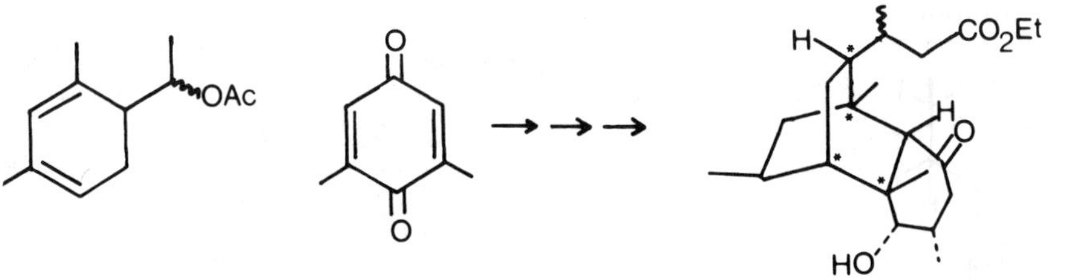

(78) (79) (80)

This compound contains the chiral centers at C(5), C(7), C(8), and C(10) (*) found in quassin (11). Grieco and his co-workers have also used the Diels-Alder approach to synthesize (83) in several steps from the product of (81) and (82) [117, 118]. In this case, all the chiral centers of (11) have been

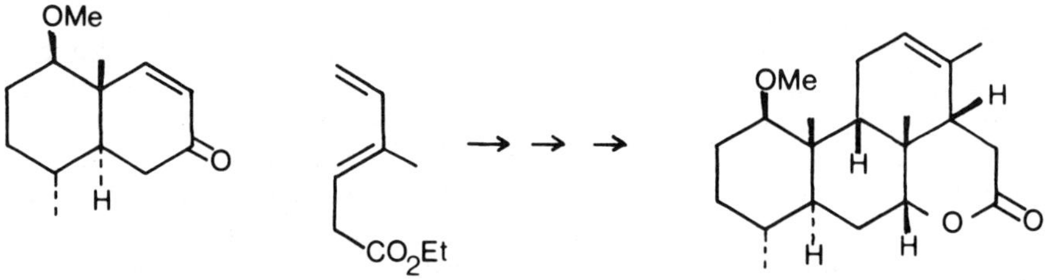

(81) (82) (83)

established except C(9). Grieco has recently used a similar method to synthesize another quassinoid, dl-castelanolide [119].

In approaches more directly applicable to a total syntheses of (55), one group [120] elected to elaborate an A-B ring system while two other groups have synthesized model BCE ring systems. The latter two approaches have provided (84) [121] and (85) [122], both of which contain the epoxymethano bridge from C(8) to C(13), the hydroxyl groups at C(11) and C(12), and several of the required contiguous chiral centers.

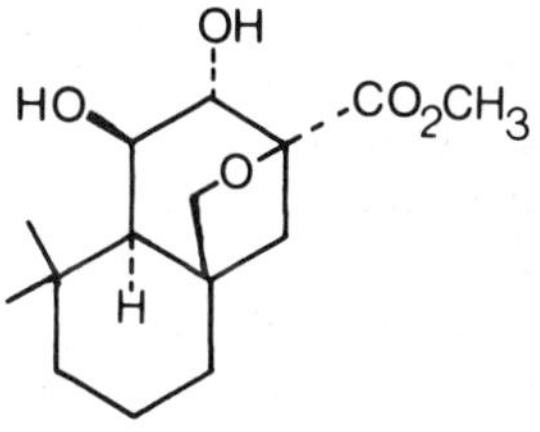

(84) 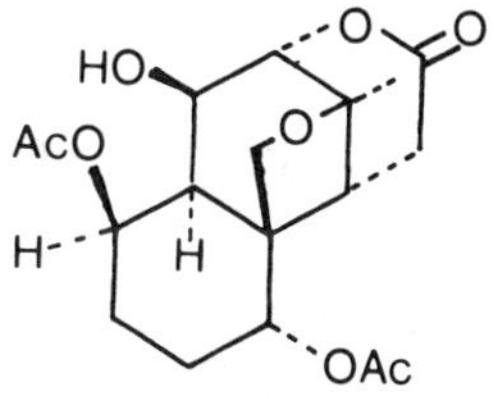 (85)

One other novel approach to the synthesis of (55) and related quassinoids is based on the fact that quassinoids are degraded triterpenes. Dias and his co-workers are attempting to convert cholic acid derivatives into quassinoid skeletons [123]. They have been successful in cleaving the D ring of the steroid skeleton with subsequent formation of the lactone moiety to give, for example, (86) [123c, d, f, g]. They have also been able to convert the A ring into a diosphenol as in (87) [123a].

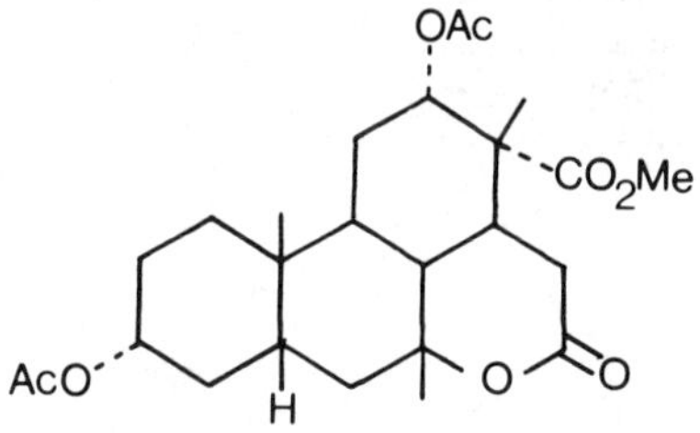

(86) 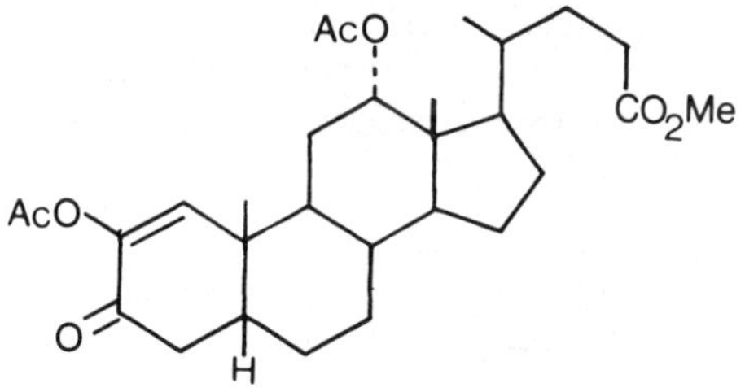 (87)

D. Clinicial Trials

Bruceantin (55) is currently undergoing phase II clinical trials under the auspices of the NCI, and there is not yet much information available about its efficacy as a potential chemotherapeutic agent. Preclinical toxicological studies in dogs and monkeys have been carried out [124], and the major toxic effects were found to be gastrointestinal toxicity and hepatic toxicity. Some other minor side effects were also seen, but all effects were found to be reversible and noncumulative.

The results of three phase I studies have been published [125, 126, 141]. In two of these studies, the major dose-limiting toxicity was found to be hypotension, which required careful monitoring of blood pressure. On a 5-day schedule of administration, cumulative myelotoxicity was also noted [125]. Febrile reactions, gastrointestinal toxicity, and some skin problems were found in both studies, but were treatable and reversible. In the third study using a weekly schedule, the dose-limiting effect was severe gastrointestinal toxicity [141]. The severity of the gastrointestinal toxicity was increased in patients with hepatic metastases. No significant therapeutic activity has been noted in these early studies.

Bruceantin (55) was found to produce no partial nor complete responses in a phase II clinical trial in patients with refractory metastatic breast carcinomas [142]. The patients involved had received previous treatments with other chemotherapeutic agents, and all experienced toxic side effects due to bruceantin (55), particularly hypotension and gastrointestinal toxicity.

IV. SUMMARY

During the last 25 years, investigations of plant extracts guided by biological activity against animal tumor systems have yielded a large number of potential antitumor agents with diverse structures. Only a few of the naturally occurring tumor-inhibitory compounds or their derivatives, such as the *Vinca* alkaloids and the podophyllotoxin lignan derivatives, have proven useful in the clinic. However, several plant-derived agents, such as tripdiolide (8) [25], homoharringtonine (15) [36], and macrocyclic trichothecenes related to baccharin (88) [127, 128], are still in early stages of development, while others, including bruceantin (55) [103] and maytansine (28) [12, 58] are currently undergoing clinical trials [14].

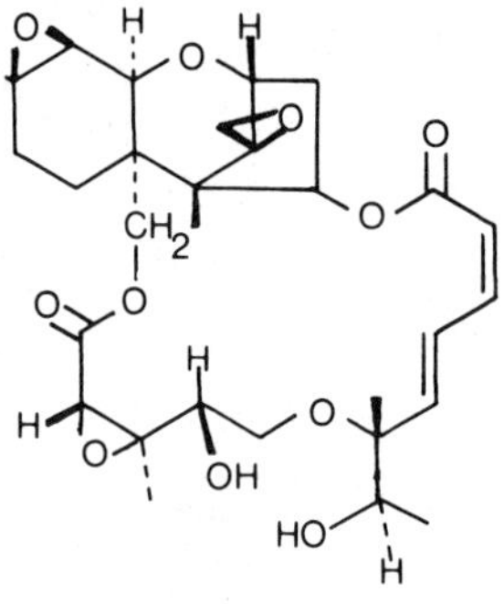

(88)

Since only a small percentage of known plant species have been investigated to date, it is likely that many new potential tumor-inhibitory plant principles are yet to be isolated. The continued development of such principles will also provide an increased understanding of the mechanisms of tumor inhibition, thus leading to the design and synthesis of more effective antineoplastic agents.

REFERENCES

1. J. L. Hartwell, Lloydia, 30: 379 (1967); 31: 71 (1968); 32: 79, 153, 247 (1969); 33: 98, 288 (1970); 34: 103, 204, 310, 386 (1971).
2. J. L. Hartwell, Cancer Treat. Rep., 60: 1031 (1976).
3. J. L. Hartwell and A. W. Schrecker, Fortschr. Chem. Org. Naturst., 15: 83 (1958).
4. S. A. Schepartz, Cancer Treat. Rep., 60: 975 (1976).
5. R. E. Perdue, Jr., Cancer Treat. Rep., 60: 987 (1976).
6. R. W. Spjut and R. E. Perdue, Jr., Cancer Treat. Rep., 60: 979 (1976).
7. R. I. Geran, N. H. Greenberg, M. M. McDonald, A. M. Schumacher, and B. J. Abbott, Cancer Chemother. Rep., Part 3, 3: 1 (1972).
8. D. Statz and F. B. Coon, Cancer Treat. Rep., 60: 999 (1976).
9. M. E. Wall, M. C. Wani, and H. Taylor, Cancer Treat. Rep., 60: 1011 (1976).
10. S. M. Kupchan, R. W. Britton, J. A. Lacadie, M. F. Ziegler, and C. W. Sigel, J. Org. Chem., 40: 648 (1975).
11. S. M. Kupchan, A. P. Davies, S. J. Barboutis, H. K. Schoes, and A. L. Burlingame, J. Am. Chem. Soc., 89: 5718 (1967).
12. S. M. Kupchan, Y. Komoda, A. R. Branfman, A. T. Sneden, W. A. Court, G. J. Thomas, H. P. J. Hintz, R. M. Smith, A. Karim, G. A. Howie, A. K. Verma, Y. Nagao, R. G. Dailey, Jr., V. A. Zimmerly, and W. C. Sumner, Jr., J. Org. Chem., 42: 2439 (1977).
13. B. J. Abbott, Cancer Treat. Rep., 60: 1007 (1976).
14. J. Douros and M. Suffness, Cancer Chemother. Pharmacol., 1: 91 (1978).
15. G. A. Cordell and N. R. Farnsworth, Lloydia, 40: 1 (1977).
16. H. Stähelin, Eur. J. Cancer, 9: 215 (1973).
17. H. Stähelin, Eur. J. Cancer, 6: 303 (1970).
18. S. K. Carter and R. B. Livingston, Cancer Treat. Rep., 60: 1141 (1976).
19. G. Mathe' and L. M. van Putten, Cancer Chemother. Pharmacol., 1: 5 (1978).
20. P. A. Radice, P. A. Bunn, Jr., and D. C. Ihde, Cancer Treat. Rep., 63: 1231 (1979).
21. S. M. Kupchan, A. L. Dessertine, B. T. Blaylock, and R. F. Bryan, J. Org. Chem., 39: 2477 (1974).
22. S. M. Kupchan, R. J. Hemingway, D. Werner, A. Karim, A. T. McPhail, and G. A. Sim, J. Am. Chem. Soc., 90: 3596 (1968).

23. G. R. Pettit, J. C. Budzinski, G. M. Cragg, P. Brown, and L. D. Johnston, J. Med. Chem., 17: 1013 (1974).
24. M. C. Wani, H. L. Taylor, M. E. Wall, P. Coggan, and A. T. McPhail, J. Am. Chem. Soc., 93: 2325 (1971).
25. S. M. Kupchan, W. A. Court, R. G. Dailey, Jr., C. J. Gilmore, and R. F. Bryan, J. Am. Chem. Soc., 94: 7194 (1972).
26. N. R. Lomax and V. L. Narayanan, Chemical Structures of Interest to the Division of Cancer Treatment, National Cancer Institute, Bethesda, Md., January 1979.
27. S. M. Kupchan, C. W. Sigel, L. J. Guttman, R. J. Restivo, and R. F. Bryan, J. Am. Chem. Soc., 95: 1353 (1972).
28. E. Schwenk, Arzneimittelforschung, 12: 1143 (1962).
29. J. Polonsky, Fortschr. Chem. Org. Naturst., 30: 101 (1973).
30. M. E. Wall and M. C. Wani, Annu. Rev. Pharmacol. Toxicol., 17: 177 (1977).
31. M. Tomita, H. Furukawa, S.-T. Lu, and S. M. Kupchan, Chem. Pharm. Bull. (Tokyo), 15: 959 (1967).
32. S. M. Sieber, J. A. R. Mead, and R. H. Adamson, Cancer Treat. Rep., 60: 1127 (1976).
33. J. T. Liemert, M. P. Corder, T. E. Elliott, and J. M. Lovett, Cancer Treat. Rep., 64: 1389 (1980).
34. M. E. Wall, M. C. Wani, C. E. Cook, K. H. Palmer, A. T. McPhail, and G. A. Sim, J. Am. Chem. Soc., 88: 3888 (1966).
35. J. W. Loder, Aust. J. Chem., 19: 1947 (1966).
36. R. G. Powell, D. Weisleder, C. R. Smith, Jr., and I. A. Wolff, Tetrahedron Lett., 4081 (1969).
37. S. M. Kupchan, Intra-Sci. Chem. Rep., 8: 57 (1973).
38. S. M. Kupchan, Cancer Treat. Rep., 60: 1115 (1976).
39. S. M. Kupchan, D. C. Fessler, M. A. Eakin, and T. J. Giacobbe, Science, 168: 376 (1970).
40. C. H. Smith, J. Larner, A. M. Thomas, and S. M. Kupchan, Biochim. Biophys. Acta, 276: 94 (1972).
41. S. M. Kupchan, A. Karim, and C. Marcks, J. Org. Chem., 34: 3912 (1969).
42. R. L. Hanson, H. A. Lardy, and S. M. Kupchan, Science, 168: 378 (1970).
43. E. Fujita, T. Fujita, H. Katayama, M. Shibuya, and T. Shingu, J. Chem. Soc. (C), 1674 (1970).
44. E. Fujita, Y. Nagao, K. Kaneko, S. Nakazawa, and H. Kuroda, Chem. Pharm. Bull. (Tokyo), 24: 2118 (1976).
45. I. H. Hall, K.-H. Lee, E. C. Mar, C. O. Starnes, and T. G. Waddell, J. Med. Chem., 20: 333 (1977).
46. S. B. Horwitz, in Antibiotics III: Mechanism of Action of Antimicrobial and Antitumor Agents (J. W. Corcoran and F. E. Hahn, eds.), Springer-Verlag, New York, 1975, pp. 48-57.

47. R. K.-Y. Zee-Cheng and C. C. Cheng, J. Pharm. Sci., 59: 1630 (1970).
48. F. R. Stermitz, K. A. Larson, and D. K. Kim, J. Med. Chem., 16: 939 (1973).
49. R. L. Noble, C. T. Beer, and J. H. Cutts, Biochem. Pharmacol., 1: 347 (1958).
50. G. H. Svoboda, J. Pharm. Sci., 47: 834 (1958).
51. R. L. Noble, C. T. Beer, and J. H. Cutts, Ann. N.Y. Acad. Sci., 76: 882 (1958).
52. I. S. Johnson, H. F. Wright, and G. H. Svoboda, J. Lab. Clin. Med., 54: 830 (1959).
53. G. H. Svoboda, Lloydia, 24: 173 (1961).
54. N. Neuss, M. Gorman, H. E. Boaz, and N. J. Cone, J. Am. Chem. Soc., 84: 1509 (1962).
55. J. W. Moncrief and W. N. Lipscomb, J. Am. Chem. Soc., 87: 4963 (1965).
56. I. S. Johnson, J. G. Armstrong, M. Gorman, and J. P. Burnett, Jr., Cancer Res., 23: 1390 (1963).
57. W. A. Creasey, in Antineoplastic and Immunosuppressive Agents, Part II (A. C. Sartorelli and D. G. Johns, eds.), Springer-Verlag, New York, 1975, p. 670.
58. S. M. Kupchan, Y. Komoda, W. A. Court, G. J. Thomas, R. M. Smith, A. Karim, G. J. Gilmore, R. C. Haltiwanger, and R. F. Bryan, J. Am. Chem. Soc., 95: 1354 (1972).
59. S. M. Kupchan, A. T. Sneden, A. R. Branfman, G. A. Howie, L. I. Rebhun, W. E. McIvor, R. W. Wang, and T. C. Schnaitman, J. Med. Chem., 21: 31 (1978).
60. S. M. Sieber, M. K. Wolpert, R. H. Adamson, R. L. Cysyk, V. H. Bono, and D. G. Johns, in Comparative Leukemia Research 1975 (J. Clemmensen and D. S. Yohn, eds.), Bibl. Haemt., 1976, p. 495.
61. A. T. Sneden and G. L. Beemsterboer, J. Nat. Prod., 43: 637 (1980).
62. M. C. Wani, H. L. Taylor, and M. E. Wall, J. Chem. Soc., Chem. Commun., 390 (1973).
63. R. G. Powell, D. Weisleder, and C. R. Smith, Jr., J. Org. Chem., 46: 4398 (1981).
64. M. Asai, E. Mizuta, M. Izawa, K. Haibara, and T. Kishi, Tetrahedron, 35: 1079 (1979).
65. M. Izawa, S. Tanida, and M. Asai, J. Antibiot., 34: 496 (1981).
66. S. Remillard, L. I. Rebhun, G. A. Howie, and S. M. Kupchan, Science, 189: 1002 (1975).
67. T. Schnaitman, L. I. Rebhun, and S. M. Kupchan, J. Cell. Biol., 68: 388a (1975).

68. F. Mandelbaum-Schavit, M. K. Wolpert-Defilippes, and D. G. Johns, Biochem. Biophys. Res. Commun., 12: 47 (1976).
69. B. Bhattacharyya and J. Wolff, FEBS Lett., 75: 159 (1977).
70. M. K. Wolpert-DeFilippes, R. H. Adamson, R. L. Cysyk, and D. G. Johns, Biochem. Pharmacol., 24: 751 (1975).
71. M. K. Wolpert-DeFilippes, V. H. Bono, Jr., R. L. Dion, and D. G. Johns, Biochem. Pharmacol., 24: 1735 (1975).
72. P. N. Rao, E. J. Freireich, M. L. Smith, and T. L. Loo, Cancer Res., 39: 3152 (1979).
73. O. Alabaster and M. Cassidy, J. Natl. Cancer Inst., 60: 649 (1978).
74. J. W. Lown, K. C. Majumdar, A. I. Meyers, and A. Hecht, Bioorg. Chem., 6: 453 (1977).
75. K. Ootsu, Y. Kozai, M. Takeuchi, S. Ikeyama, K. Igaraschi, K. Tsukamoto, Y. Sugino, T. Tashiro, S. Tsukagoshi, and Y. Sakurai, Cancer Res., 40: 1707 (1980).
76. E. Higashide, M. Asai, K. Ootsu, S. Tanida, Y. Kozai, T. Hasegawa, T. Kishi, Y. Sugino, and M. Yoneda, Nature, 270: 721 (1977).
77. S. Tanida, M. Izawa, and T. Hasegawa, J. Antibiot., 34: 489 (1981).
78. N. Nakahama, M. Izawa, M. Asai, M. Kida, and T. Kishi, J. Antibiot., 34: 1581 (1981).
79. (a) E. J. Corey, L. O. Weigel, A. R. Chamberlin, H. Cho, and D. H. Hua, J. Am. Chem. Soc., 102: 6613 (1980); (b) E. J. Corey, L. O. Weigel, A. R. Chamberlin, and B. Lipshutz, J. Am. Chem. Soc., 102: 1439 (1980); (c) E. J. Corey, L. O. Weigel, D. Floyd, and M. G. Bock, J. Am. Chem. Soc., 100: 2916 (1978); (d) E. J. Corey, M. G. Bock, A. P. Kozikowski, A. V. Rama Rao, D. Floyd, and B. Lipshutz, Tetrahedron Lett., 1051 (1978); (e) E. J. Corey, H. E. Wetter, A. P. Kozikowski, and A. V. Rama Rao, Tetrahedron Lett., 777 (1977); (f) E. J. Corey and M. G. Bock, Tetrahedron Lett., 2643 (1975).
80. (a) A. I. Meyers, P. J. Reider, and A. L. Campbell, J. Am. Chem. Soc., 102: 6597 (1980); (b) A. I. Meyers, D. L. Comins, D. M. Roland, R. Henning, and K. Shimizu, J. Am. Chem. Soc., 101: 7104 (1979); (c) A. I. Meyers, D. M. Roland, D. L. Comins, R. Henning, M. P. Fleming, and K. Shimizu, J. Am. Chem. Soc., 101: 4732 (1979); (d) A. I. Meyers, K. Tomioka, D. M. Roland, and D. Comins, Tetrahedron Lett., 1375 (1978); (e) J. M. Kane and A. I. Meyers, Tetrahedron Lett., 771 (1977); (f) A. I. Meyers and R. S. Brinkmeyer, Tetrahedron Lett., 1749 (1975); (g) A. I. Meyers, C. C. Shaw, D. Horne, L. M. Trefonas, and R. J. Majeste, Tetrahedron Lett., 1745 (1975); (h) A. I. Meyers and C. C. Shaw, Tetrahedron Lett., 717 (1974).
81. (a) R. Bonjouklian and B. Ganem, Carbohydr. Res., 76: 245 (1979); (b) R. Bonjouklian and B. Ganem, Tetrahedron Lett., 2835 (1977); (c) J. E. Foy and B. Ganem, Tetrahedron Lett., 775 (1977).

82. (a) P.-T. Ho, Can. J. Chem., 58: 861 (1980); (b) P.-T. Ho, Can. J. Chem., 58: 858 (1980); (c) O. E. Edwards and P.-T. Ho, Can. J. Chem., 55: 371 (1977).
83. (a) G. Gormley, Jr., Y. Y. Chan, and J. Fried, J. Org. Chem., 45: 1447 (1980); (b) W. J. Elliott and J. Fried, J. Org. Chem., 41: 2469 (1976).
84. E. Götschi, F. Schneider, H. Wagner, and K. Bernauer, Helv. Chim. Acta, 60: 1416 (1977).
85. (a) M. Isobe, M. Kitamura, and T. Goto, Tetrahedron Lett., 239 (1981); (b) M. Isobe, M. Kitamura, and T. Goto, Tetrahedron Lett., 3465 (1979).
86. M. Samson, P. DeClercq, H. De Wilde, and M. Vandewalle, Tetrahedron Lett., 3195 (1977).
87. D. H. R. Barton, S. D. Gero, and C. D. Maycock, J. Chem. Soc., Chem. Commun., 1089 (1980).
88. N. Hashimoto, K. Matsumura, M. Motohashi, K. Ootsu, Y. Kozai, and T. Kishi, 177th Natl. Meet. Am. Chem. Soc., Honolulu, 1979; Abstr. Med. Sec. 26.
89. R. T. Eagan, J. N. Ingle, J. Rubin, S. Frytak, and C. G. Moertel, J. Natl. Cancer Inst., 60: 93 (1978).
90. F. Cabanillas, V. Rodriguez, S. W. Hall, M. A. Burgess, B. G. Bodey, and E. J. Freireich, Cancer Treat. Rep., 62: 425 (1978).
91. B. A. Chabner, A. S. Levine, B. L. Johnson, and R. C. Young, Cancer Treat. Rep., 62: 429 (1978).
92. R. H. Blum and T. Kahlert, Cancer Treat. Rep., 62: 435 (1978).
93. A. P. Chahinian, C. Nogeire, T. Ohnuma, M. L. Greenberg, M. Sivak, I. S. Jaffrey, and J. F. Holland, Cancer Treat. Rep., 63: 1953 (1979).
94. M. J. O'Connell, A. Shani, J. Rubin, and C. G. Moertel, Cancer Treat. Rep., 62: 1237 (1978).
95. R. T. Eagan, E. T. Creagan, N. J. Ingle, S. Frytak, and J. Rubin, Cancer Treat. Rep., 62: 1577 (1978).
96. F. Cabanillas, G. P. Bodey, M. A. Burgess, and E. J. Freireich, Cancer Treat. Rep., 63: 507 (1979).
97. E. T. Creagan, T. R. Fleming, J. H. Edmonson, and J. N. Ingle, Cancer Treat. Rep., 63: 2061 (1979).
98. I. S. Jaffrey, J. M. Denefrio, and P. Chahinian, Cancer Treat. Rep., 64: 193 (1980).
99. J. A. Neidhart, L. R. Laufman, C. Vaughn, and J. D. McCracken, Cancer Treat. Rep., 64: 675 (1980).
100. D. L. Ahmann, S. Frytak, L. K. Kvols, R. G. Hahn, J. H. Edmonson, H. F. Bisel, and E. T. Creagan, Cancer Treat. Rep., 64: 721 (1980).
101. S. Rosenthal, D. T. Harris, J. Horton, and J. H. Glick, Cancer Treat. Rep., 64: 1115 (1980).

102. M. E. Wall and M. C. Wani, 7th Int. Symp. Chem. Natl. Prod., IUPAC, Riga, 1970, Abstr. 614.
103. S. M. Kupchan, R. W. Britton, J. A. Lacadie, M. F. Ziegler, and C. W. Sigel, J. Org. Chem., 40: 648 (1975).
104. A. T. Sneden, in Basis for Cancer Therapy 1: Advances in Medical Oncology, Research and Education, Vol. 5 (B. W. Fox, ed.), Pergamon Press, Oxford, 1979, p. 75.
105. J. Polonsky, J. Varenne, T. Prange', and C. Pascard, Tetrahedron Lett., 1853 (1980).
106. F. A. Darwish, F. J. Evans, and J. D. Phillipson, Planta Med., 39: 232 (1980).
107. K.-H. Lee, Y. Imakura, Y. Sumida, R.-Y. Wu, I. H. Hall, and H.-C. Huang, J. Org. Chem., 44: 2180 (1979).
108. Z. Jin-Sheng, L. Long-ze, C. Zhung-liang, and Xu Ren-sheng, Planta Med., 39: 265 (1980).
109. L.-L. Liao, S. M. Kupchan, and S. B. Horwitz, Mol. Pharmacol., 12: 167 (1976).
110. I. H. Hall, K.H. Lee, S. A. ElGebaly, Y. Imakura, Y. Sumida, and R. Y. Wu, J. Pharm. Sci., 68: 883 (1979).
111. M. Fresno, A. Gonzales, D. Vasquez, and A. Jimenez, Biochim. Biophys. Acta, 518: 104 (1978).
112. S. M. Kupchan, J. A. Lacadie, G. A. Howie, and B. R. Sickles, J. Med. Chem., 19: 1130 (1976).
113. C. A. Valdenegro-Benitez, M. S. thesis, University of Virginia, 1976.
114. M. E. Wall and M. C. Wani, J. Med. Chem., 21: 1186 (1978).
115. M. Okano and K.-H. Lee, J. Org. Chem., 46: 1138 (1981).
116. N. Stojanac, A. Sood, Z. Stojanac, and Z. Valenta, Can. J. Chem., 53: 619 (1975).
117. P. A. Grieco, G. Vidari, S. Ferrino, and R. C. Haltiwanger, Tetrahedron Lett., 1619 (1980).
118. P. A. Grieco, S. Ferrino, G. Vidari, and J. C. Huffman, J. Org. Chem., 46: 1022 (1981).
119. P. A. Grieco, R. Lis, S. Ferrino, and J. Y. Jaw, J. Org. Chem., 47: 601 (1982).
120. D. L. Snitman, M.-Y. Tsai, and D. S. Watt, Syn. Commun., 8: 195 (1978).
121. O. D. Dailey, Jr. and P. L. Fuchs, J. Org. Chem., 45: 216 (1980).
122. G. A. Kraus and M. J. Taschner, J. Org. Chem., 45: 1175 (1980).
123. (a) J. R. Dias and B. Nassim, Steroids, 35: 2584 (1980); (b) J. R. Dias, R. Ramachandra, and B. Nassim, Org. Mass. Spectrom., 13: 307 (1978); (c) J. R. Dias and R. Ramachandra, J. Org. Chem., 42: 3584 (1977); (d) J. R. Dias and R. Ramachandra, Org. Prep. Proc., Int., 9: 109 (1977); (e) J. R. Dias and R. Ramachandra, Syn. Commun., 7: 293 (1977); (f) J. R. Dias and R. Ramachandra, J. Org. Chem., 42: 1613 (1977); (g) J. R. Dias and R. Ramachandra, Tetrahedron Lett., 3685 (1976).

124. T. R. Castles, R. L. Bridges, J. C. Bhandari, and C. C. Lee, Toxicol. Appl. Pharmacol., 41: 192 (1977).
125. A. V. Bedikian, M. Valdivieso, G. P. Bodey, W. K. Murphy, and E. J. Freireich, Cancer Treat. Rep., 63: 1843 (1979).
126. M. G. Garnick, R. H. Blum, G. P. Canellos, R. J. Mayer, L. Parker, A. T. Skarin, F. P. Li, I. C. Henderson, and E. Frei III, Cancer Treat. Rep., 63: 1929 (1979).
127. S. M. Kupchan, B. B. Jarvis, R. G. Dailey, Jr., W. Bright, R. F. Bryan, and Y. Shizuri, J. Am. Chem. Soc., 98: 7092 (1976).
128. S. M. Kupchan, D. R. Streelman, B. B. Jarvis, R. G. Dailey, Jr., and A. T. Sneden, J. Org. Chem., 42: 4221 (1977).
129. A. T. Sneden, W. C. Sumner, Jr., and S. M. Kupchan, J. Nat. Prod., 45: 624 (1982).
130. R. G. Powell, D. Weisleder, C. R. Smith, Jr., J. Kozlowski, and W. K. Rohwedder, J. Am. Chem. Soc., 104: 4929 (1982).
131. M. Isobe, M. Kitamura, and T. Goto, J. Am. Chem. Soc., 104: 4997 (1982).
132. M. Isobe, M. Kitamura, and T. Goto, Chem. Lett., 1907 (1982).
133. D. H. R. Barton, M. Benechie, F. Khuong-Huu, P. Potier, and V. Reyna-Pinedo, Tetrahedron Lett., 23: 651 (1982).
134. D. H. R. Barton, S. D. Gero, and C. D. Maycock, J. Chem. Soc. Perkin Trans. I: 1541 (1982).
135. H. M. Sirat, E. J. Thomas, and J. D. Wallis, J. Chem. Soc. Perkin Trans. I: 2885 (1982).
136. V. Ratanatharathorn, N. Gad-el-Mawla, H. E. Wilson, J. D. Bonnet, S. E. Rivkin, and R. Mass, Cancer Chemother. Rep., 66: 1587 (1982).
137. R. H. Creech, K. Stanley, S. E. Vogl, D. S. Ettinger, P. D. Bonomi, and O. Salazar, Cancer Chemother. Rep., 66: 1417 (1982).
138. Y. F. Liou, I. H. Hall, M. Okano, K. H. Lee, and S. G. Chaney, J. Pharm. Sci., 71: 430 (1982).
139. K. Fukumoto, M. Chihiro, Y. Shiratori, M. Ihara, T. Kametani, and T. Honda, Tetrahedron Lett., 23: 2973 (1982).
140. L. Mandell, D. E. Lee, and L. F. Courtney, J. Org. Chem., 47: 610 (1982).
141. J. Liesmann, R. J. Belt, C. D. Haas, and B. Hoogstraten, Cancer Treat. Rep., 65: 883 (1981).
142. C. L. Wiseman, H.-Y. Yap, A. Y. Bedikian, G. P. Bodey, and G. R. Blumenschein, Am. J. Clin. Oncol., 5: 389 (1982).

5

THE CHEMISTRY AND BIOCHEMISTRY OF PURINE AND PYRIMIDINE NUCLEOSIDE ANTIVIRAL AND ANTITUMOR AGENTS

PAUL F. TORRENCE

National Institute of Arthritis, Diabetes, and Digestive
and Kidney Diseases
National Institutes of Health
Bethesda, Maryland

I. INTRODUCTION

The structure of the common major constituents of DNA (thymidine, deoxycytidine, deoxyguanosine, deoxyadenosine) or RNA (uridine, cytidine, guanosine, adenosine) cannot be viewed by a chemist without the question eventually coming to mind: "What if . . . ?" Indeed, what if the 5-methyl group of thymidine were hydrogen or ethyl? What if the stereochemistry of the sugar C2' hydroxyl were of the arabino configuration rather than the ribo configuration? Such questions have served as the basis for the development of antagonists of nucleosides and nucleotides and this, in turn, has led to agents which are useful in the treatment of human viral and neoplastic disease. The ability of the chemist to manipulate the structure of the constituents of genes is, therefore, a chemotherapeutic approach of great promise; however, it is also an approach of great hazard due to the semblance of such modified nucleosides to the natural substances.

In the past decade, it has become abundantly evident, through studies on the biology of novel nucleoside analogs and through research in virus biochemistry, that at least some clinically important viruses are vulnerable to inhibition of replication by agents that do not affect the host cell [1-7]. Associated with viral replication may be enzymes with no known counterparts in the uninfected host cell, for instance, the RNA-dependent DNA polymerase (reverse transcriptase) of retroviruses. Alternatively, the virus may induce enzyme activities which are already present in the host cell: for example, herpes simplex virus induces the synthesis of a number of enzymes of nucleic acid synthesis, including a thymidine kinase, a DNA polymerase, a deoxycytidine or deoxycytidylate deaminase, a DNA polymerase, a deoxyribonuclease, and a ribonucleotide reductase [8]. These enzymes differ considerably from those found in the uninfected host cells. For instance, deoxythymidine kinase and deoxycytidine kinase activities, which apparently reside in the same enzyme molecule, are more heat stable than the host cell enzymes, are more resistant to feedback inhibition, and possess a lower pH optimum and a lower K_m value than those of the corresponding host cell enzymes [8]. These differences may be viewed as a part of a viral strategy to gain some advantage over sole reliance on host cell enzymes; however, these differences provide exploitable targets for chemotherapeutical attack.

How may the study of nucleoside analogs as inhibitors of viral replication be expected to assist the development of an effective chemotherapy of cancer? This question has been answered rather effectively by Shannon and Schabel [7]. First, cancer patients are often more susceptible to certain virus infections than the general population; furthermore, the successful aggressive use of radiation therapy and/or combination chemotherapy may further compromise the immune system. Patients with hematological malignancies are often at greatest risk. Infections from the herpes viruses, cytomegaloviruses, rubeola viruses (measles), hepatitis viruses, or papoava viruses often run a fatal course in such patients. Thus selective antiviral agents would be a valuable adjunct to cancer chemotherapy. Second, there is gathering circumstantial evidence to implicate a viral etiology in at least a few types of human cancer [9,10]. Oncogenic viruses are well established in other animals but definitive proof has thus far been lacking for the human situation. The herpes virus group is most closely associated with human neoplastic disease; thus Epstein-Barr virus may be the etiologic agent of Burkitt's lymphoma and nasopharyngeal carcinoma, whereas herpes simplex virus type 2 may be involved as a causative agent in human cervical carcinoma [10,11]. Recently, Epstein-Barr virus was again implicated in human cancer by the observation that mononucleosis (known to be caused by Epstein-Barr virus) may increase the risk of developing Hodgkin's disease [11a]. RNA tumor viruses may be linked to leukemias and lymphomas [9]. Not only may such viruses be involved in the initial transformation to the malignant state, but they may also be involved in the reinduction of leukemia in humans. Thus agents that would selectively block such viruses as the type C RNA tumor viruses could be valuable in the remission therapy of neoplastic disease [7]. Finally, there are many lessons to be learned from the biochemistry of a cell that has been enslaved by a virus. The virus may induce new proteins that are sufficiently different from those of the host cells to permit the design of specific inhibitors. Nucleoside analogs may also be employed to probe the subtle differences that may exist between virus-induced and host-programmed enzymes. As these enzymes are critical to nucleic acid metabolism, useful insights may be obtained for the development of chemotherapeutic drugs.

In contrast to the selective chemotherapy of viral diseases based on biochemical differences between virus-infected and uninfected cells, there has been no target found which could be the basis for selective cancer chemotherapy (with the exception of asparaginase, which is used to treat cancers that rely on an exogenous source of asparagine). There are, however, many distinctive biochemical differences between malignant cells and normal cells (e.g., plasminogen activator, carcinoembryonic antigen, α-fetoprotein, tumor isoenzymes, etc.). Eventually, some differences may be found that could be exploited chemically. Until such an insight is gained, we must rely on increasing the efficacy of known agents and further refining and extending the leads currently in hand as outlined in a recent article by Montgomery [12].

There exist a number of excellent monographs on the chemistry and biochemistry of nucleosides and nucleotides, such as the individual works by Scheit [13], Suhadolnik [14,15] and Henderson and Paterson [16]. The two-volume series Basic Principles in Nucleic Acid Chemistry edited by Ts'o [17] and the collective volumes edited by Zorbach and Tipson [18] and by Townsend and Tipson [19] are also quite useful, the latter especially to the practicing chemist. Individual works by Walker [20] and Hutchinson [21] in the treatise Comprehensive Organic Chemistry serve as sound introductions to the organic chemistry of nucleosides and nucleotides; however, to date the most comprehensive treatment of the organic chemistry of nucleic acids is that by Kochetkov and Budovskii [22]. The proceedings of several meetings or symposia have been published and, even though two of these contain material that is several years old, they are still quite informative [23-27].

II. NUCLEIC ACID BIOSYNTHESIS

As pointed out by Montgomery [28,29], there are at least 85 enzymatic reactions that contribute to the de novo biosynthesis of nucleic acids, and only about 14 of these steps are known to be blocked by metabolite analogs or their metabolic products. An abbreviated scheme of the major pathways of de novo nucleic acid biosynthesis is presented in Fig. 5.1. Frequent reference to these conversions will be made during the subsequent discussion of the biological activity of nucleoside analogs. It may be noted that purine nucleoside metabolism is relatively uncomplicated compared to pyrimidine nucleotides [30]. Pyrimidine deoxyribonucleotides, as an example, are interconverted, hydrolyzed, phosphorylated, deaminated, and methylated, whereas purine nucleotides are involved only in hydrolysis and phosphate transfer reactions [16].

III. 5-SUBSTITUTED PYRIMIDINE NUCLEOSIDES*

One of the most active areas of nucleoside chemistry and biochemistry is 5-substituted pyrimidine nucleosides (Fig. 5.2). Thymidine and deoxycytidine analogs are of interest for two major reasons; the inhibition of tumor growth and the selective blocking of viral replication.

Thymidine (1), a 5-substituted pyrimidine nucleoside, is of current clinical interest [32] because it has beneficial clinical actions in combination with other agents. For example, it is a "rescue agent" for methotrexate or 5-fluoro-2'-deoxyuridine toxicity; it increases the sensitivity of tumor cells to araC; it potentiates the antitumor activities of 5-fluorouracil and cyclophosphamide. Thymidine also shows some promise as an anticancer agent when it is administered by itself in high dosage by continuous infusion. This method of administration is mandated by the solubility characteristics of thymidine and the necessity of obtaining rather high ($\sim 10^{-3}$ M) plasma concentrations. In this regard, depot forms of thymidine have been synthesized and studied as an alternative method of administration [33]. In cell culture, tumor cells can be killed outright by excess thymidine since they are more sensitive than normal cells to nutritional restrictions. The substantive mechanism involved in this cell-killing and antitumor effect is the conversion of thymidine to its 5'-triphosphate and subsequent feedback inhibition of ribonucelotide reductase, the enzyme responsible for the conversion of CDP to dCDP.

*For a discussion of the chemistry of 5-substituted pyrimidine nucleosides, the reader is referred to the recent review by Bradshaw and Hutchinson [31].

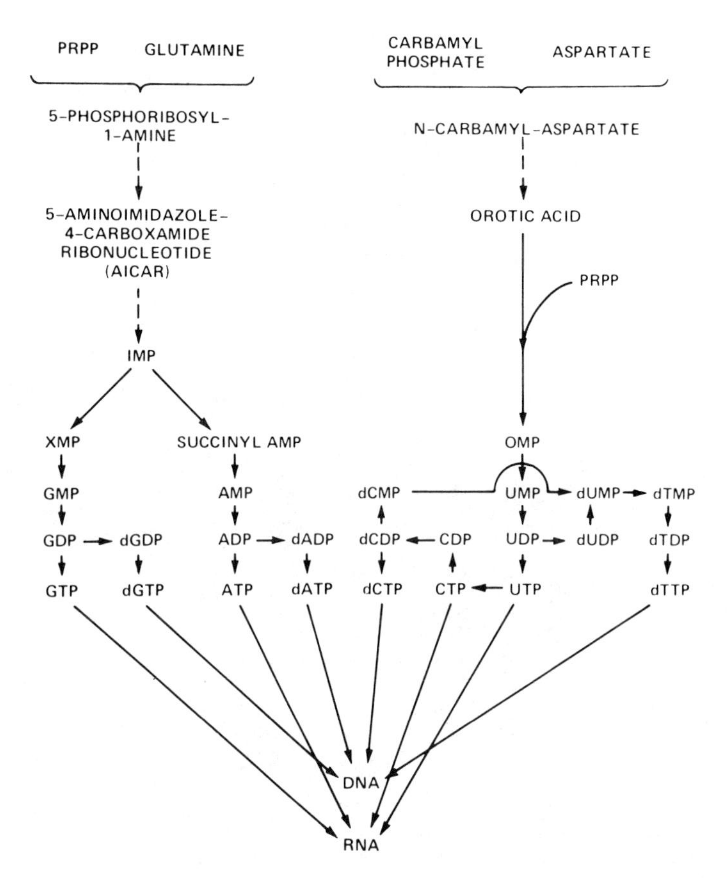

FIGURE 5.1 De novo biosynthesis of nucleic acids. (From Ref. 5.)

The potential of 5-substituted pyrimidine nucleosides as cancer chemomotherapeutic agents is based on 5-fluorouracil [34, 35]. The cytotoxic and tumor inhibitory properties of 5-fluorouracil is a matter of current debate. One school of thought is that 5-fluorouracil is converted to the 5-monophosphate of 5'-fluoro-2'-deoxyuridine (2), which inhibits DNA synthesis by blockade of thymidylate synthetase [37-37]. A second school of thought [38, 39] suggests that 5-fluorouracil is incorporated into RNA via 5-fluorouridine and that the antitumor effect is effected through base-pair transformations and changes in RNA structure, processing, and modification (e.g., methylation) [40, 41]. In vitro the conclusion has been reached that the ability of 5-fluoro-2'-deoxyuridine to halt growth of L1210 cells is correlated with its ability to inhibit thymidylate synthetase [42]. Both of those mechanisms of toxicity are mediated by the lethal synthesis of the nucleosides 5-fluoro-2'-deoxyuridine (2) or its riboside counterpart, 5-fluorouridine.

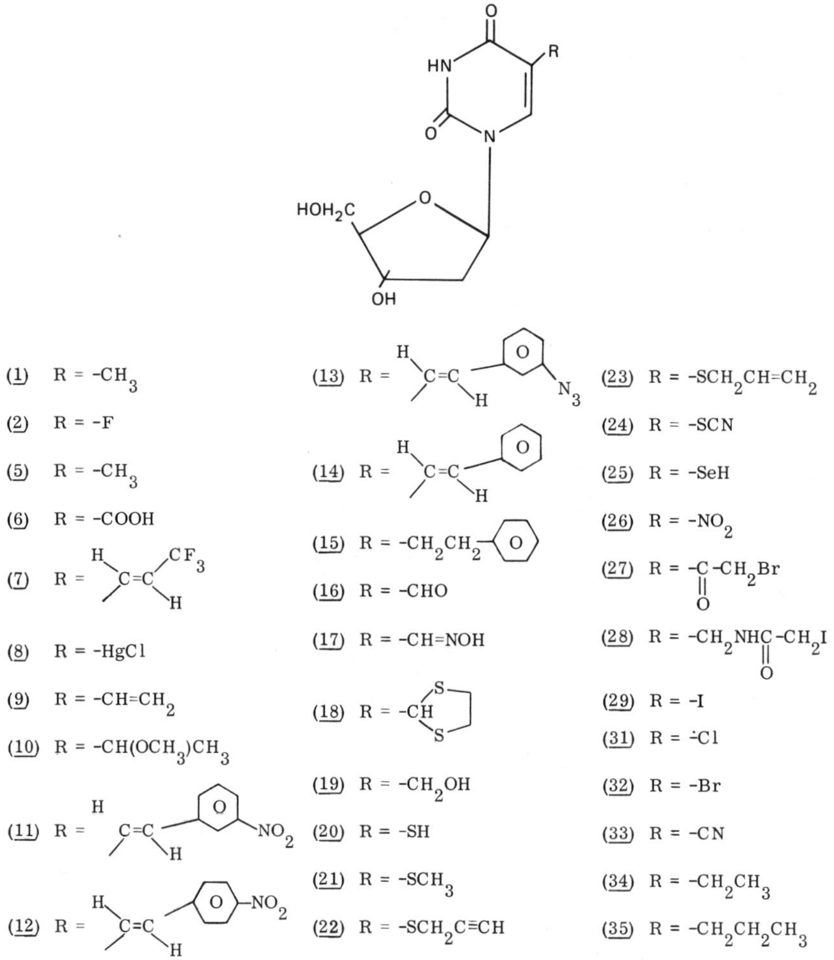

(1) R = $-CH_3$

(2) R = -F

(5) R = $-CH_3$

(6) R = -COOH

(7) R = $(H)C{=}C(H)CF_3$

(8) R = -HgCl

(9) R = $-CH{=}CH_2$

(10) R = $-CH(OCH_3)CH_3$

(11) R = $(H)C{=}C(H)-\langle O \rangle-NO_2$

(12) R = $(H)C{=}C(H)-\langle O \rangle-NO_2$

(13) R = $(H)C{=}C(H)-\langle O \rangle-N_3$

(14) R = $(H)C{=}C(H)-\langle O \rangle$

(15) R = $-CH_2CH_2-\langle O \rangle$

(16) R = -CHO

(17) R = -CH=NOH

(18) R = $-CH\langle S,S \rangle$

(19) R = $-CH_2OH$

(20) R = -SH

(21) R = $-SCH_3$

(22) R = $-SCH_2C{\equiv}CH$

(23) R = $-SCH_2CH{=}CH_2$

(24) R = -SCN

(25) R = -SeH

(26) R = $-NO_2$

(27) R = $-C(=O)-CH_2Br$

(28) R = $-CH_2NHC(=O)-CH_2I$

(29) R = -I

(31) R = -Cl

(32) R = -Br

(33) R = -CN

(34) R = $-CH_2CH_3$

(35) R = $-CH_2CH_2CH_3$

FIGURE 5.2 Some 5-substituted pyrimidine nucleosides with antiviral and/or antitumor activity.

5-Fluorouracil itself is most valuable in the treatment of carcinoma of the breast and of the gastrointestinal tract, and may be of some use in the topical treatment of skin malignancies and cancer of the cervix or ovary. The best responses are obtained when 5-fluorouracil is employed in combination chemotherapy. Its activity is restricted to solid tumors [43].

Contrary to expectation, the nucleoside 5'-fluoro-2'-deoxyuridine (2), to which 5-fluorouracil is anabolized, is not superior to 5-fluorouracil itself as a cancer chemotherapeutic agent. This is due to its rapid cleavage to base and sugar by the ubiquitous thymidine and uridine phosphorylases. This degradation is faster than its conversion to the lethal 5-fluoro-2'-deoxyuridine 5'-monophosphate [44].

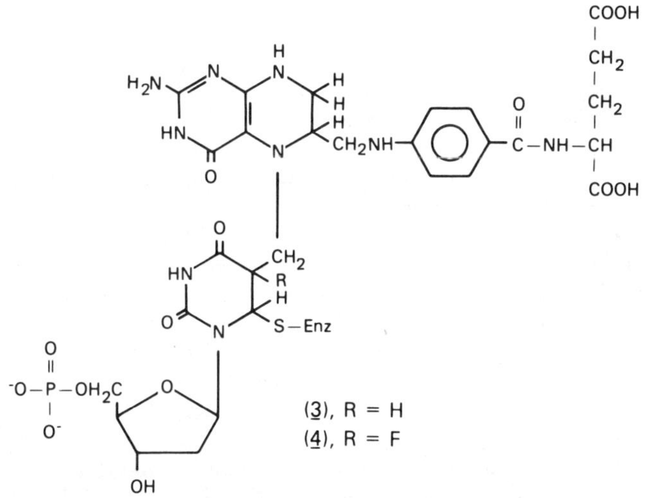

FIGURE 5.3 Intermediates in the conversion of dUMP to TMP by thymidylate synthetase or the inhibition of thymidylate synthetase by FdUMP.

To understand the mechanism by which 5-fluoro-2'-deoxyuridine 5'-monophosphate (FdUMP) inhibits thymidylate synthetase and leads to a "thymineless" death [45], it is necessary to consider the mechanism by which 2'-deoxyuridine 5'-monophosphate (dUMP) is converted to thymidine 5'-monophosphate (dTMP) (Fig. 5.3). The reaction [40] first involves reversible complex formation between the enzyme and the substrate (dUMP). In a second step, the 5-carbon of the pyrimidine ring of dUMP is alkylated by the one-carbon donor, N^5,N^{10}-methylenetetrahydrofolic acid, to give the intermediate (3). An internal redox reaction then occurs to give dTMP and the oxidized cofactor, 7,8-dihydrofolic acid. Concurrent with the C-5 alkylation is the addition of the SH group of a cysteine residue of thymidylate synthetase [47].

The effective inhibition of thymidylate synthetase by FdUMP requires the presence of tetrahydrofolic acid; in its absence, binding is weak and reversible. FdUMP, in the presence of tetrahydrofolic acid, reacts as does dUMP to give the covalent complex (4) (Fig. 5.3); however, in contrast to the intermediate (3), arising from dUMP, (4) cannot be decomposed since the C-F bond cannot be broken. The covalent complex, (4), slowly undergoes reversion to FdUMP and tetrahydrofolic acid ($t_{1/2} \sim 10$hr) [46].

A considerable simplification in the synthesis of 5-fluoropyrimidine nucleosides, previously available only by de novo construction of the base followed by base-sugar condensation, has come from the use of trifluoromethyl hypofluorite [48-51]. The reaction of 2',3',5'-tri-O-acetyluridine with trifluoromethylhypofluorite (CF_3OF) in chloroform gives a 6-alkoxy-5-fluoro-5,6-dihydropyrimidine adduct that undergoes base-catalyzed elimination of alcohol to give the 5-fluoropyrimidine nucleoside.

The substitution of fluorine for hydrogen led to the synthesis [52, 53] of 5-trifluoromethyl-2'-deoxyuridine [(5), trifluorothymidine] which possesses both antitumor and antiviral activities [54]. The original synthesis of trifluorothymine, the required base for the above enzymatic synthesis of the nucleoside, was shortened to one step by Mertes and Saheb [55], who found that triflurorthymine could be generated from 5-carboxyluracil and sulfur tetrafluoride. A chemical synthesis of (5) was reported soon after [56]. Kobayashi et al. [57] reported that nucleosides such as (5), trifluoromethylcytidine, or trifluoromethyl-araC could be prepared in moderate to good yields by reaction of a properly protected 5-halopyrimidine nucleoside with a trifluoromethyl-copper complex. By similar methodology, 6- or 8-substituted purine nucleosides were obtained.

While trifluorothymidine (5) has produced some objective responses in the combination chemotherapy of certain neoplastic diseases, especially pediatric neuroblastoma, it has found a wider application as a topical antiviral agent for the treatment of herpes simplex eye infections. In fact, it has been concluded that (5) may be the best antiviral agent evaluated to date for the treatment of ocular herpes virus diseases [54].

Trifluorothymidine (5) is converted to the 5'-mono- and then to the 5'-triphosphate by cells and is incorporated into cellular DNA in keeping with the similarity in steric bulk between the trifluoromethyl group and the methyl group. Trifluorothymidine is also incorporated into the DNA of vaccinia virus; when 2% of the vaccinia DNA thymidine residues are replaced by (5), the virions become noninfective. In addition, vaccinia DNA containing (5) is smaller in size (52S and 39S contrasted with 70S) than normal vaccinia DNA. As a result, there is faulty transcription of late viral mRNAs which translate to faulty virion proteins [54, 55].

A second important mechanism of action of trifluorothymidine is potent irreversible inhibition of thymidylate synthetase [59] by its 5'-monophosphate. This irreversible inactivation arises from the inherent instability of the C-5 pyrimidine trifluoromethyl group of (5). Under mildly basic conditions, (5) hydrolyzes to 5-carboxy-2'-deoxyuridine (6) [53]. According to Santi and Sakai [60], this solvolysis of the CF_3 group of (5) occurs via nucleophilic attack at pyrimidine C-6. This labilizes the CF_3 group by generating a negative charge at pyrimidine C-5. A series of elimination-addition reactions then occur to give (6). Santi [46] has found that thymidylate synthetase from *Lactobacillus casei* catalyzes the release of fluoride from the 5'-monophosphate of (5) and gives rise to a product with a ultraviolet (UV) spectrum similar to 5-acyl-substituted 2'-deoxyuridine.

It is considered [54] that the cytotoxicity and antitumor properties of (5) are due chiefly to its inhibition of thymidylate synthetase, whereas its antiviral properties are ascribable primarily to its incorporation into viral DNA. The former conclusion has been further reinforced [42].

Wataya et al. [61] effectively extended the CF_3 group by vinylogous conjugation in the 5'-monophosphate of *trans*-5-(3,3,3-trifluoro-1-propenyl)-2'-deoxyuridine (7), which inactivates thymidylate synthetase by a mechanism similar to that which obtains in the case of trifluorothymidine. A putative advantage of this approach may be the ability to extend the CF_3 reactive functionality until it is in a suitable position to covalently bind to some nucleophile of a given enzyme according to the general formula of Fig. 5.4.

The synthesis of compound (7), as well as a variety of other 5-substi- tuted pyrimidine nucleoside may undergo palladium metal exchange, and the oped by Bergstrom and co-workers [62-64], who exploited the established [65] 5-mecuration of uracil and cytosine derivatives. A 5-mercuri-substituted pyrimidine nuceloside may undergo palladium metal exchange, and the resultant organopalladium intermediate can be reacted with an alkene, for instance, to yield a 5-alkenyl pyrimidine nucleoside (9). As another example, reaction of 5-chloromercuri-2'-deoxyuridine (8) with Li_2PdCl_4 and ethylene in methanol gave 5-(1-methoxyethyl)-2'-deoxyuridine (10) which can be converted to 5-ethyl-2'-deoxyuridine [64] in 57% yield. Quite a number of 5-substituted pyrimidine nucleosides have been prepared by this approach; recently, Bigge et al. [66] extended this reaction to the direct synthesis of various 5-substituted styryl derivatives of 2'-deoxyuridine and its 5'-monophosphate. Some of these latter styryl nucleosides and nucleotides [3-nitrostyryl (11), 4-nitrostyryl (12), 3-adizostyryl (13), styryl (14), and the reduced derivative phenylethyl (15)] showed moderate antiviral activity and, at somewhat higher concentrations, could inhibit the growth of L1210 cells in culture [69]. In addition, the 5'-monophosphate of 5(E)-(3-azidostyryl)-2'-deoxyuridine (13) is a photoactivated inhibitor of thymidylate synthetase and a light-dependent inhibitor of vaccinia virus replication and the replication of L1210 and human lymphoblastoid cells [68]. The intermediacy of a nitrene is supported by the available experimental evidence.

Uracil and its derivatives react with formaldehyde under acidic or basic conditions to give the 5-hydroxymethyluracil derivatives, which can be oxidized (with MnO_2) to the 5-formyluracils [69-71]. The 5'-monophosphate of 5-formyl-2'-deoxyuridine (16) was found to be a potent irreversible inhibitor of thymidylate synthetase [72-75]. It is of interest that the monophosphate of (16) was designed [76] as a multisubstrate inhibitor of thymidylate synthetase due to the known reactivity of tetrahydrofolic acid with carbonyl compounds. 5-Formyl-2'-deoxyuridine has been reported to be a rather potent inhibitor of viral replication (pseudorabies, vaccinia, and herpes simplex viruses) but was not very selective since it blocked DNA

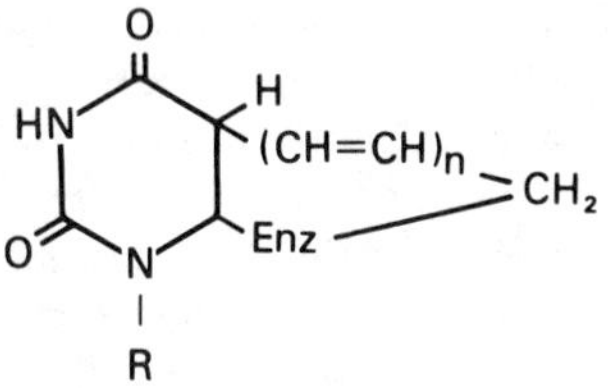

FIGURE 5.4 Putative intermediate in the reaction of the 5'-monophosphate of (5) (n = 0) or (7) (n = 1) with thymidylate synthetase.

synthesis and cell growth at concentrations closely approximating those required for inhibition of viral replication [75, 77, 78]. The 5'-monophosphate oxime and the dithiolane derivatives of (16), specifically (17) and (18), were competitive inhibitors of thymidylate synthetase, albeit roughly 10 times less potent than the monophosphate of (16) [75]. The dithiolane (18), however, did not inhibit virus replication, nor was it cytotoxic; on the other hand, the oxime (17) was equipotent to (16) as an inhibitor or herpes simplex virus replication, but was 25 times less cytotoxic than (16). In addition, (17) was also 100 times less effective than (16) as an inhibitor of vaccinia virus replication. As is the case for 5-nitro-2'-deoxyuridine (see below), strong inhibition of thymidylate synthetase seems to be associated with cytotoxicity and antivaccinia virus activity but not antiherpesvirus activity.

5-Hydroxymethyl-2-'deoxyuridine (19), the intermediate to (16), has demonstrated antiviral [79] and cytotoxic properties [80], but the antiviral action was devoid of selectivity [79].

Bardos and co-workers have synthesized 5-mercaptopyrimidine nucleosides by two separate approaches: (1) classical base-sugar condensation, and (2) addition of methyl hypobromite in methanol followed by reaction of the resulting adduct with sodium disulfide [81-85]. Such 5-mercaptopyrimidine nucleosides are endowed with a variety of biological activities [84]. At the polynucleotide level, partially thiolated polycytidylic acid is a potent inhibitor of reverse transcriptase [85] and has been administered to patients with leukemia [86]. Of particular interest is 5-mercapto-2'-deoxyuridine (20), which possesses antineoplastic activity [87, 88] and is a potent reversible inhibitor of thymidylate synthetase [89]. Although (20) is virtually inactive as an inhibitor of herpes simplex virus, the 5-methyl derivative (21) possesses significant antiherpes virus activity. Two congeners of (21), the 5-propargyl (22) and 5-allyl (23) derivatives, prepared by selective 5-alkylation of (20), also show significant antiviral activity. Compounds (22) and (23) may also be regarded as isosteres of the previously reported 5-propynyloxy- and 5-allyloxy-2'-deoxyuridines, which also are active antivirals (vide infra).

A thymidine analog which may be considered closely related to the above 5-mercapto- and 5-S-alkyl pyrimidine nucleosides is 5-thiocyano-2'-deoxyuridine (24), which is readily prepared by the action of chlorothiocyanogen (ClSCN) on 2'-deoxyuridine [90-92]. Compound (24) can be easily reduced to (20) by the action of mercaptoethanol, dithiothretitol, or glutathione [91]. It may even be possible that (24) may be transformed in the cell to (20) since its biological activities are in many respects similar to those of (20). Compound (24) can block the replication of several tumor cell lines in vitro (e.g., KB, L5178y, and L1210) [42, 91], and inhibits the growth of viruses in vitro (herpes and vaccinia virus) [93] or in vivo (vaccinia virus) [94]. Although ascertained only by labeling and reversal studies in cell cultures [91, 93, 95], inhibition of thymidylate synthetase is at least one mechanism of action of (24). Although there seems to be no doubt that thymidylate synthetase inhibition is responsible for the antiproliferative effects of (24) [42], it remains to be established that this is primarily responsible for its antiviral action. It may be worthwhile to point out that 2', 3', 5'-tri-O-acetyl-5-thiocyanouridine is able to inactivate vesicular stomatitis virus extracellularly [93] and that both (24) and the uridine congener, 5-thiocyanouridine, are cytocidal to the parasites Schistosoma mansoni and Brugia pahangi (J. J. Jaffe and P. F. Torrence, unpublished observations, 1975). It seems possible that such thiocyano compounds may have some biological effects not directly related to nucleic acid metabolism.

As a further extension of the study of 5-mercaptopyrimidine nucelosides, several 5-selenium-substituted uracil derivatives were prepared [96] by addition of methyl hypobromite to the pyrimidine 5, 6 double bond followed by reaction with sodium diselenide. The 5-hydroselenopyrimidines could be obtained easily by reduction with dithiothreitol. 5-Hydroseleno-2'-deoxyuridylic acid (25) was (in the presence of excess thiols) as potent an inhibitor of thymidylate synthetase as (20) itself; however, compound (25) was less active than (20) in the inhibition of growth of L1210 cells [96].

Recently, 5-nitropyrimidine derivatives have become of interest for their biological activities. The first nitropyrimidine nucleoside to be synthesized was the ribonucleoside 5-nitrouridine. Nitration of 2', 3', 5'-tri-O-(3, 5-dinitrobenzoyl)uridine with nitric acid [97] gave, after saponification, 5-nitrouridine, which also has been synthesized by the mercuric cyanide-nitromethane condensation [98]. Analogous nitration approaches to 5-nitro-2'-deoxyuridine (26), however, resulted only in glycoside bond cleavage (G. F. Huang and P. F. Torrence, unpublished observations, 1976) [99]. A 1% yield on the di-O-toluyl ester of (26 was realized when 5-nitrouracilylmercury was reacted with the appropriately protected 2'-deoxy-D-ribofuranosyl chloride [99]. Kluepfel et al. [100] reported the preparation of (26) using a nucleoside deoxyribosyltransferase from Lactobacillus; however, the first practical chemical synthesis of (26) and its 5'-monophosphate was achieved [101] using nitronium tetrafluoroborate in sulfolane, a reagent originated by Kuhn and Olah [102]. 5-Nitro-2'-deoxycytidine and its 5'-monophosphate were also obtained, albeit in poor yield, when the latter reagent was used [103].

5-Nitro-2'-deoxyuridine (26) exhibits potent in vitro antiviral activity toward herpes simplex virus and vaccinia virus [100, 104]; in addition, it is quite cytotoxic to a number of cells grown in culture [42, 105]. The nitronucleoside, (26), is not active against virus strains that do not induce thymidine kinase in the host cell [104] or in a cell line that is deficient in the same enzyme [105], suggesting that conversion to the 5'-monophosphate may be necessary for its antiviral activity. The incorporation of labeled 2'-deoxyuridine into the DNA of uninfected primary rabbit kidney cells is blocked by (26) at a much lower concentration than is the incorporation of labeled thymidine [104]; furthermore, the antivaccinia virus activity and the cytotoxicity of (26) are antagonized by low concentrations of thymidine [104, 105]. These data suggested that in the intact cell, (26) may owe its antiviral activity and cytotoxic effects to a blockade of thymidylate synthetase. Indeed, the 5'-monophosphate of (26) has been found to be a potent mechanism-based inhibitor of purified thymidylate synthetase of *Lactobacillus casei* [106-108]. A variety of evidence from model studies, kinetics, isotope effects, and actual isolation of the complex of the monophosphate of (26) with enzyme has provided strong evidence for the formation of the intermediate pictured in Fig. 5.5 [109, 110]. Finally, as pointed out by Washtien et al. [105], (26) differs in several important ways from 5-fluoro-2'-deoxyuridine; the base 5-nitrouracil is not toxic; the inhibition of thymidylate synthetase by the monophosphate of (26) does not require folate cofactor; it seems to have no other cellular target aside from thymidylate synthetase.

The 5'-monophosphate of 5-(α-bromoacetyl)-2'-deoxyuridine (27) has been reported [111] as an active-site directed irreversible inhibitor of thymidylate synthetase with a K_i value of 4.1 μM compared to a K_i value of 0.014 μM for the monophosphate of (2) and a K_i value of 68 μM for the 5'-monophosphate of the earlier reported [112] 5-(iodoacetamido)methyl nucleoside (28). The mechanism by which the nucleotide of (27) inactivates thymidylate synthetase is unknown; however, some interesting possibilities are represented in Fig. 5.6.

We have dealt to a considerable extent with thymidylate synthetase inhibitors, the prototype of which was 5-fluoro-2'-deoxyuridine (2), a potent and clinically useful antineoplastic agent. Although many of the compounds thus far considered have both antiviral and antitumor properties, most of them cannot be regarded as highly selective in their antiviral activity since they block thymidylate synthetase, an enzyme essential for replication of normal cells. From this point on, the emphasis will shift away from such agents to the goal of obtaining a nucleoside analog (or analogs) capable of halting nucleic acid replication in the virus-infected cell without interfering with metabolism of the uninfected host cell.

When nucleoside analogs are considered as antiviral agents, clearly the prototype or "lead" compound is 5-iodo-2'-deoxyuridine [113-115] (29), which was originally synthesized by Prusoff [116] and shown to possess in

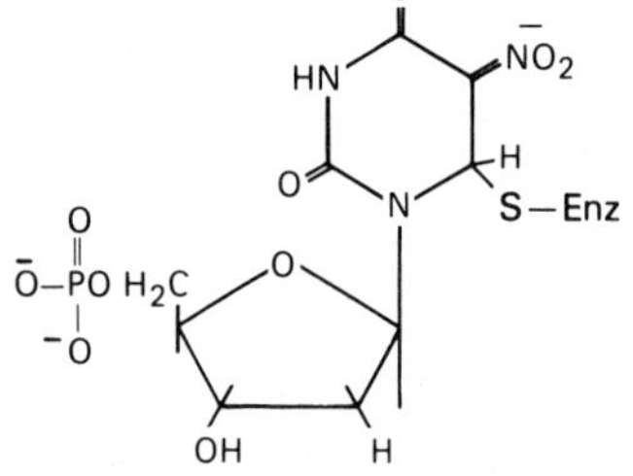

FIGURE 5.5 Covalent adduct involved in the inactivation of thymidylate synthetase by 5-nitro-2'-deoxyuridine 5'-monophosphate.

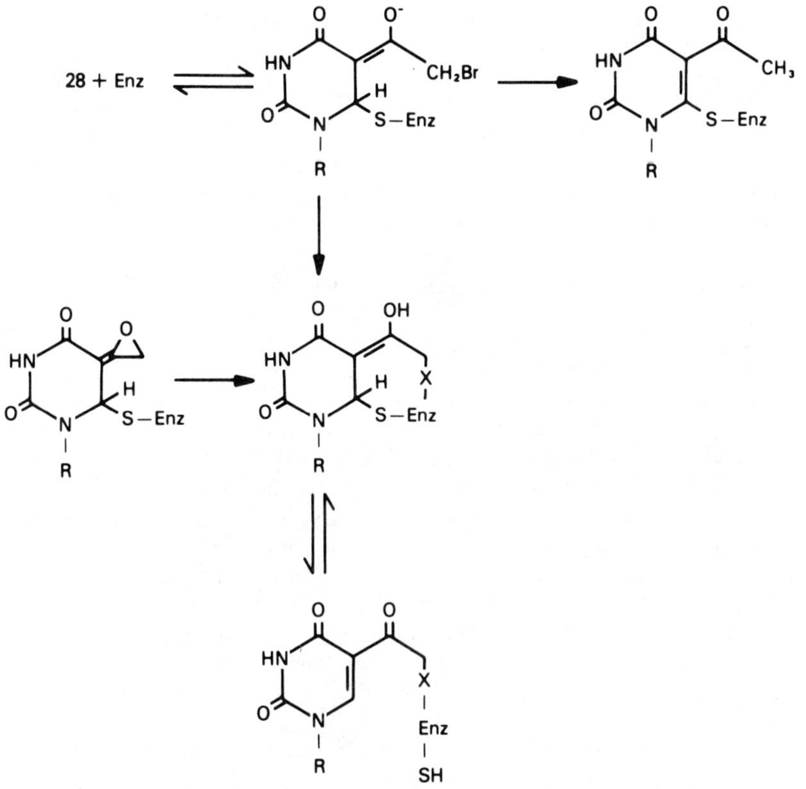

FIGURE 5.6 Some hypothetical intermediates in the inactivation of thymidylate synthetase by 5-(α-bromoacetyl)-2'-deoxyuridine 5'-monophosphate. (From Ref. 111.)

vitro and in vivo antiviral activity [117-120]. 5-Iodo-2'-deoxyuridine (29) shows greatest antiviral activity against DNA viruses, the most important of which is herpes virus. 5-Iodo-2'-deoxyuridine is approved by the U.S. Food and Drug Administration (FDA) for use in the topical treatment of herpes simplex eye infections [7]. In addition, compound (29) has given beneficial results in the chemotherapy of herpes genitalis, herpes zoster, herpes labialis, herpetic whitlow, and various other mucocutaneous herpetic infections. Systemic use of (29) is not indicated in any viral infection; in fact, two separate studies have shown (29) to have unacceptable toxicities and, moreover, to be ineffective in the prevention of death from biopsy proven herpes simplex encephalitis [7].

5-Iodo-2'-deoxyuridine (29) may exert its antiviral or other biological effects through a number of mechanisms. Compound (29) is readily phosphorylated in cells to its 5'-mono-, di-, and triphosphates and these nucleotides can act as competitive inhibitors of the enzymes that normally utilize the corresponding thymidine nucleotides or thymidine itself; second, the 5'-triphosphate of (29) exhibits feedback inhibition of ribonucleotide reductase, thymidine kinase, and deoxycytidylate deaminase. In addition, a highly significant aspect of the action of (29) is its incorporation into DNA; this has been held responsible for its antiviral activity. Substitution of iodine for the methyl of thymidine may affect replication, transcription, and the binding of DNA to proteins. When incorporated into DNA, (29) increases DNA fragility and thus can result in a decrease in virus infectivity. In addition, (29) is incorporated into the DNA of bacteria or eukaryotic cells, and it acts as a radiosensitizer.

The facile incorporation of (29) into DNA is the cause of a number of problems associated with its clinical use. 5-Iodo-2'-deoxyuridine posseses the important limitations of mutagenicity, embryotoxicity, teratogenicity, and the ability to activate latent oncogenic viruses. As pointed out by Prusoff et al. [114], the use of (29) or other agents that are incorporated into DNA should be restricted to the treatment of diseases with high mortality or great morbidity. Thus, while (29) has demonstrated the possibility of selective chemotherapy of viral diseases, it is still far from being the ideal antiviral agent.

In an attempt to provide antiviral agents that would not be incorporated into DNA, Prusoff and colleages have prepared a series of nucleosides that would not be expected to be phosphorylated by thymidine kinase. The most interesting of this series of 5'-amino-5'-deoxyribonucleosides is 5-iodo-5'-amino-2',5'-dideoxyuridine (30) [115] (Fig. 5.7). Two separate synthetic

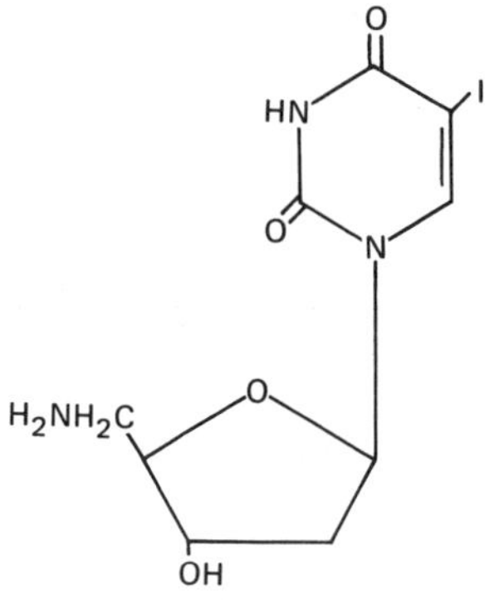

O
HN
I
O
N
O
H_2NH_2C
OH

(30)

FIGURE 5.7 Chemical structure of 5-iodo-5'-amino-2,5'-dideoxyuridine.

approaches have been used in the preparation of (30). In one approach [121], displacement with azide on the tosyl group of 5'-O-tosyl-2'-deoxyuridine gave 5'-azido-2'-, 5'-dideoxyuridine which could be catalytically reduced to 5'-amino'2-, 5'-dideoxyuridine. Mercuration with mercuric acetate gave the 5-mercuri nucleoside, which was converted to (30) by treatment with iodine in ethanol. In a second approach [122], (29) was 5'-tosylated and then converted to 5-iodo-5'-azido-2', 5'-dideoxyuridine with lithium azide. This intermediate was transformed to (30) using the triphenylphosphine procedure of Mungall et al. [123].

Compound (30) is less active as an antiherpes virus agent in cell culture than (29); however, (30) is far less cytotoxic than either of the latter nucleosides [115]. The specificity of antiviral action of (30) has been attributed to the fact that it is a substrate for the herpes virus-induced thymidine kinase but is not a substrate for host cell thymidine kinase [115]. This phosphorylation of (30) leads to its conversion to the triphosphate, which is then incorporated into the viral and host DNA in the infected cell.*

The two other possible 5-halogeno-2'-deoxyuridines,† 5-chloro- and 5-bromo-2'-deoxyuridine (31) and (32), also exhibit antiviral activity against DNA viruses and retroviruses and can inhibit cellular proliferation as well [7]. These analogs are, however, not very specific in their antiviral action; for instance, the 5-bromo analog (32) is extensively incorporated into the genetic material of both viruses and cells. Antiviral and anticellular activities of (32) have often been related to the incorporation of (32) into DNA and attendant modification of transcription, translation, and DNA-repressor protein interactions [113, 114]. It is, however, curious that cell lines may be isolated in which 100% of the DNA thymine has been replaced by 5-bromouracil and that such lines are perfectly viable (when grown in the dark) [125]. Less is known of the origins of the biological activity of 5-chloro-2'-deoxyuridine (31). It may, as is the case of (32) and (29), be acting as a feedback or competitive inhibitor of some of the enzymes of thymidine metabolism.

5-Cyano-2'-deoxyuridine (33) and its derivatives have been prepared by a number of methods, including condensation reactions and modifications of various uridines of 2'-deoxyuridines. Watanabe and Fox [98] prepared the tribenzoate of 5-cyanouridine using the mercuric cyanide-nitromethane condensation procedure. Bleaky et al. [127] reacted persilylated 5-iodo-2'-deoxyuridine with cuprous cyanide to obtain a 4% yield of the deoxy analog (33). Using chemistry developed by Ueda et al. [128], Torrence et al. [129] obtained a 45% yield of (33) by reaction of 3', 5'-di-O-acetyl-5-bromo-2'-deoxyuridine with potassium cyanide in DMSO containing potassium

*The in vitro incorporation of the phosphoramidate linkage into nucleic acids was noted first by Letsinger et al. [124].

†The unstable halogen asatine (^{211}At) has also been incorporated in a nucleoside structure. 5-Astato-2'-deoxyuridine was reported by Rossler et al. [126].

acetate. Hampton et al. [130] reported a 75% yield of (33) by treatment of 5-iodo-2'-deoxyuridine with KCN and dicyclohexyl-18-crown-6 in DMF.

From a steric viewpoint, the cyano group most closely approximates either a chloro or bromo substituent [131]. Furthermore, since the inductive and resonance effects of the cyano group are substantial [131], it was of interest to determine whether 5-cyano-2'-deoxyuridine (33) would act similar to 2'-deoxyuridines with strong electron-withdrawing substituents such as fluoro (2), trifluoromethyl (5) and nitro (26) which act at an early stage of DNA biosynthesis (thymidylate synthetase) or whether it might act as does the bromo- or chloro-2'-deoxyuridine (31) and (32), at later stages of DNA biosynthesis. Of additional interest was the consideration that the 5'-monophosphate of (33) might act as a mechanism-based thymidylate synthetase inhibitor through a ketenimine intermediate represented in Fig. 5.8.

5-Cyano-2'-deoxyuridine (33) is an effective inhibitor of the replication of vaccinia virus, although it is not as effective as (29) or (32). Biochemical studies [95, 133] suggested that the antiviral activities of (33) may be due to its phosphorylation and subsequent inhibition of thymidylate synthetase. Although Chang et al. [132] could find no evidence for irreversible enzyme inhibition by the 5'-monophosphate of (33), thus ruling out the possibility shown in Fig. 5.8, the monophosphate of (33) was a potent competitive inhibitor of thymidylate synthetase from *L. casei* with a K_i value of 0.55 μM.

A different theoretical approach to the problem of the incorporation of nucleoside antivirals into host cell DNA [134, 135] is exemplified by 5-ethyl-2'-deoxyuridine (34) [136]. The hypothesis was offered that since mutagenic and other adverse consequences of fraudulent nucleosides may be due to base mispairing during replication or transcription of the DNA containing the altered nucleotide, then such consequenses might be considerably reduced with an analog that closely resembled the natural nucleoside (thymidine) in its keto-enol tautomeric equilibrium and therefore its base-pairing properties. One such analog is 5-ethyl-2'-deoxyuridine (34), a

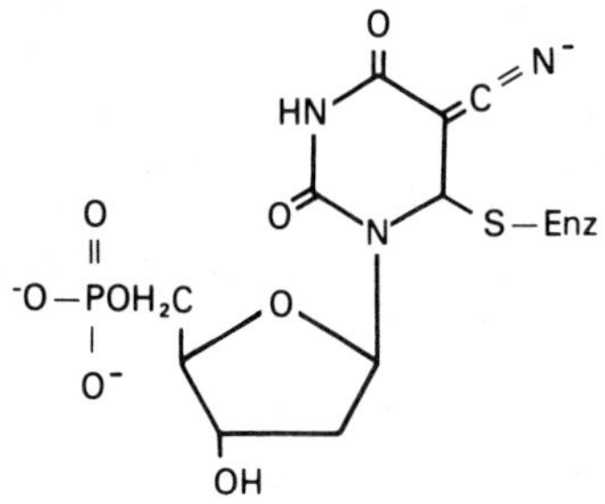

FIGURE 5.8 Potential intermediate resulting from the interaction of 5-cyano-2'-deoxyuridine 5'-monophosphate with thymidylate synthetase. (From Ref. 132.)

potent and selective antiviral agent in cull culture and animal models. Beneficial effects have also been claimed in the treatment of human viral diseases. [7]. Incorporation of (34) into DNA is not mutagenic and may not induce activation of oncogenic viruses.

While the mutagenic potential of thymidine analogs has been related to shifts in keto-enol tautomerism of the N3-hydrogen and C4-carbonyl groups or the pK_a of the N3-hydrogen, recent studies suggest that factors other than tautomerism, such as base stacking characteristics, may be primarily responsible for mispairing during replication or transcription [137-139].

Another 5-alkylpyrimidine nucleoside which shows an antiherpes virus activity comparable to (34) is 5-propyl-2'-deoxyuridine (35) [140-143].

A number of other 5-substituted-2'-deoxyuridines have been synthesized and shown to possess potent and selective antiherpes virus activity (Table 5.1). The most remarkable aspect of these various nucleosides is their lack of toxicity toward the uninfected host cell. The term "antiviral index" has been defined as the concentration of a nucleoside analog required to effect a 50% reduction in virus cytopathogenicity divided by the concentration of nucleoside needed to inhibit the growth of host cell by 30% [153]. By this definition, the higher the antiviral index, the more selective is the antiviral agent in question. Under terms of this definition, De Clercq et al. [153] reported the following antiviral indices for several nucleoside antivirals: 5-iodo-2'-deoxyuridine (29), 27; 5-trifluoromethyl-2'-deoxyuridine (5), 1.7; 1-(β-D-arabinofuranosyl)adenine (araA), 16; 1-(β-D-arabinofuranosyl)thymine (araT), $\geq$ 600; 5-ethyl-2'-deoxyuridine (34), 143; acycloguanosine, 1250; (E)-5-(2-bromovinyl)-2'-deoxyuridine (45), > 7000. This latter compound, (E)-5-(2-bromovinyl)-2'-deoxyuridine (45) is one of the most selective and most active (in cell culture) antiviral agents reported to date. While (45) also has shown in vivo antiviral activity in animal models [153], its usefulness as a clinical antiviral agent remains to be ascertained.

The selectivity of (45) as an antiherpes virus agent may be determined at two different levels of DNA biosynthesis. First, thymidine kinaseless mutants of herpes simplex virus type 1 [154] and in vitro studies with thymidine kinase itself suggest that (45) is preferentially phosphorylated by the herpes virus-induced enzyme as compared to the host cell kinase [155]. Second, the 5'-triphosphate of (45) preferentially inhibited (competitively with thmidine triphosphate) the purified DNA polymerase of herpes simplex virus type 1 as compared to human DNA polymerase α, β and γ [155].

When 2'-deoxyuridine derivatives are converted to the corresponding 2'-deoxycytidine analogs, a further specificity of antiviral action may be achieved. This is due to the fact that, in addition to herpes virus-induced deoxypyrimidine nucleoside kinase and DNA polymerase, herpes virus induces two other enzymes, deoxycytidine deaminase and deoxycytidylate deaminase [156, 157]. To the extent that these viral-induced enzymes may be preferentially inhibited by 2'-deoxycytidine nucleosides or nucleotides,

TABLE 5.1 5-Substituted 2'-Deoxyuridines with Selective Antiherpes Virus Activity

Compound	R	Minimum effective concentration[a]
5-Methylthiomethyl-2'-deoxyuridine (37) [144, 145]	$-CH_2SCH_3$	4
5-Mercaptomethyl-2'-deoxyuridine (36) [146]	$-CH_2SH$	3
5-Azidomethyl-2'-deoxyuridine (38) [144, 147]	$-CH_2N_3$	0.7
5-Methylamino-2'-deoxyuridine (39) [148]	$-NHCH_3$	2.5
5-Ethylamino-2'-deoxyuridine (40) [148]	$-NHCH_2CH_3$	-
5-Propynyloxy-2'-deoxyuridine (41) [149]	$-OCH_2C{\equiv}CH$	0.7
5-Cyanomethyleneoxy-2'-deoxyuridine (42) [150]	$-OCH_2C{\equiv}N$	-
5-Methoxymethyl-2'-deoxyuridine (43 [151]	$-CH_2OCH_3$	2
5-Vinyl-2'-deoxyuridine (44) [152]	$-CH{=}CH_2$	0.04
E-5-(Bromovinyl)-2'-deoxyuridine (45) [153]	$(H)C{=}C(Br)(H)$	0.007
E-5-(Iodovinyl)-2'-deoxyuridine (46) [153]	$(H)C{=}C(I)(H)$	0.01
5-Allyl-2'-deoxyuridine (47) [141]	$-CH_2CH{=}CH_2$	-
5-Methylsulfonylmethyl-2'-deoxyuridine (48) [145]	$-CH_2-S(=O)_2-CH_3$	4

[a]Concentration (μg/mL) required to effect a 50% reduction in cytopathogencity of herpes simples virus type 1 in cell culture.

then the virus-infected cell may be exposed to a greater concentration of the corresponding inhibitory 2'-deoxyuridine congener. Additionally, after selective phosphorylation by the viral-induced deoxypyrimidine nucleoside kinase (thymidine kinase), a differential effect on virus-infected versus uninfected cell may be obtained due to the different properties of deoxycytidine deaminase as compared to deoxycytidylate deaminase. For instance, 5-bromo-2'-deoxycytidine (49) (Fig. 5.9) is phosphorylated to 5-monophosphate in extracts of herpes simplex virus type 1-infected cells, but not in extracts of uninfected cells [158]. Compound (49) is a comparatively poor substrate of deoxycytidine deaminase so that in an uninfected cell, relatively little of (49) is converted to the rather toxic 5-bromo-2'-deoxyuridine (32). However, the 5'-monophosphate of (49) is a quite effective substrate of deoxycytidylate deaminase and lethal levels of the monophosphate of (32) are generated in the virus-infected cell. If, as pointed out by De Clercq and Torrence [5], herpes simplex-1 virus also codes for a deoxycytidine deaminase, then both possible pathways may obtain. Several other 2'-deoxycytidine analogs have been reported to possess a higher degree of selectivity in their natural action than the corresponding 2'-deoxyuridine derivatives. These include 5-nitro-2'-deoxycytidine (50) and 5-ethynyl-2'-deoxycytidine (51) [152] (Fig. 5.9).

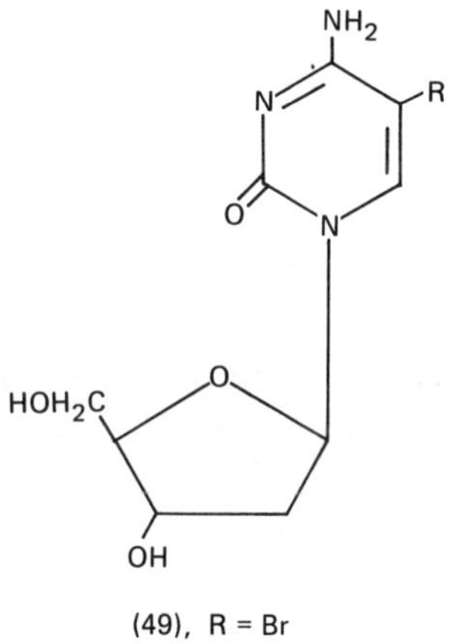

(49), R = Br
(50), R = NO_2
(51), R = -C≡CH

FIGURE 5.9 Some 21-Deoxycytidine Analogs.

IV. NUCLEOSIDE ANALOGS ARISING FROM INVERSION OF CONFIGURATION AT RIBOSE C2

A. AraA [9-(β-D-Arabinofuranosyl)adenine, Spongoadenosine, Vidarabine, Vira-A] (7, 159-165)

AraA is a naturally occurring nucleoside that was chemically synthesized before it was isolated from nature (*Streptomyces antibioticus*). Successful approaches to the synthesis of araA have included: (1) conversion of 9-β-D-lyxofuranosyl)adenine and then cleavage to araA [166, 167]; (2) condensation of tri-O-benzoyl-D-arabinofuranosyl halide with benzoyladenine [168, 169]; (3) via 8,2'-anhydroadenine [170, 171] (Fig. 5.10); (4) via D-arabinofurano[1',2':4,5]oxazolidine 2-thione [172] (Fig. 5.10); (5) from 5-amino-4-cyano-1-β-D-arabinofuranosylimidazole [173].

AraA has demonstrated antitumor activity in mice [161] and has been used in the treatment of patients with chronic myelogenous leukemia in acute blast crisis [174], but its greatest utility to date has been as an antiviral agent [7, 159, 167]; it was the first systematically active antiviral agent to be approved by the FDA for use in humans. AraA possesses significant activity against many DNA viruses, including herpes simplex virus, vaccinia virus, cytomegalovirus, and varicella zoster virus; in addition, araA inhibits the multiplication of several oncogenic RNA viruses such as Rous sarcoma virus or gross murine leukemia virus.

The most dramatic proof of araA's clinical efficacy was reported in a collaborative, double-blind, placebo-controlled study [175]. AraA reduced the mortality of biopsy-proven herpes simplex encephalitis from 70% to 28%; moreover, survivors who had been on araA treatment had reduced neurological sequelae. AraA is also highly effective in the treatment of herpes simplex keratitis and keratouveitis and may have usefulness in the therapy of herpes simplex virus and varicella zoster virus-induced infections of immunocompromised cancer patients [7, 159, 160]. Most recently, the combination of araA and interferon produced the first effective elimination of the carrier state of hepatitis-B [176]. Neonatal herpes simplex infections, both disseminated and those with central nervous system involvement, responds favorably to araA [177, 178].

In the cell, araA is converted to the 5'-mono-, di-, and triphosphates. Ara-adenosine triphosphate (ATP) is an inhibitor of DNA polymerase and is also incorporated into DNA; these two mechanisms are often presumed to be primarily responsible for its antiviral action [162-165]. Some degree of selectivity of action may be afforded by the fact that araATP inhibits the herpes simplex virus-induced DNA polymerase to a greater extent than the cellular DNA polymerase α and β [179]. A nucleotide-independent toxicity of araA involves the irreversible inhibition of *S*-adenosylhomocysteine hydrolase [180]. Additional effects of araA and its nucleotides include inhibition of ribonucleotide reductase, inhibition of the poly(A) polymerase that is responsible for posttranscriptional addition of poly(A) to mRNAs, and

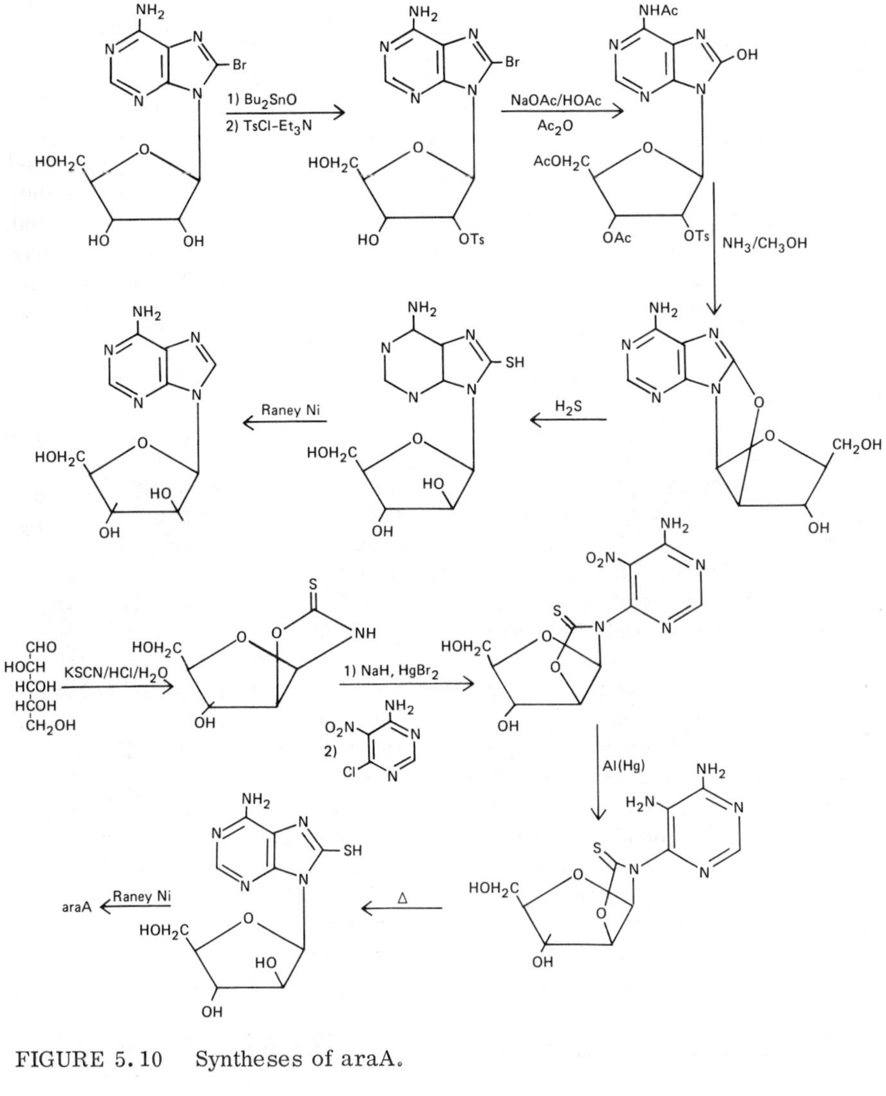

FIGURE 5.10 Syntheses of araA.

termination of DNA synthesis by incorporation at the growing 3'-terminus [162-165].

AraA is quickly deaminated [7, 159-165] in the whole animal or cell to 1-(β-D-arabinofuranosyl)hypoxanthine (araHX), which, at least in cell culture, is a less potent antiviral agent. There is considerable interest in the use of adenosine deaminase inhibitors to prevent this inactivation of araA. Inhibitors of adenosine deaminases, such as EHNA, coformycin, or 2'-deoxycoformycin (see Sec. X), definitely increase the cell toxicity and antiviral activity of adenosine analogs such as araA or cordycepin [162-165]. However, as noted in Sec. X, it is not clear that adenosine deaminase is an enzyme that can be inhibited with impunity since its deficiency leads to profound immunodeficiency and since it may be involved in detoxification of the normal metabolites 2'-deoxyadenosine and adenosine.

Of the various analogs and derivatives of araA that have been reported, a few are of special interest. The 5'-monophosphate of araA, araAMP, has greater water solubility than araA itself, and since it is only slowly dephosphorylated in vivo, it is protected against the action of adenosine deaminase and has a longer serum half-life than araA [7, 159, 166]. AraAMP may also be taken up as the nucleotide by the cell [164]. For these reasons, some clinical trials of araAMP have been pursued [7]. A carbocyclic analog of araA, referred to as C-araA (cyclaradine), (±)-9-[2α, 3B-dihydroxy-4α-(hydroxymethyl)cyclopent-1α-yl]adenine, is deaminase, nucleoside phosphorylase, and hydrolase resistant, and possesses significant in vitro and in vivo activity [7, 181]. Another adenosine deaminase resistant analog of araA is 2-fluoroaraA (9-β-D-arabinofuranosyl-2-fluoroadenine) [182], which possesses potent antitumor and antiviral activities [183, 184]. The α-anomers of araA and ara-8-aza are also resistant to deaminases; however, although these compounds are active in vitro, they are not effective in vivo against systemic herpes virus infections in mice [7, 185]. Other araA derivatives or analogs with reportedly significant in vitro and/or in vivo antiviral activity include 9(β-D-arabinofuranosyl)adenosine-5'-phosphate-1-oxide [160, 186]; N'-[9-(β-D-arabinofuranosyl)-9H-purin-6-yl]-N,N-dimethylformamidine, [187], 9-(β-D-arabinofuranosyl)adenine cyclic-3'-,5'-hydrogen phosphate (cyclic araAMP) [188, 190], 9-(β-D-arabinofuranosyl)-N^6-hydroxyadenine (araHA) [191], the deaminase-resistant 2'-azido-2'-deoxy-β-D-arabinofuranosyladenine [192], and 2,6-diamino-9-(β-D-arabinofuranosyl)purine [193], which is converted in vivo to araG [9-(β-D-arabinofuranosyl)guanine] and which also possesses significant antiherpes virus and antivaccinia virus activity [193].

B. AraC [1-(β-D-Arabinofuranosyl)cytosine, Cytosine Arabinoside, Cytarabine] [7, 159, 163-165, 194]

The nucleoside antimetabolite, araC, is of considerable value in the primary treatment of acute myelogenous leukemias, especially when it is used in combination chemotherapy [43, 195]. It is also useful as second-line therapy of acute lymphoblastic leukemia and non-Hodgkin's lymphomas. While araC blocks the replication of DNA viruses (and some RNA viruses) in vitro and in vivo, its therapeutic to toxic ratio approaches unity. In addition, its potent immunosuppressive property makes it unlikely that it will be useful as an antiviral agent in humans; indeed, araC exacerbated the course of disseminated herpes zoster [196], which responds favorably to araA chemotherapy.

The mechanism of cytotoxic action of araC is not completely understood [159, 163-165, 194]. It has been established that araA exerts its cell-killing action in the S phase of cell multiplication and that it must be phosphorylated by nucleoside and nucleotide kinases to the 5'-triphosphate, araCTP. AraCTP is a potent competitive inhibitor (with respect to dCTP) of eukaryotic DNA polymerase [197, 198]. In addition, araC is incorporated into DNA; Kufe et al. found a highly significant relationship ($p < 0.0001$) between the incorporation of araC into DNA of L1210 cells and clonogenic survival [199]. Inhibition of ribonucleotide reductase by araCTP has been considered as another possible target of araC, but this mode of action has been deemed unimportant since araCTP does not inhibit the reductase at concentrations in which it is found in araC-treated cells; moreover, toxic levels of araC do not deplete any of the deoxyribonucleotide pools [164]. AraC and its nucleotides also inhibit sialic acid metabolism [200].

A major limitation [159, 163-165, 194] of the therapeutic usefulness of araC may be its rapid deamination to the noncytotoxic araU [1-(β-D-arabinofuranosyl)uracil]. The enzyme cytidine deaminase, which accomplishes this inactivation, is present at high levels in human erythrocytes, liver, and kidney. Approaches to this problem have included the synthesis of araC analogs or derivatives resistant to deamination (see below) or development of inhibitors of cytidine deaminase.

One of the most useful members of this latter category is tetrahydrouridine [201, 202] (THU) (Fig. 5.11) which can be regarded as a transition-state analog inhibitor of cytidine deaminase. As consequences of this inhibition, THU markedly increases the incorporation of 2'-deoxycytidine into normal or neoplastic tissues in the mouse and also selectively increases

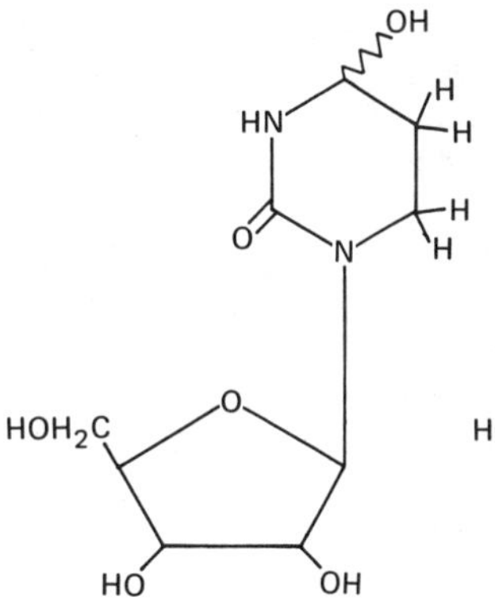

THU

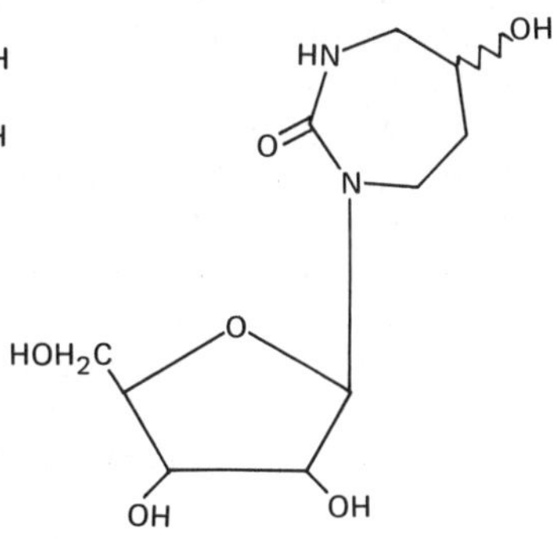

(52)

FIGURE 5.11 Structure of cytidine deaminase inhibitors.

the level of araCTP in leukemia cells [163-165]. Noting that the potent adenosine deaminase inhibitors coformycin and 2'-deoxycoformycin have a seven-membered ring as well as a hydroxyl situated two carbons distant from the nearest ring nitrogen of the aglycon, Marquez et al. [203,204] synthesized 1,3-deazepin-2-one ribonucleosides by condensation of silylated 1,3-deazepin-2-one nucleosides with 2,3,5,tri-O-benzoyl-D-ribofuranosyl bromide followed by sodium borohydride reduction and debenzoylation. One of the diastereomeric deazepinone products (52) (Fig. 5.11) was found to be 10 times more potent than THU as an inhibitor of cytidine deaminase.

In general, araC or its analogs may be synthesized (Fig. 5.12) by any of five different approaches: (I) base-sugar condensation; (II) inversion of configuration at ribose C2'; (III) amination of an araU derivative; (IV) elaboration of a sugar derivative; and (V) direct modification of araC itself. The application of method I is exemplified by the condensation of 5-O-benzoyl-3-O-acetyl-2-azido-2-deoxy-D-arabinofuranosyl chloride with silylated cytosine to give the α and β anomers of 1-(2'-azido-2'-deoxy-β-D-arabinofuranosyl)cytosine (53), which could be reduced to 1-(2'-azido-2'-amino-2'-deoxy-β-D-arabinofuranosyl)cytosine (54) [205]. Both of these araC analogs were found to be resistant to the action of cytidine deaminase, both analogs were markedly cytotoxic to various human and mouse cell lines, and both could cure L1210 leukemia in mice. Treatment of cytidine with phosphorus oxychloride in ethyl acetate and one equivalent of water gave rise to O^2,2'-cyclocytidine [206], itself of interest as a depot form of araC. Cleavage of O^2,2'-cyclocytidine to araC with mild aqueous base thus illustrates method II. A similar approach employed the reaction of α-acetoxyisobutyryl chloride with ribonucleosides [207]. Combination of methods I and II is illustrated by the synthesis of araC achieved by mercuric bromide catalyzed condensation of N^4-acetylbis(trimethylsilyl)cytosine with 1-chloro-2-O-acetyl-3-O-p-tolylsulfonyl-5-O-(ethoxycarbonyl)-D-xylofuranose to yield compound (55), which is converted by base hydrolysis (through the ribo epoxide) to araC [208]. The first synthesis of araFC [209] [1-(β-D-arabinofuranosyl)5-fluorocytosine], (56), which is of interest as an antileukemic agent [210], involved consecutive pyrimidine-4 thiation, S-methylation, and subsequent displacement with liquid ammonia, starting from the intermediate acetylated araFU. Method IV can be illustrated with the Sanchez-Orgel synthesis [211], which employs unprotected sugars. Reaction of D-arabinose with cyanamide and ammonia gives the aminooxazoline (57), which can be reacted with cyanoacetylene to give after hydrolysis, araC. Finally, to present an example of method V, trifluoromethyl hypofluorite reacts with N-2',3',5'-tetraacetylarabinofuranosylcytosine to give, after decomposition, of intermediates, araFC in good yield [212].

The araC derivatives araFC and anhydro-araC (58) (cyclotidine) [213] show excellent antitumor activity in vivo and thus are currently in clinical

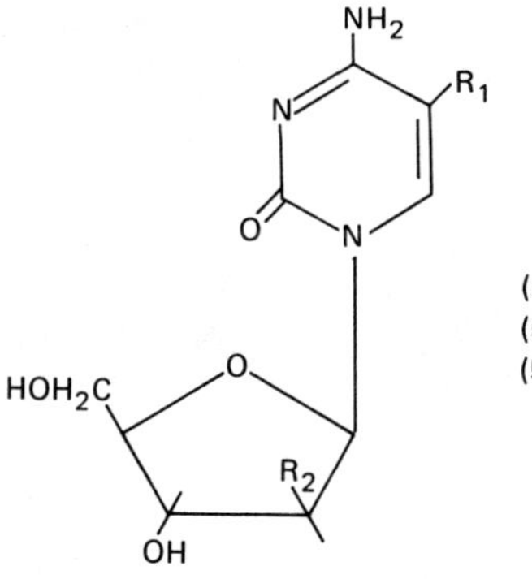

NH2
R1
N
O
N
HOH2C
O
R2
OH

(53), $R_1 = H$; $R_2 = N_3$
(54), $R_1 = H$; $R_2 = NH_2$
(56), $R_1 = F$; $R_2 = OH$

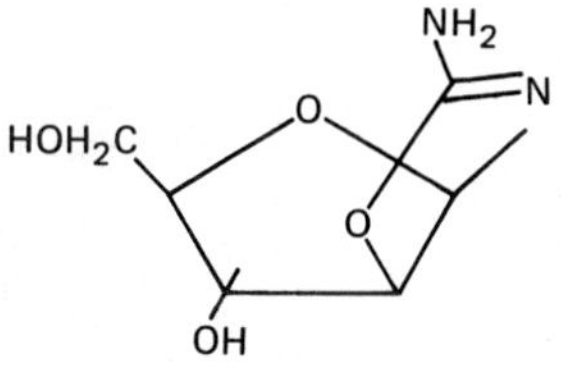

NH2
N
HOH2C
O
O
OH

(57)

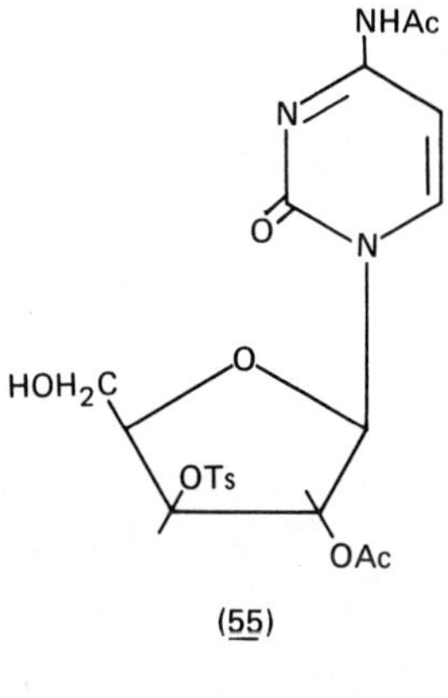

NHAc
N
O
N
HOH2C
O
OTs
OAc

(55)

NH
R
N
N
O
HOH2C
O
OH

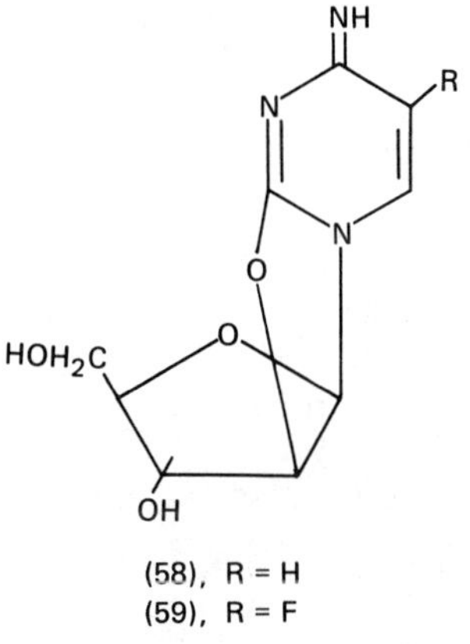

(58), R = H
(59), R = F

FIGURE 5.12 Some araC derivatives and some intermediates in their syntheses.

trial as is anhydro-araFC [214], the cyclonucleoside depot form of araFC. Some selected examples of araC analogs of interest include the following (Fig. 5.13):

1. 2'-Fluoro-5-iodoaracytosine (59) [215], a potent and selective inhibitor of herpes virus replication [216].
2. 5-Azacytosine arabinoside (60), which is an analog of both araC and 5-azacytidine and which showed greater efficacy in the mouse L1210 leukemia system than does either parent compound [217].

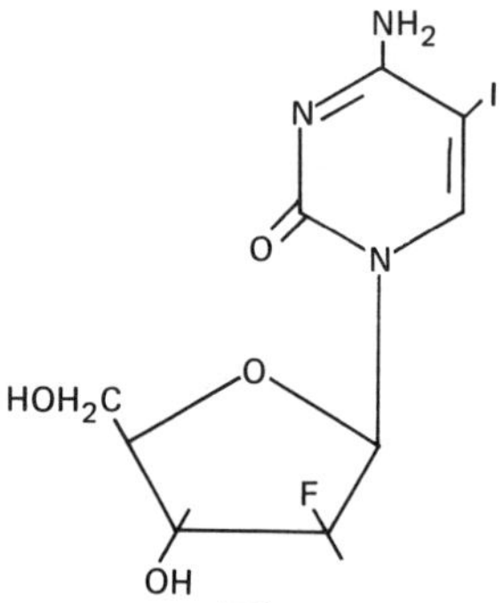

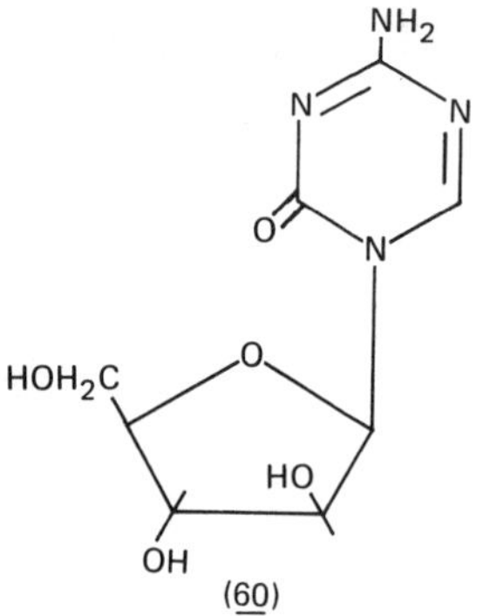

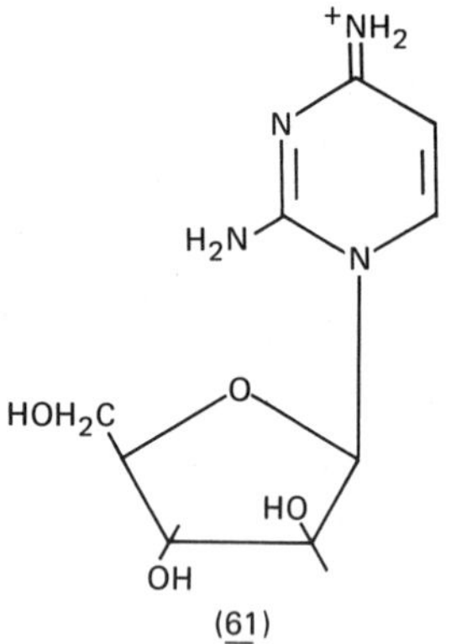

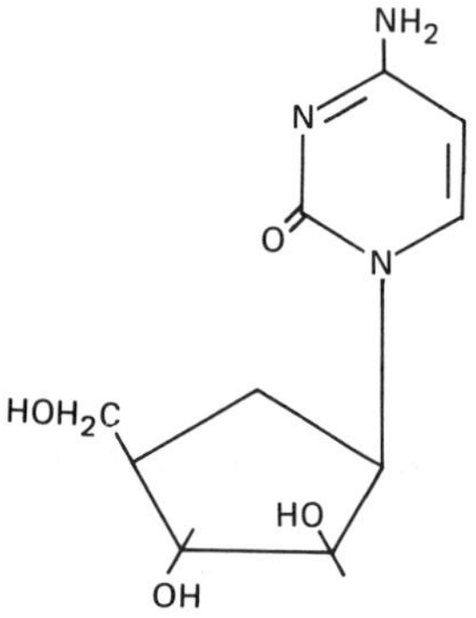

FIGURE 5.13 AraC analogs

3. 1-(β-D-Arabinofuranosyl)-2-amino-1,4(2H)-iminopyrimidine (araAIPy), a deaminase-resistant depot form of araC which effected a cure in the L1210 mouse leukemia system [218].
4. A deaminase-resistant carbocyclic analog of araC, C-araC (62), which is active against L1210 leukemia [219].
5. The other pyrimidine 5-halogenated (5-Cl, 5-Br, 5-I) derivatives of araC as well as 5-methyl araC, all of which possess significant antiviral activity and may be depot forms of the corresponding uracil nucleosides [220-222].
6. The α anomer of araC, α-araC, which suppresses Gross murine leukemia virus replication in mouse embryo cells [7].

C. AraU [1-(β-D-Arabinofuranosyl)uracil, Spongouridine] and AraT [1-(β-D-arabinofuranosyl)thymine, Spongothymidine] and Their Analogs [7,159]

A number of 5-substituted uracil arabinonucleosides have been synthesized and evaluated for antiviral activity. The best known is araT, which selectively blocks the replication of herpes simplex virus [223], varicella zoster virus [224], equine herpes virus [225], and Epstein-Barr virus [226]. AraT is virtually devoid of cytotoxic effects toward the uninfected cell [223,224]; thus such uracil arabinonucleosides are devoid of antitumor activities. Since the 5'-triphosphate of araT inhibits both viral and mammalian DNA polymerases [227], it is assumed that the specificity of action of araT arises completely from the fact that it is phosphorylated much more extensively in the viral-infected cell due to viral induction of deoxypyrimidine kinase [224,228,229]. As is the cases for other arabinonucleosides, araT may be incorporated into DNA [230]. The parent arabinonucleoside, araU, long considered to be pharmacologically inert, is also able to inhibit the growth of herpes simplex in cell culture [231].

Inspection of the data of Table 5.2 reveals that, in contrast to the C-5-substituted pyrimidine 2'-deoxyribonucleosides situation, from a large variety of functional groups, only a few gave rise to active antiviral agents. The mechanistic origin of these differeing structure-activity dependencies is not known; however, these differences may suggest either a fundamental difference in the activation of the arabinonucleosides compared to the 2'-deoxyribonucleosides, or a difference in the mechanism of inhibition of virus growth by the arabinonucleosides versus the deoxyribonucleosides.

Similar to the synthesis of araC and its analogs, a wide variety of synthetic approaches have been employed to prepare the various analogs listed in Table 5.2. For instance, Ueda et al. [237] used the previously observed thiocyanation of uridine derivatives [90,91] and their reductive cleavage to obtain a series of 5-alkylthio and 5-methylsulfonyl arabinonucleosides (Fig. 5.14).

TABLE 5.2 Antiviral Activity of 5-Substituted Uracil Arabinonucleosides

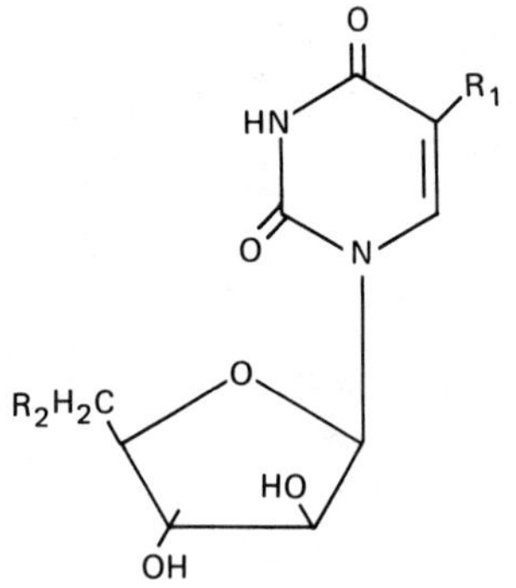

R_1	R_2	Antiviral activity	References
H	OH	+	231
CH_3	OH	++	223
CH_2CH_3	OH	++	232-234
$CH_2CH_2CH_3$	OH	+	234
$CH_2CH_2CH_2CH_3$	OH	+	234
$OCH_2C{\equiv}CH$	OH	+	235
NO_2	OH	-	235
CH	OH	-	235
OH	OH	-	235
SCN	OH	++	91, 236
SCH_3	OH	+	237
SCH_2CH_3	OH	-	237
$SCH_2CH_2CH_3$	OH	-	237
SO_2CH_3	OH	-	237
$CH{=}CH_2$	OH	++	238
$CH{=}CH{-}CH_3$	OH	+	238
$CH{=}CH{-}CH_2{-}CH_3$	OH	-	238
Cl	OH	++	239, 240
Br	OH	++	239, 240

TABLE 5.2 (Continued)

I	OH	++	221, 239, 240
H	N_3	-	239
H	NH_2	-	239
CH_3	N_3	-	239
CH_3	NH_2	-	239
Br	N_3	-	239
Br	NH_2	-	239
I	N_3	-	239
T	NH_2	-	239

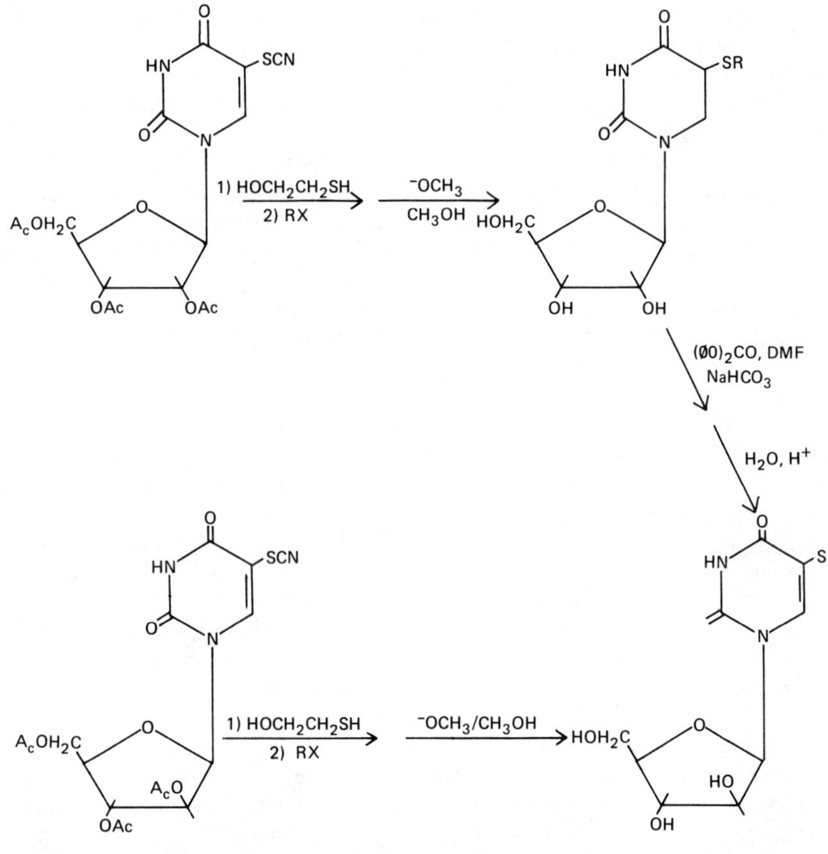

O
HN
SCN
O
N
O
A_cOH_2C
OAc
OAc
1) $HOCH_2CH_2SH$
2) RX
$^-OCH_3$
CH_3OH
O
HN
SR
O
N
HOH_2C
O
OH
OH
$(\emptyset O)_2CO$, DMF
$NaHCO_3$
H_2O, H^+
O
HN
SCN
O
N
A_cOH_2C
O
A_cO
OAc
1) $HOCH_2CH_2SH$
2) RX
$^-OCH_3/CH_3OH$
O
HN
SR
N
HOH_2C
O
HO
OH

FIGURE 5.14 Synthesis of 5-alkthiopyrimidine arabinonucleosides from 5-thiocyanopyrimidine nucleoside precursors.

V. AZAPYRIMIDINE NUCLEOSIDES

A. 6-Azauridine

In addition to activity against several experimental tumors, the nucleoside 6-azauridine possesses antiviral activity against a wide variety of RNA and DNA viruses with strongest activity against dengue, lymphocytic choriomenigitis, and subacute sclerosing panencephalitis viruses, rather moderate activity against vaccinia virus, and borderline activity against herpesvirus [241]. In clinical trial, 6-azauridine failed to block vaccination "takes," whereas 5-iodo-2'-deoxyuridine did [242]. Benefit has been claimed in the treatment of herpes eye infections with systemic administration of the 2',3',5'-triacetate of 6-azauridine [243,244]. Although 6-azauridine is under investigation for its effect on psoriasis and polycythemia vera, the opinion has been advanced that its use as an antiviral agent may be limited by its toxicity and low potency [1].

Prerequisite to the antiviral activity of 6-azauridine is its phosphorylation to 6-azauridine 5'-monophosphate by the enzyme uridine kinase [241]. This phosphorylation step may serve as a basis for some selectivity against certain viruses such as Rous sarcoma virus, which may induce synthesis of uridine kinase in the host cell.

The primary site of action of 6-azauridine may be the inhibition of orotidylic acid decarboxylase by its 5'-monophosphate [241]. Thus RNA synthesis is inhibited by a cutoff of a supply of UMP from orotidine 5'-monophosphate. A molecular basis for the inhibition of orotidylic acid decarboxylase by 6-azauridine 5'-monophosphate has been provided by the studies of Saenger and colleagues [245,246]. Consideration of x-ray structure analyses and conformational energy computations showed that orotidine 5'-monophosphate is in the syn glycosidic linkage conformation (Fig. 5.15) and has the rare trans-gauche orientation about the C(4')-C(5') bond (Fig. 5.16). During the process of decarboxylation, the base moiety must rotate from syn to anti, and the C(4')-C(5') bond must change from trans-gauche to gauche-gauche to correspond eventually to the uridine 5'-monophosphate product (Fig. 5.17). 6-Azauridine 5'-monophosphate itself possesses a syn glycosidic bond conformation and the uncommon trans-gauche conformation about the C(4')-C(5') bond (Figs. 5.15 and 5.16). Thus the behavior of 6-azauridine 5'-monophosphate as an inhibitor of orotidylic acid decarboxylase is due to its conformational similarity to the substrate. Saenger et al. [246] have further suggested that the enzyme recognizes orotidine 5'-monophosphate by at least two key functional groups: the carboxyl group and the 5'-monophosphate group. Since the 5'-monophosphate groups of both substrate and inhibitor are bound at the same enzyme location, it appears that the pyrimidine C-2 carbonyl of 6-azauridine 5'-monophosphate may mimic the 6-carboxyl group of orotidine 5'-monophosphate.

Until quite recently, the view was held that 6-azauridine is not converted in the cell to the 5'-di- or 5'-triphosphate [241]; however, Rodaway and Marcus [247] have presented evidence to the contrary. They found

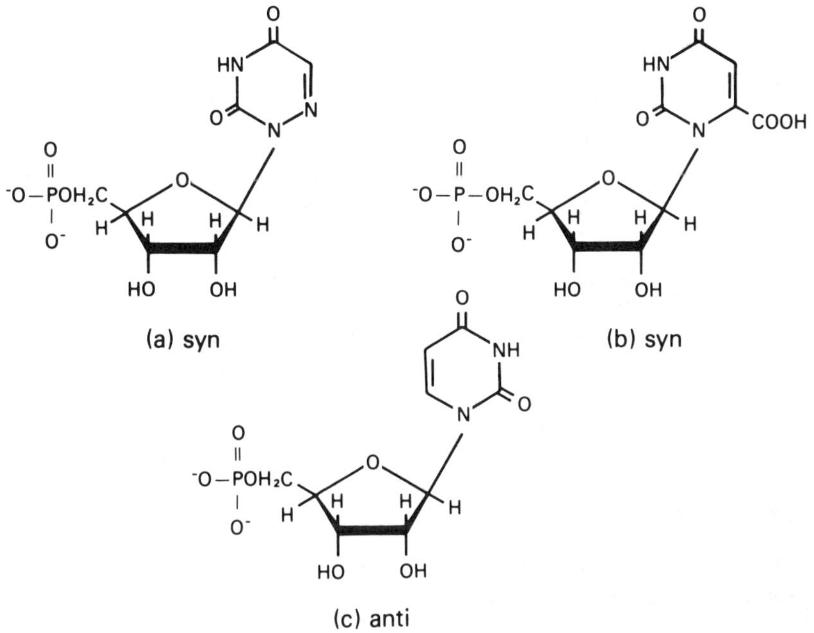

FIGURE 5.15 Favored orientations about the glycosidic linkage for (a) 6-azauridine 5'-monophosphate, (b) orotidine 5'-monophosphate, and (c) uridine 5'-monophosphate.

that 6-azauridine was converted to the 5'-triphosphate and incorporated into RNA in wheat embryonic axis. This finding opens the possibility that 6-azauridine may have other varied effects on cells in vitro enzyme systems [241] such as RNA polymerase and polynucleotide phosphorylase have been shown to be inhibited by 6-azauridine tri- and diphosphate, respectively.

B. 5-Azacytidine [1-(β-D-Ribofuranosyl)-5-azacytidine] [241,248-250]

5-Azacytidine was, like 6-azauridine, first synthesized [251] by consensing 2,3,5-tri-O-acetyl-β-D-ribofuranosyl isocyanate with 2-methylisourea to give 1-(2',3',5'-tri-O-acetyl-β-D-ribofuranosyl)-4-methoxy-2-oxo-1,2-dihydro-1,3,5-triazine. Treatment of this intermediate with methanolic ammonia gave 5-azacytidine which also has been isolated from cultures of Streptoverticillium ladakanus [252]. Direct glycosylation of silyated 5-azacytosine also has been used for preparation of 5-azacytidine and similar nucleosides [253-255].

5-Azacytidine is a promising drug for the treatment of patients with acute myelogenous leukemia that is refractory to standard therapy [43,248,

O
O
$C_{3'}$
$H_{5'}$
$H_{5''}$
$H_{4'}$

gauche-gauche

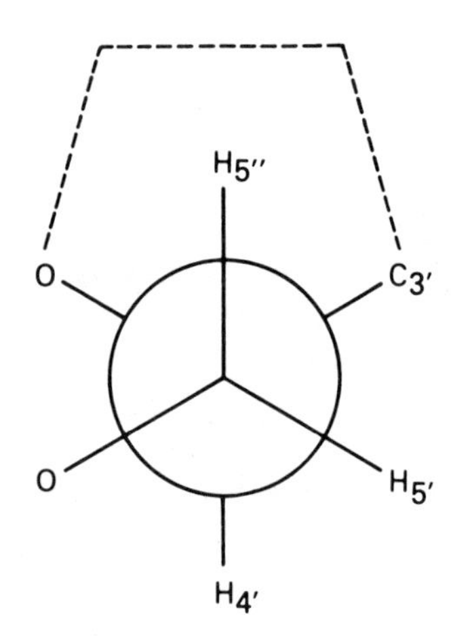

FIGURE 5.16 Newman projections for rotamers about the C(4')-C(5') bond. The rotamer not presented is gauche-trans.

249]. A remission rate of 20% has been obtained with this drug. 5-Azacytidine is currently being evaluated in combination chemotherapy with other agents such as β-2'-deoxythioguanosine. This latter combination produced a remission rate of 29% in refractory acute myelogenous leukemia [256].

The biological activity of 5-azacytidine has been ascribed to its interference with nucleic acid metabolism [241,248-251,257]. 5-Azacytidine is phosphorylated by cellular kinases to 5'-mono-, di-, and triphosphates; indeed, development of resistance to 5-azacytidine cytotoxicity is associated with depletion of uridine kinase activity. It is through the 5'-triphosphate, however, that 5-azacytidine probably exerts its primary biological effects since 5-azacytidine is incorporated into mRNA and tRNA and modifies it so that it is nonfunctional in protein synthesis. 5-Azacytidine also inhibits the maturation of 28S and 18S, but not 38S, rRNA. Polysome degradation is accelerated by 5-azacytidine, and, as a result, protein synthesis is inhibited. Synthesis of 4S and 5S RNA is inhibited by 5-azacytidine, which incorporated into those species of RNA. 5-Azacytidine also blocks methylation of 4S RNA with the greatest effect on the formation of N^2-methylguanosine and N^2,N^2-dimethylguanosine [258]. Alteration in states of differentiation has also been associated with the incorporation of 5-azacytidine into DNA, which apparently alters DNA methylation patterns [259]. The incorporation of thymidine into DNA is also blocked by 5-azacytidine. 5-Azacytidine also alters the synthesis and activity of induced liver enzymes as well as the enzymes of polyamine metabolism, and, as the 5'-monophosphate, may inhibit orotidylic acid decarboxylase.

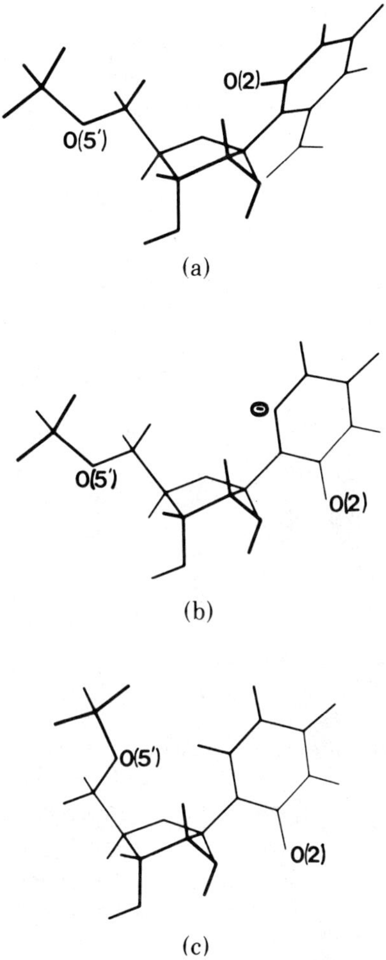

(a)

(b)

(c)

FIGURE 5.17 Represented here are successional conformational changes that occur during the decarboxylation of orotidine 5'-monophosphate (a) to give uridine 5'-monophosphate product (c). (From Ref. 246.)

A chemical basis for the biological effects of 5-azacytidine relates to the inherent instability of the sym-triazine ring [241]. The hydrolytic behavior [260-262] of azacytidine is detailed in Fig. 5.18. The hypothesis has been advanced that after the incorporation of 5-azacytidine into RNA, reactions similar to those of Fig. 5.18 spontaneously occur, giving rise to nonfunctional RNA [241,250,260].

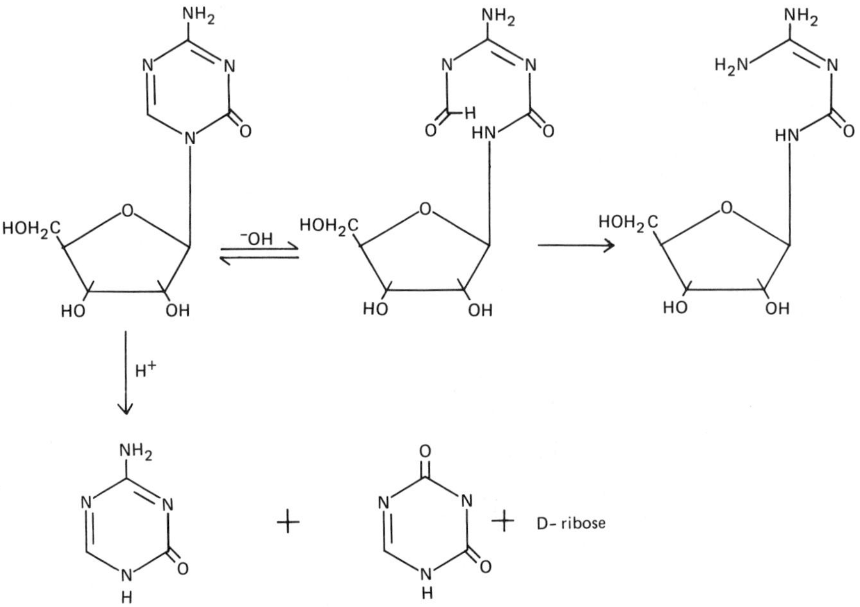

FIGURE 5.18 Hydrolysis of 5-azacytidine.

At least two derivatives of 5-azacytidine are of interest for their biological properties.

1. The analog, 2'-deoxy-5-azacytidine, is as effective an inhibitor of protein synthesis in bacteria as is 5-azacytidine itself; in addition, it is incorporated into DNA. A prerequisite for the biological activity of 2'-deoxy-5-azacytidine appears to be its deamination by cytidine deaminase to give 2'-deoxy-5-azauridine which may be hydrolyzed to 5-azauracil [241].
2. In order to eliminate the problem of solution instability of 5-azacytidine, Beisler et al. [263-265] prepared 5,6-dihydro-5-azacytidine by sodium borohydride reduction of 5-azacytidine or appropriately blocked derivatives. This dihydro congener was more stable than the parent 5-azacytidine, retained significant antitumor activity, and was similar to 5-azacytidine in its mode of action [258].

VI. RIBAVIRIN AND RELATED NUCLEOSIDES

The nucleoside ribavirin [(63), Fig. 5.19, virazole, 1-β-D-ribofuranosyl-1,2,4-triazole-3-carboxamide], first prepared by Witkowski et al. [266], has been described [267, 268] as a broad-spectrum antiviral agent with activity against both RNA and DNA viruses. Influenza viruses have the greatest sensitivity to ribavirin, and this is the basis of several clinical trials with the agent (vide infra). Poxviruses, herpesviruses, and RNA tumor viruses also respond well to ribavirin in vitro. With regard to the latter virus group, it was found that combination of various cytoreductive anticancer agents with ribavirin to inhibit the inducing virus effected a significant reduction of viral titer and an increase in survival time in leukemia AKR mice [268a]. Of interest is the observation [269, 270] that ribavirin was effective in reducing anti-DNA antibodies and proteinuria and prolonging survival of mice with an autoimmune syndrome similar to the human disease systemic lupus ertythematosus.

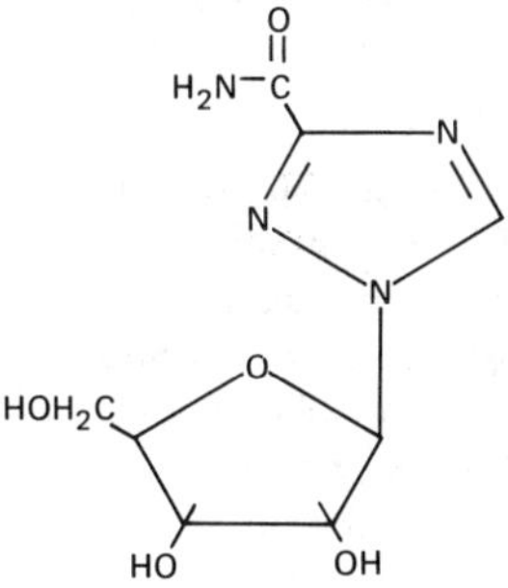

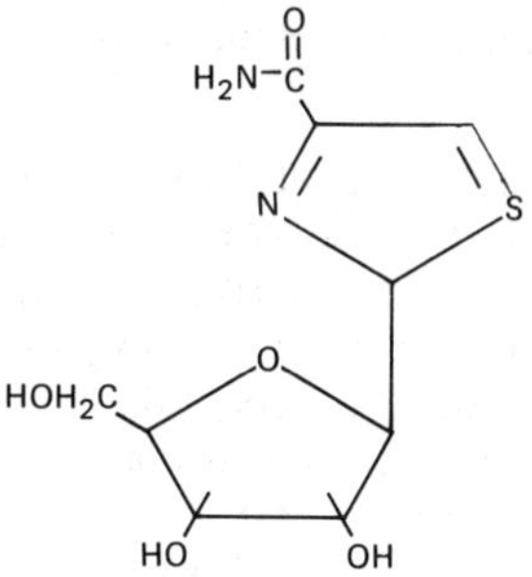

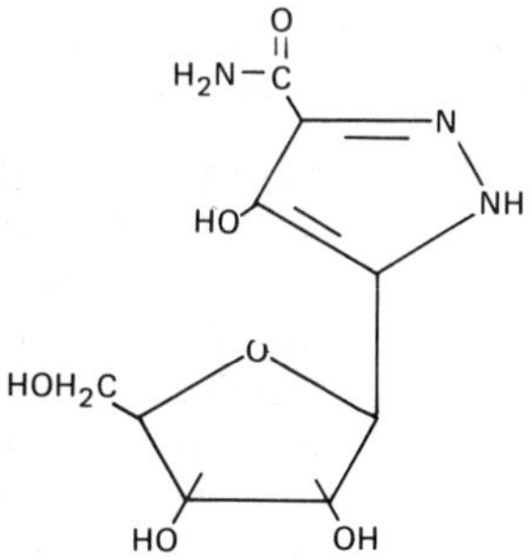

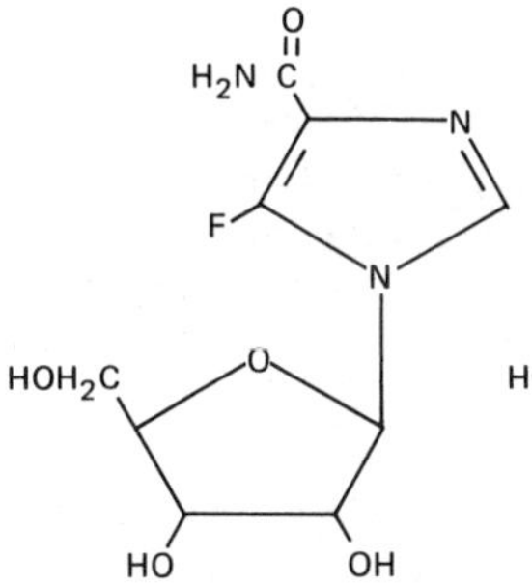

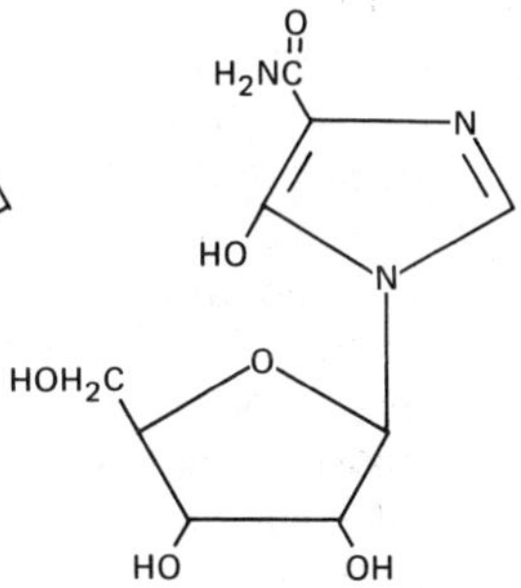

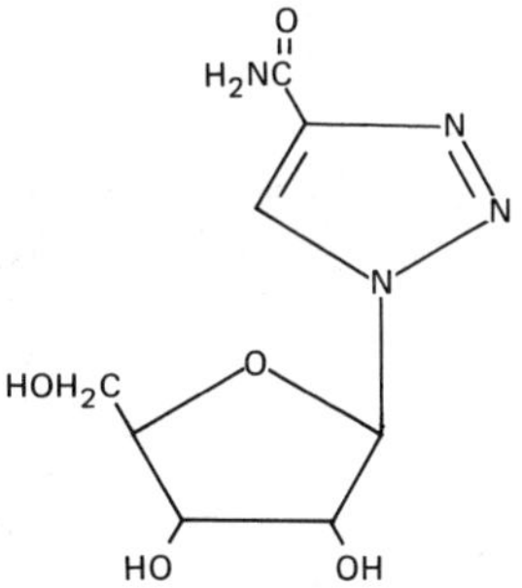

FIGURE 5.19 Ribavirin and some of its congeners with significant antiviral activity.

Clinical studies on the effect of ribavirin on the course of influenza have yielded mixed results [268]. Among controlled studies, two have reported some clinical efficacy of ribavirin against influenza. Rivavirin has been reported to have some clinical efficacy in acute type A hepatitis, herpes zoster, herpetic gingivostomatitis, herpes genitalis, and measles. While a number of clinical trials involving ribavirin are ongoing, it is particularly interesting that it is also being evaluated for the chemotherapy of the deadly Lassa fever [271].

Ribavirin is rapidly taken up by cells by a facilitated transport mechanism [268]. It is metabolized to the deaminated form, 1-β-D-ribofuranosyl-1,2,4-triazole-3-carboxylic acid, and the corresponding deaminated free base. Other major metabolic products include the ribavirin heterocyclic base (1,2,4-triazole-3-carboxamide) and the 5'-mono-, di-, and triphosphates. The notion has been advanced that in humans ribavirin may be converted by the liver to some active, but yet unidentified metabolic product [268].

The mechanism of ribavirin action may be polyvalent in nature [268, 272]. A number of significant biochemical events have been attributed to this nucleoside and are outlined below.

1. The geometry [273] of ribavirin's carboxamide group has suggested a similarity to guanosine, and indeed, for certain viruses (e.g., measles), ribavirin activity is reversed by guanosine and xanthosine, but much less effectively by inosine [274]. The intracellular metabolite of ribavirin, ribavirin 5'-monophosphate, inhibits the enzyme inosine monophosphate (IMP) dehydrogenase [274,275], which converts IMP to xanthosine 5'-monophosphate, which is a supply of guanosine 5'-monophosphate. This inhibition results in a significant reduction in the guanylate pool.
2. Ribavirin has been reported to inhibit the synthesis of DNA and RNA in uninfected cells at concentrations corresponding closely to the concentration required for inhibition of virus proliferation [268]. In this light, the antiviral action of ribavirin would not be truly selective but would result from a general depression of all (host and virus-specified) nucleic acid synthesis. However, Drach et al. [276] found that ribavirin inhibited thymidine uptake, and when DNA biosynthesis was monitored by means other than incorporation of tritiated thymidine, the effect of ribavirin on DNA synthesis was much less pronounced.
3. Although a number of investigators have questioned the specificity of ribavirin action against a number of viruses, there is a considerable amount of data to indicate that ribavirin may be a specific inhibitor of influenza virus [268]. For instance, synthesis of influenza A virus-induced polypeptides were inhibited by ribavirin in cell culture, but there was no effect on synthesis of host cell proteins [277]. While host cell DNA or RNA polymerases were

not significantly inhibited by ribavirin 5'-triphosphate [268, 275], the RNA-dependent RNA polymerase of influenza virus was. At the same time, ribavirin 5'-triphpsphate had little effect on vesicular stomatitis virus RNA polymerase [278].

4. Most recently, it has been found that ribavirin is a potent inhibitor of the 5'-terminal guanylation of in vitro synthesized uncapped mRNA [272]. This inhibition of mRNA capping would lead to accumulation of mRNAs of considerably reduced efficiency in protein synthesis.

A number of ribavirin analogs have been evaluated for their antiviral activity, and these structure-activity studies have shown that the structural features required for antiviral activity are relatively stringent. These studies have been lucidly detailed elsewhere [279]; the following points will serve to summarize (Fig. 5.19).

1. Alteration of the β-D-ribofuranosyl moiety of ribavirin to 2'-deoxy-β-D-ribofuranosyl, α- or β-D-arabinofuranosyl, 2-deoxy-α-D-lyxofuranosyl, α-L-arabinopyranosyl, 3-deoxy-β-D-*erythro*-pentofuranosyl, β-D-pucofuranosyl, 6-deoxy-β-D-*erthyro*hex-5-enofuran-2-ulosyl, 5'-deoxy-β-D-ribofuranosyl, and 5'-amino-5'-deoxy-β-D-ribofuranosyl resulted in loss of antiviral activity. In addition, 5'-O-substituted ribavirin derivatives (5'-O-nitrate and 5'-O-sulfamate) as well as analogs in which 3'-OH group was replaced with amino or the 2'- or 3'-OH groups were methylated were without activity [279]. In the case of the latter two analogs, this lack of activity has been related to lack of 5'-phosphorylation by the cell [280].
2. Substitution of various groups (NH_2, NO_2, CH_3, SH) at the 5-position of ribavirin produced analogs devoid of antiviral activity [279].
3. Of several thiazole analogs of ribavirin, only one, 2-β-D-ribofuranosylthiazole-4-carboxamide (64), was significantly active, albeit less so than ribavirin, against herpes, parainfluenza, and rhinovirus in vitro [279].
4. The nucleoside antibiotic pyrazomycin [pyrazofurin, (65)] has significant in vitro broad-spectrum antiviral activity [268, 279], but this nucleoside is too toxic to be considered as a practical antiviral agent; however, pyrazofurin has been used in clinical trials against various neoplasms. Here too, toxicity seems to be a limiting factor. Pyrazofurin is converted in cells to the 5'-monophosphate, which is an inhibitor of orotidylate decarboxylase. It also inhibits aminoimidazole carboxamide ribonucleotide transformylase [15]. Other pyrazoles, glycosylated on nitrogen, are devoid of significant antiviral activity [279].

5. In regard to ribavirin analogs derived from imidazole, the most interesting is 5-fluoro-1-β-ribofuranosylimidazole-4-carboxamide (66), which possesses a broad-spectrum antiviral activity less potent than that of ribavirin [281]. Other 5-halogenated derivatives possess even less activity. The naturally occurring nucleoside, bredinin [15], (67), also possesses some antiherpes virus and antivaccinia virus activity in experimental rheumatoid arthritis [282].
6. The isomeric triazole nucleoside 1-β-D-ribofuranosyl-1,2,3-triazole-4-carboxamide shows weak activity against vaccinia virus, whereas the bredinin-related derivative, 5-hydroxy-1-β-D-ribofuranosyl-1,2,3-triazole-4-carboxamide (68), has significant in vitro activity against measles virus [279].
7. One rather simple chemical derivative or ribavirin is also of interest: the 2',3',5'-triacetate. In certain in vivo situations at least, this product of ribavirin may show greater antiviral activity than its ribavirin parent [282].

These studies suggest an absolute requirement for the 4-carboxamido group and D-ribose as the glycosyl moiety for full expression of antiviral activity. In addition, the findings with the 1,2,3-triazole analogs and the data on the imidazole analogs suggest the possible necessity of an electron-rich hydrogen-bonding substituent at the heterocyclic ring position corresponding to 5 in ribavirin [279].

VII. ALIPHATIC (ACYCLIC) NUCLEOSIDE ANALOGS

In the past several years, two nucleoside analogs with extensively altered sugar moieties have been reported to possess potent antiviral activity. These two analogs are (S)-9-(2,3-dihydroxypropyl)adenine [283] [(S)-DHPA] and 9-(2-hydroxyethoxymethyl)guanine [284,285] (acycloguanosine, acyclovir). Their close structural resemblance to adenosine and guanosine, respectively, is conveyed by Fig. 5.20. A third aliphatic nucleoside analog is EHNA [erthro-9(2-hydroxy-3-nonyl)adenine], which shows moderate in vitro activity [286] but is without in vivo activity against herpes virus [7, 286].

Acycloguanosine is a potent inhibitor ($ID_{50} \sim 0.1\ \mu M$) of herpes simplex virus type 1 in cell culture and is also highly inhibitory to the replication of herpes simplex type 2, varicella zoster, and Epstein-Barr viruses [4,7]. It shows little or no activity against vaccinia virus, adenovirus, or a number of RNA viruses [4,7]. Acycloguanosine is virtually without toxicity to the uninfected cell in vitro; however, not much data on the in vivo pharmacology of this nucleoside analog has been published. Clinical trials of this new agent are just beginning: a 3% ointment of acycloguanosine showed efficacy against herpes keratitis in a controlled study; a preliminary and uncontrolled study showed that acycloguanosine may arrest infection

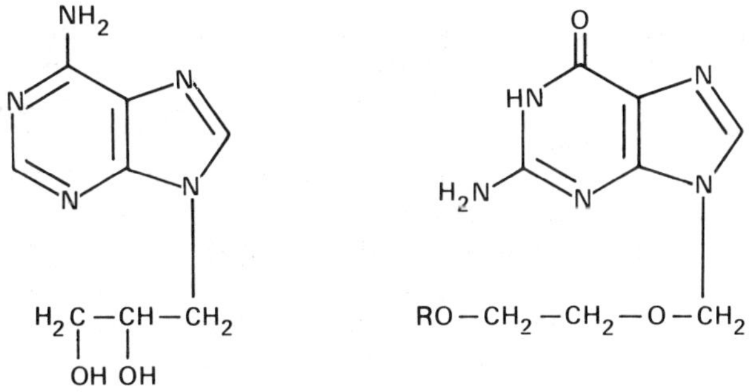

(S)-DHPA
(S)-9-(2,3-DIHYDROXYPROPYL) ADENINE

R = H, ACYCLOGUANOSINE
9-(2-HYDROXYETHOXYMETHYL) GUANINE
R = $PO(OH)_2$, Acyclo GMP

FIGURE 5.20 Structure of (S)-DHPA and acycloguanosine and its 5'-monophosphate.

from cutaneous or systemic herpes zoster or herpes simplex in patients having received a recent bone marrow transplant or in patients with cancer [4]. Controlled clinical trials with acycloguanosine are in progress for herpes simplex encephalitis, genitalis, and labialis [4].

Herpes virus-encoded thymidine kinase converts acycloguanosine to its monophosphate; this conversion occurs in extracts of herpes virus-infected cell at a rate of 30-120 times faster than it does in uninfected cell extracts [287]. Further, the resulting acycloGMP is converted to the di- and triphosphate. The latter is an effective inhibitor of the herpes virus-induced DNA polymerase, which is inhibited 2-50 times more strongly than is the mammalian DNA polymerase [285,288,289].

Barrio et al. [290] have recently reported a general approach for the synthesis of such open-chain nucleoside analogs. This procedure involves the alkylation of 2-chloro-6-iodopurine with iodomethyl [(trimethylsilyl)-oxy]ether followed first by replacement of the 6-iodo group by hydroxy with the use of potassium carbonate in dioxane and finally generation of acycloguanosine by treatment with ammonia under pressure. Similar procedures were used to synthesize the corresponding acyclic analogs of adenine and cytosine.

The second aliphatic nucleoside analog of particular interest is (S)-DHPA. In contrast to acycloguanosine, (S)-DHPA shows broad-spectrum antiviral activity against a variety of RNA and DNA viruses [283]. (S)-DHPA also appears quite selective in its antiviral action since it does not inhibit host cell DNA, RNA, or protein synthesis or impair cell viability unless extremely high concentrations are used [283]. This nucleoside analog also shows in vivo activity. (S)-DHPA is not a substrate for adenosine deaminase; in fact, it strongly inhibits this enzyme. Nothing so far is known regarding its mode of action or the basis of its antiviral selectivity.

De Clercq and Holy [291] conducted a structure-activity study of various analogs of (S)-DHPA and found that the antiviral activity of (S)-DHPA was rather unique and depended on at least three factors: presence of the adenine base; presence of the 2,3-dihydroxypropyl substitutent at the purine 9-position; the absolute configuration of the molecule.

VIII. PYRROLOPYRIMIDINE NUCLEOSIDES [14,15]

Three pyrrolopyrimidine nucleosides have been the subject of considerable chemical and biochemical research since their discovery about two decades ago. They are tubercidin (sparsomycin A, 7-deazaadenosine), sangivamycin, and toyocamycin (uramycin, vengicide) (Fig. 5.21). These three nucleosides possess antifungal and antibacterial properties are are potent cytotoxins to mammalian cells. Inhibition of virus growth by these nucleoside antibiotics also has been reported, but the inhibition was not selective.

Of the above three nucleosides, the most intensively studied from a clinical viewpoint has been tubercidin (69). Since tubercidin is an extremely toxic compound when administered intravenously, its direct systemic use has not been possible. When used topically, tubercidin has shown some efficacy in the treatment of various cutaneous neoplasms (e.g., basal cell carcinoma, squamous cell carcinoma, etc.) [292]. Tubercidin has the property of being rapidly and efficiently absorbed by mammalian red blood cells where it is sequestered by conversion to the 5'-triphosphate. This phenomenon has been exploited in order to reduce tubercidin's toxicity; thus tubercidin has been absorbed in vitro into erythrocytes of blood. After plasmapheresis, the erythrocytes are then returned to the donor. This same property helps make possible an effective treatment of schistosomiasis in mice and monkeys [293]. In mammalian hosts, many parasites are unable to synthesize the purine ring de novo and must therefore rely upon salvage pathways to supply their purine requirements. Furthermore, the adult stage of Schistosoma mansoni feeds in erythrocytes. These two facts, coupled with the efficient uptake of tubercidin by red blood cells, permits a targeted delivery or an agent to which the parasites are particularly sensitive [293].

Tubercidin has a variety of effects on cellular biochemistry [14,15]. In the cell, tubercidin is converted to the 5'-triphosphate, which is incorporated into both RNA and DNA. Relative to the latter phenomenon, it has been found that tubercidin 5'-di- and triphosphates are substrates for ribonucleotide reductase. Tubercidin is not degraded to the free base, 7-deazaadenine, by adenosine phosphorylase and it is not deaminated by adenosine

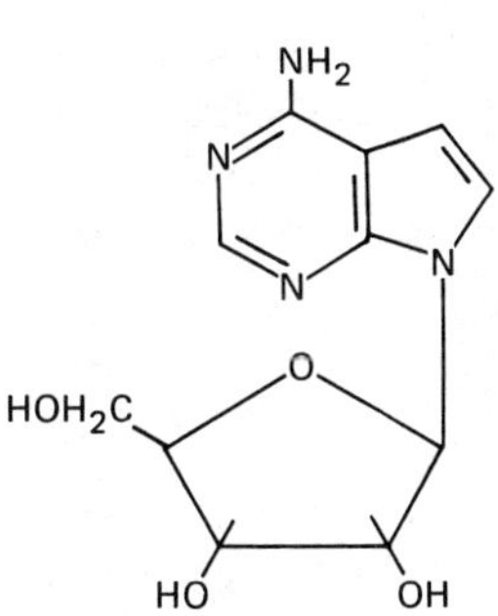

Tubercidin
(69)

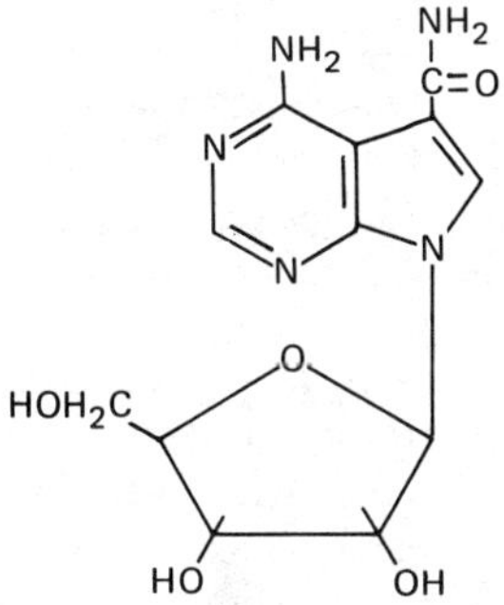

Sangivamycin
(70)

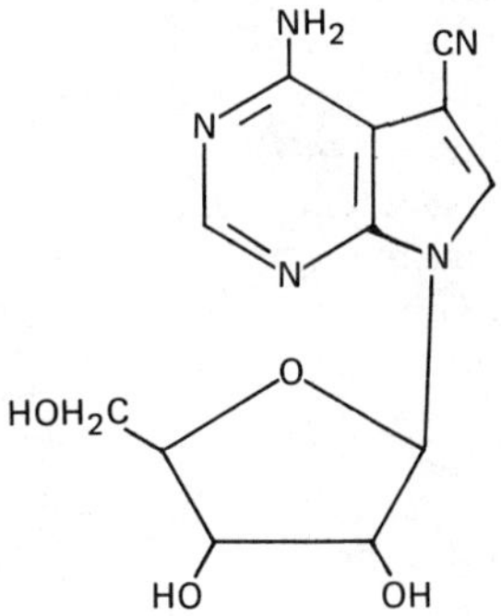

Toyocamycin
(71)

FIGURE 5.21 Structures of the pyrrolopyrimidine nucleosides.

deaminase. The 5'-triphosphate of tubercidin is inhibitory with respect to ATP or dATP for a number of RNA or DNA polymerizing enzymes, and this results in a reduced rate of nucleic acid synthesis for all classes of DNA and RNA. In the presence of tubercidin, the rate of synthesis of poly(A^+)-mRNA is dramatically reduced, and this is believed to be the basis for the potent inhibition of cell multiplication ($IC_{50} \sim 10^{-8}$ M). Tubercidin also blocks protein synthesis, methylation of tRNA, processing of rRNA, de novo purine synthesis, glucose utilization, and mitochondrial respiration.

Both sangivamycin (70) and toyocamycin (71) are converted in the cell to the 5'-mono-, di-, and triphosphates and are subsequently incorporated into RNA [14, 15]. For the case of toyocamycin, at least, this incorporation into RNA results in a inhibition of rRNA maturation. As is true for tubercidin, toyocamycin and sangivamycin are multifaceted in their effects in cellular reactions, and it is difficult to ascribe their biological effects to inhibition of any one particular biochemical event.

A pyrrolopyrimidine nucleoside of current interest is queuosine (72) (nucleoside Q) (Fig. 5.22). This hypermodified nucleoside occupies the first position of the anticodon of several tRNAs, including $tRNA^{Tyr}$, $tRNA^{Asp}$, $tRNA^{Asn}$, and $tRNA^{His}$ [294-298]. The enzyme tRNA-guanine transglycolase, found in animal sera and amniotic fluid [299], catalyzes the specific removal of guanine from the first anticodon position of the tRNAs above and effects its replacement with Q base (queuine) or Q-base precursors (7-cyano-7-deazaguanine or 7-aminomethyl-7-deazaguanine) [300-302]. No polynucleotide chain scission occurs during this reaction. The above-mentioned tRNAs are almost completely substituted with Q or Q* (hexose-containing Q derivatives) in normal mammalian cells [303, 304], but Q-deficient tRNA has been found in reticulocytes [296, 305, 306], fetal and regenerating liver [305, 306], germ-free mice maintained on a defined diet [307], and in certain tumors [298, 303, 304, 308, 309]. When Q base (queuine) is given in continuous infusion to Ehrlich ascities tumor-bearing mice, there results a decrease in tumor growth [310]. It was suggested, on the basis of these and other data, that a deficiency of nucleoside Q may favor tumor growth.

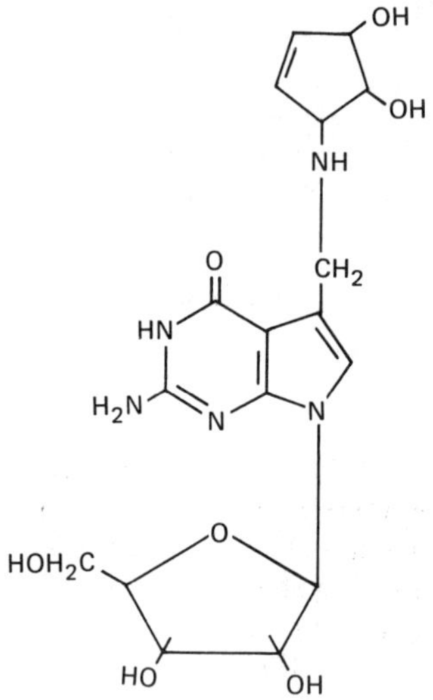

FIGURE 5.22 Structure of queuosine.

IX. NUCLEOSIDES AND THEIR DERIVATIVES AS METHYLATION INHIBITORS

With few exceptions, the mRNAs of eukaryotes and plant and animal viruses contain a 5'-terminal blocked structure, referred to as 5' "cap" (Fig. 5.23) [311-313]. This unique structure sets such RNAs apart from the prokaryotic polycistronic mRNAs, which contain only 5'-triphosphate termini. The positively charged 7'-methylguanosine of the cap structure gives the 5'-terminus a polar character that is important for its interaction with ribosomal proteins. The 5', 5'-triphosphate bridge imparts flexibility to the 7-methylguanosine residue: nuclear magnetic resonance studies of m^7GpppA^mpAp suggest that the 7-methylguanosine is intercalated between the two adenine bases [314].

In general, uncapped mRNAs are poorly translated in cell-free protein synthesis systems, such uncapped RNAs do not bind well to 40S initiation complexes. In addition, the cap structure may influence the mRNA's

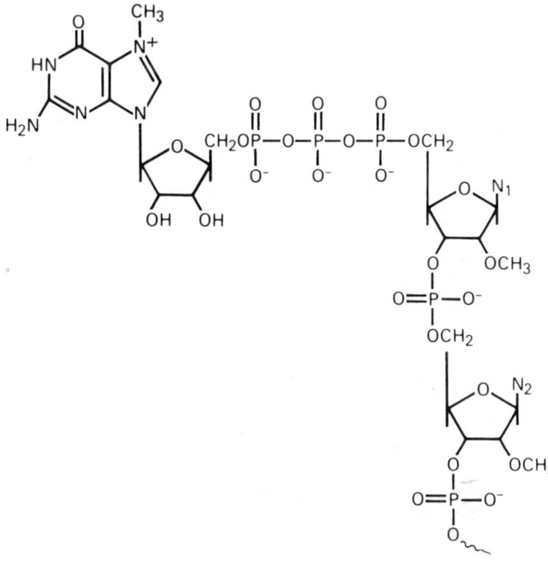

FIGURE 5.23 A general structure of 5'-blocked and methylated "cap" structure of eukaryotic or viral RNAs. The 2'-O-methyl group of the ribose of base N_2 may or may not be present. For viral mRNAs, the 5'-penultimate base (N_1) is always a purine, which may or may not be methylated. When the 5'-penultimate base is adenine, it is usually methylated. For eukaryotic mRNAs, N_1 and N_2 may be adenine, N^6-methyladenine, guanine, cytosine, or uracil. Sindbis virus RNA is exceptional in that a small proportion of 3-methylguanosine may be found at the 5'-terminus.

lifetime by conferring resistance to the action of nucleases, especially exonucleases, which degrade the RNA from the 5'-end [313].

For viruses, at least three different pathways can be used to generate a capped structure [313]. For reovirus (Fig. 5.24) or vaccinia virus, the GTP that forms the m^7G cap donates only its α phosphate to the 5'-5'-triphosphate bridge; the first nucleotide in the chain initiated by the RNA polymerase donates the other two phosphates. In vesicular stomatitis virus, the reverse situation obtains since the GTP that gives rise to the m^7G donates two ($\alpha + \beta$) phosphates to the triphosphate bridge. For influenza virus, the origin of the cap structure is completely unique: a portion of the host cell RNA, specifically the 5'-terminus (10-15 nucleotides), is cannibalized for capping of the influenza mRNA [315, 316]. The details of cell mRNA cap biosynthesis are less well understood, but at least some aspects must be similar to that of reovirus or vaccinia virus since guanyltransferase and methyltransferase activities similar to the virion-associated enzymes, have been found in mammalian cells. Methylation and cap formation occurs at the level of heterogeneous nuclear RNA during or shortly

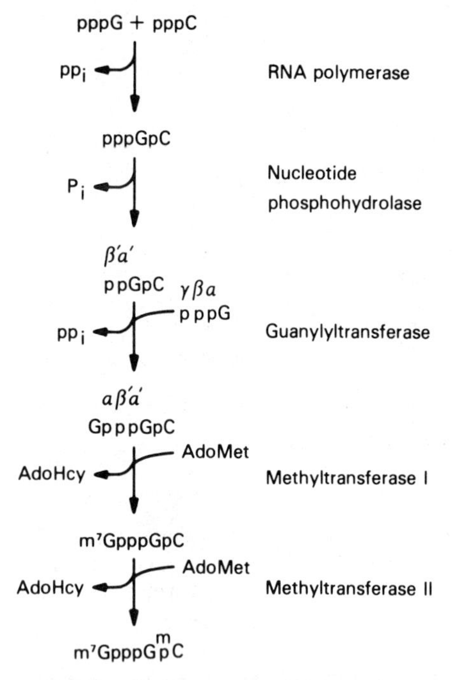

FIGURE 5.24 Mechanism of reovirus mRNA "cap" biosynthesis by viral-associated enzymes. AdoMet is S-adenosylmethionine, and AdoHcy is S-adenosylhomocysteine in mammals.

after transcription, and the cap structures are conserved during processing to mRNA.

Borchardt [317] has pointed out several approaches to the development of inhibitors of S-adenosylmethionine-dependent methyltransferases. These include (Fig. 5.25): (i) inhibition of adenosyltransferase; (ii) inhibition of S-adenosylmethionine-dependent methyltransferase by S-adenosylmethione analogs; (iii) inhibition of S-adenosylmethionine-dependent methyltransferases by exploiting the S-adenosylmethionine regulatory mechanism (Fig. 5.25) with either S-adenosylhomocysteine analogs that would bind to specific methyltransferases or with compounds that would interfere with S-adenosylhomocysteine metabolism to raise its intracellular concentration, thereby blocking the methyltransferase by product inhibition.

A general synthetic approach to S-adenosylhomosysteine analogs is illustrated in Fig. 5.26 for the specific example of 5'-deoxy-5'-(isobutylthio)-3-deazaadenosine (73) [318]. The starting nucleoside for this synthesis, 3-deazaadenosine (74), was first prepared by condensation of 4-chloroimidazo[4, 5-c]pyridine with 1, 2, 3, 5-tetra-O-acetyl-β-D-ribofuranose [319]. Deblocking the acetyl protecting groups with alcoholic ammonia gave 4-chloro-1-(β-D-ribofuranosyl)imidazo[4, 5-c]pyridine, which was treated with hydrazine and then Raney nickel to give the desired 3-deazaadenosine. One disadvantage of this approach was that the intermediate 6-chloro-3-deazapurine riboside was relatively unreactive toward nucleophilic substitution due to higher electron density at C-6 compared to the

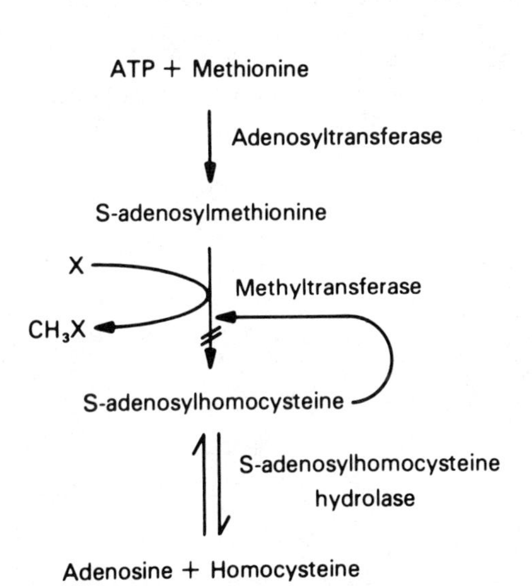

FIGURE 5.25 Regulation and metabolism of S-adenosylmethionine and S-adenosylhomocysteine in mammals.

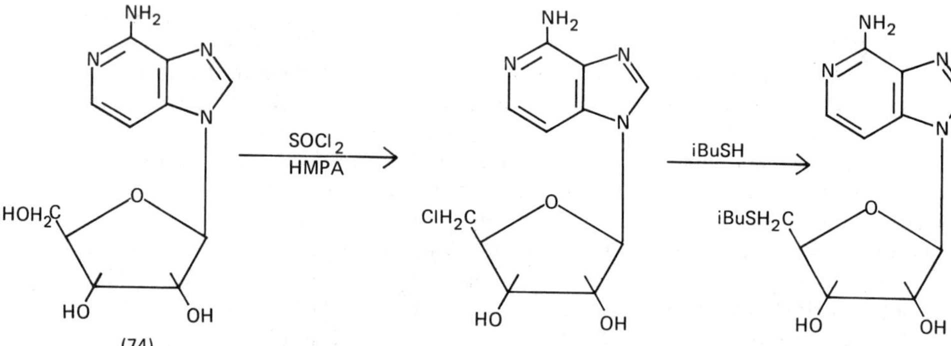

FIGURE 5.26 Synthesis of 5'-deoxy-5'-(isobutylthio)-3-deazaadenosine.

corresponding 6-chloropurine. This problem was overcome [320] by introduction of a replaceable electron-withdrawing chlorine atom at C-4 (corresponding to C-2 of the purine ring). Thus trimethylsilylated 4,6-dichloro-imidazo[4,5-c]pyridine was condensed with 2,3,5-tri-O-benzoyl-D-ribofuranosyl bromide to give both anomers of the 1-riboside (Fig. 5.27). A considerable improvement in this reaction was claimed when the fusion method of base-sugar condensation was used [321].

Structure-activity studies of S-adenosylhomocysteine binding to the enzyme S-adenosylhomocysteine hydrolase have shown that the enzyme is quite specific [317]; 3-deazaadenosyl-L-homocysteine was the only analog that possessed substrate properties. The adenosine analog 3-deazaadenosine (74) as well as 5'-deoxy-5'-isobutylthio-3-deazaadenosine (73) were

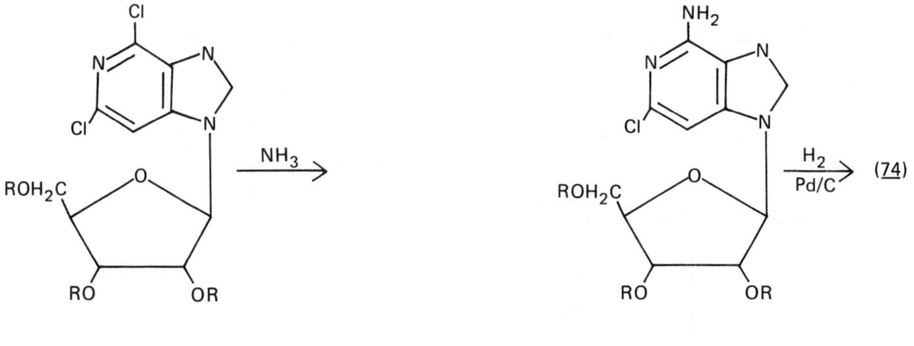

R = Bz or Ac

FIGURE 5.27 Intermediates in the synthesis of 3-deazaadenosine.

both good inhibitors of S-adenosylhomocysteine hydrolase. 3-Deazaadenosine (74) and (73) both showed antiviral activity against Rous sarcoma virus and Gross murine leukemia virus. It has been, however, difficult to ascertain whether or not the antiviral activities of 3-deazaadenine and (73) are related to an inhibition of viral mRNA cap methylation as a primary event, since these nucleoside analogs are not very specific in their actions. For instance, 3-deazaadenosine inhibits macrophage phagocytosis, leukocyte chemotaxis, histamine release, phospholipid methylation, protein carboxymethylation, and lymphocyte mitogenesis [317].

The nucleoside antibiotic cordycepin (3'-deoxyadenosine) is cytotoxic to a strain (WI-L2) of cultured human lymphoblasts. One root of this lymphocytoxicity appears to be the conversion of cordycepin to the 3'-deoxy analogs of S-adenosylmethionine and S-adenosylhomocysteine, which then inhibits nucleic acid methylation [322]. Adenine arabinoside (araA) and 2'-deoxyadenosine also have been shown to be apparent suicide inhibitors of S-adenosylhomocysteine hydrolase from the same human lymphoblast cell [323]. These studies suggest a nucleotide-independent mechanism of toxicity for cordycepin, 2'-deoxyadenosine, and adenine arabinoside and further suggest that inhibitors of enzymes involved in S-adenosylmethionine metabolism and/or methylation need not be obvious structural analogs of S-adenosylmethionine or its metabolites.

The S-adenosylhomocysteine analogs, S-tubercidinyl-L-homocysteine, Sinefungin, and 5'-deoxy-5'-(isobutylthio)adenosine (Fig. 5.28), inhibit the replication of herpes simplex, vaccinia virus, and polyoma virus, and block the transformation of cells induced by Rous sarcoma virus and mouse sarcoma virus [317, 324]. These analogs have been shown to inhibit methyltransferases of various kinds, including mRNA methylases, tRNA methylases, catechol-O-methyltransferase, and protein carboxymethyltransferases. Indeed, 5'-deoxy-5'-(isobutylthio)adenosine, for example, has been shown to inhibit the methylation of mRNA, especially the cap structure. The biological effects of these analogs are not restricted to inhibition of virus growth since such nucleosides also exhibit antimitotic and antiparasitic activities, and inhibit polyamine biosynthesis [325] and phospholipid methylation [326].

Thus, while it is clear that the exact mechanism of action of these agents may be difficult to define, it is clear that such analogs of S-adenosylhomocysteine can have dramatic biological effects. Whether or not these effects are mediated through inhibition of S-adenosylhomocysteine hydrolase or direct inhibition of S-adenosylmethionine-dependent methyltransferases, these lead compounds may provide additional structures which may specifically inhibit viral replication or modulate cellular metabolism in some useful manner.

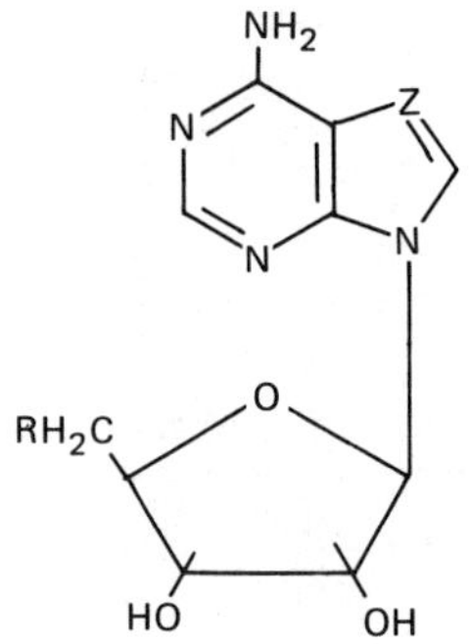

Structure	Z	R
S-adenosylmethionine	N	$^{+}S(CH_3)CH_2CH_2CH(NH_2)COOH$
S-adenosylhomocysteine	N	$SCH_2CH_2CH(NH_2)COOH$
S-tubercidinyl-L-homocysteine	CH	$SCH_2CH_2CH(NH_2)COOH$
5'-deoxy-5'-(isobutylthio)adenosine (SIBA)	N	$SCH_2CH(CH_3)_2$
sinefungin	N	$CH(NH_2)CH_2CH_2CH(NH_2)COOH$

FIGURE 5.28 Structures of *S*-adenosylmethionine and *S*-adenosylhomocysteine and its analogs.

X. CONCLUSIONS

We have seen that pruine and pyrimidine nucleoside analogs, by incorporation into nucleic acids or by modification of the activity of the enzymes of nucleic acid biosynthesis, provide some of the most powerful and useful inhibitors of viral replication and neoplastic tissue growth. A great contributor to this success has been the synthesis of novel nucleoside structures and the use of such nucleosides as probes to gain a greater appreciation of the fundamental principles involved in the biochemistry of virus replication and the regulation and growth of the cell. Close cooperation among chemists, biochemists, and virologists will continue to provide in nucleoside analogs useful in the treatment of viral and neoplastic diseases. Obviously, progress on the latter front would come more rapidly if some target enzyme unique to the neoplastic cell could be identified. Nonetheless, some encouragement may be taken from the field of antiviral chemotherapy where a combination of serendipity and rational design have been major factors in the discovery of selective antiviral agents. While serendipity may determine the specific chemical structure that is eventually found to be the most selective inhibitor of, for instance, herpes virus replication, there is no doubt that through accumulation and interpretation of chemical and biochemical evidence, the general structure that will be a selective inhibitor has been defined. It is reasonable to suspect that a similar enlightenment process may be possible with the problem of cancer chemotherapy, tempered by the relative greater difficulties of ascertaining the differences between a neoplastic cell and a normal cell compared to those determining the differences between a virus-infected cell and an uninfected cell.

One area where some activity should, and probably will, be concentrated is the problem of catabolism of nucleoside analogs. For instance, the potential usefulness of a number of 5-substituted pyrimidine nucleosides has been considerably compromised by the enzyme thymidine phosphorylase, which catalyzes the reversible reaction of phosphate and thymidine to 2-deoxyribose-1-phosphate and thymine. One approach to this problem would be the design and synthesis of modified analogs which would be resistant to cleavage by this enzyme and still retain activity against other target enzymes such as thymidylate synthetase. Of interest in this regard is the report [327] from Bardos's laboratory that 1-(2-deoxy-β-D-ribofuranosyl)-5-methylmercapto-2-pyrimidinone possesses significant anti-herpesvirus activity, but due to the absence of a C4 oxygen, may be resistant to cleavage by thymidine phosphorylase. A second approach, based on the work of Baker and colleagues and suggested by Santi [46], would be to find an inhibitor of thymidine phosphorylase. One possible candidate in this regard is 5-benzyluracil.

Another area in which some activity may be expected is that of cell regulation by low-molecular-weight nucleotides. One such example is an oligonucleotide referred to as 2, 5A [5-O-triphosphoryladenylyl(2'→5')-adenylyl(2'→5')adenosine], which is unique in that it is the first naturally occurring oligonucleotide with 2', 5'-phosphodiester bonds [328]. This material is formed in extracts of interferon-treated cells upon incubation with double-stranded RNA or in intact cells after interferon treatment and viral infection. This oligonucleotide, 2, 5A, is an extremely potent and reversible inhibitor of protein synthesis and acts by activation of a latent endonucleases that degrades mRNA. There is also evidence which suggests that the role of 2, 5A may not be limited to interferon treatment, but that it may have some more general role in cell regulation [329, 330]. This unique oligonucleotide therefore provides an entirely new lead to mechanisms to modulate cellular activities.

The science of the synthesis and evaluation of the biological activities of nucleosides and nucleotides has been proceeding for about three decades. In this time, studies of nucleoside analogs have made many important contributions to our understanding of cellular biochemistry and to the treatment of disease. With the expected continued advances in the chemistry of nucleoside analogs coupled with the information to be gained through the sometimes revolutionary advances in the fields of biochemistry and molecular biology, we can confidently expect that the next three decades will see contributions of nucleoside and nucleotide analogs to the chemotherapy of diseases that will dramatically exceed those of the last three.

ACKNOWLEDGMENTS

The author is indebted to Glenda M. Torrence for her invaluable assistance in the preparation of this manuscript and to Ian and Jessica Torrence for their understanding and patience.

REFERENCES

1. W. H. Prusoff and P. H. Fischer, in Nucleoside Analogues, Chemistry, Biology and Medical Applications (R. T. Walker, E. De Clercq, and F. Eckstein, eds.), Plenum Press, New York, 1979, pp. 281-318.
2. W. H. Prusoff, M. S. Chen, P. H. Fischer, T.-S. Lin, T. T. Shiau, and R. F. Schinazi, Adv. Ophthalmol., 38: 3-16 (1979).
3. R. J. Whitley and C. A. Alford, South. Med. J., 71: 1134-1140 (1978).
4. M. S. Hirsch and M. N. Swartz, N. Engl. J. Med., 302: 903-907, 949-953 (1980).
5. E. De Clercq and P. F. Torrence, J. Carbohyd., Nucleosides, Nucleotides, 5: 187-224 (1978).
6. E. De Clercq, Arch. Int. Physiol. Biochem., 87: 353-395 (1979).
7. W. M. Shannon and F. M. Schabel, Jr., Pharmacol. Ther., 11: 263-390 (1980).
8. S. Kit, Pharmacol. Ther., 4: 501-585 (1979).
9. R. C. Gallo, in Modern Trends in Human Leukemia III (R. Neth, R. C. Gallo, P.-H. Hofschneider, and K. Mannweiler, eds.), Springer-Verlag, New York, 1979, pp. 7-24.
10. A. S. Evans (ed.), Viral Infections of Humans, Plenum Press, New York, 1976.
11. S. E. Luria, J. E. Darnell, Jr., D. Baltimore, and A. C. Campbell, General Virology, IIIrd ed., Wiley, New York, 1978.

11a. W. Gutensohn and P. Cole, N. Engl. J. Med., 304: 135-140 (1981).

12. J. A. Montgomery, J. Med. Chem., 23: 1063-1067 (1980).
13. K. H. Scheit, Nucletodide Analogues, Wiley, New York, 1980.
14. R. J. Suhadolnik, Nucleoside Antibiotics, Wiley, New York, 1970.
15. R. J. Suhadolnik, Nucleosides as Biological Probes, Wiley, New York, 1979.
16. J. F. Henderson and A. R. P. Paterson, Nucleotide Metabolism, Academic Press, New York, 1973.

17. P. O. P. Ts'o (ed.), Basic Principles in Nucleic Acid Chemistry, Vols. I and II, Academic Press, New York, 1974.
18. W. W. Zorbach and R. S. Tipson (eds.), Synthetic Procedures in Nucleic Acid Chemistry, Wiley, New York, 1968.
19. L. B. Townsend and R. S. Tipson (eds.), Nucleic Acid Chemistry, Parts 1 and 2, Wiley, New York, 1978.
20. R. T. Walker, in Comprehensive Organic Chemistry, Vol. VI (D. Barton and W. D. Ollis, eds), Pergamon Press, Oxford, 1979, pp. 53-104.
21. D. W. Hutchinson, Comprehensive Organic Chemistry, Vol. VI, (D. Barton and W. D. Ollis, eds.), Pergamon Press, Oxford, 1979, pp. 105-145.
22. N. K. Kochetkov and E. I. Budovskii, Organic Chemistry of Nucleic Acids, Plenum Press, New York, 1972.
23. R. E. Harmon, R. K. Robins, and L. B. Townsend (eds.), Chemistry and Biology of Nucleosides and Nucleotides, Academic Press, New York, 1978.
24. A. Bloch (ed.), Chemistry, Biology and Clinical Uses of Nucleoside Analogs, Ann. N.Y. Acad. Sci., 255 (1975).
25. R. T. Walker, E. De Clercq, and F. Eckstein (eds.), Nucleoside Analogues, Chemistry, Biology and Medical Applications, Plenum Press, New York, 1979.
26. A. C. Sartorelli and D. G. Johns (eds.), in Handbook of Experimental Pharmacology, Vol. 38, Springer-Verlag, New York, 1974.
27. G. J. Galasso, R. C. Merigan, and R. A. Buchanan (eds.), Antiviral Agents and Viral Diseases of Man, Raven Press, New York, 1979.
28. J. A. Montgomery, Prog. Med. Chem., 7, pt. 1, 69-123 (1970).
29. J. A. Montgomery, R. D. Elliott, P. W. Allan, L. M. Rose, and L. L. Bennett, Jr., Adv. Enzyme Regul., 17: 419-435 (1979).
30. L. L. Bennett, Jr., J. A. Montgomery, R. W. Brockman, and Y. F. Shealy, Adv. Enzyme Regul., 16: 255-271 (1978).
31. T. K. Bradshaw and D. W. Hutchinson, Chem. Soc. Rev., 6: 43-62 (1977).
32. D. S. Martin, R. L. Stolgi, R. C. Sawyer, R. Nayak, S. Speigelman, C. W. Young, and T. Woodcock, Cancer, 45: 1117-1128 (1980).
33. W. Ensminger and A. Rosowsky, Proc. Am. Assoc. Cancer Res., 18: 109 (1977).
34. C. Heidelberger, N. K. Chaudhuri, P. Dannenberg, D. Mooren, L. Griesbach, R. Duschinsky, R. J. Schnitzer, E. Pleven, and T. Scheiner, Nature, 179: 663-666 (1957).
35. C. Heidelberger, in Handbook of Experimental Pharmacology, Vol. 38, Pt. II (A. C. Sartorelli and D. G. Johns, eds.), Springer-Verlag, New York, 1974, pp. 193-231.
36. C. Heidelberger, Prog. Nucleic Acid Res. Mol. Biol., 4: 1-50 (1965).

37. P. V. Danenberg, Biochim. Biophys. Acta, 497: 73-92 (1977).
38. S. Spiegelman, R. Sawyer, R. Nayak, E. Ritzi, R. Stolfi, and D. Martin, Proc. Natl. Acad. Sci. USA, 77: 4966-4970 (1980).
39. S. Spiegelman, R. Nayak, R. Sawyer, R. Stolfi, and D. Martin, Cancer, 45: 1129-1134 (1980).
40. R. I. Glazer and K. D. Hartman, Mol. Pharmacol., 17: 245-249 (1980).
41. R. I. Glazer and M. Legraverend, Mol. Pharmacol., 17: 279-282 (1980).
42. J. Balzarini, E. De Clercq, P. F. Torrence, M. P. Mertes. J. S. Park, C. L. Schmidt, D. Shugar, P. J. Barr, A. S. Jones, G. Verhelst and R. T. Walker, Biochem. Pharmacol., 31: 1089-1095 (1982).
43. C. M. Haskell, in Cancer Treatment (C. M. Haskell, ed.), W. B. Saunders, Philadelphia, 1980, pp. 53-123.
44. A. Rossi, in Nucleoside Analogues, Chemistry, Biology and Medical Applications (R. T. Walker, E. De Clercq, and F. Eckstein, eds.), Plenum Press, New York, 1979, pp. 409-444.
45. S. S. Cohen, Ann. N.Y. Acad. Sci., 186: 292-301 (1971).
46. D. V. Santi, J. Med. Chem., 23: 103-111 (1980).
47. T. I. Kalman, Biochemistry, 10: 2567-2573 (1971).
48. M. J. Robins and S. R. Naik, J. Am. Chem. Soc., 93: 5277-5278 (1971).
49. M. J. Robins and S. R. Naik, J. Chem. Soc., Chem. Commun., 18-19 (1972).
50. M. J. Robins, G. Ramani, and M. MacCoss, Can. J. Chem., 53: 1302-1306 (1975).
51. M. J. Robins, M. MacCoss, S. R. Naik, and G. Ramani, J. Am. Chem. Soc., 98: 7381-7390 (1976).
52. C. Heidelberger, D. Parsons, and D. C. Remy, J. Am. Chem. Soc., 84: 3597-3598 (1962).
53. C. Heidelberger, D. G. Parsons, and D. C. Remy, J. Med. Chem., 7: 1-5 (1964).
54. C. Heidelberger and D. H. King, Pharmacol. Ther., 6: 427-442 (1979).
55. M. P. Mertes and S. E. Saheb, J. Pharm. Sci., 52: 508-509 (1963).
56. K. J. Ryan, E. M. Acton, and L. Goodman, J. Org. Chem., 31: 1181-1184 (1966).
57. Y. Kobayashi, K. Yamamoto, T. Asai, M. Nakano, and I. Kumadaki, J. Chem. Soc., Perkin Trans. I, 275-2761 (1980).
58. C. Heidelberger, Ann. N.Y. Acad. Sci., 255: 317-325 (1975).
59. P. Reyes and C. Heidelberger, Mol. Pharmacol., 1: 14-30 (1965).
60. D. V. Santi and T. T. Sakai, Biochemistry, 10: 3598-3607 (1971).
61. Y. Wataya, A. Matsuda, D. V. Santi, D. E. Bergstrom, and J. L. Ruth, J. Med. Chem., 22: 339-340 (1979).
62. D. E. Bergstrom and J. L. Ruth, J. Am. Chem. Soc., 98: 1587-1589 (1976).

63. J. L. Ruth and D. E. Bergstrom, J. Org. Chem., 43: 2870-2876 (1978).
64. D. E. Bergstrom and M. K. Ogawa, J. Am. Chem. Soc., 100: 8106-8112 (1978).
65. R. M. K. Dale, D. C. Livingston, and D. C. Ward, Proc. Natl. Acad. Sci. USA, 70: 2238-2242 (1973).
66. C. F. Bigge, P. Kalaritis, J. R. Deck, and M. P. Mertes, J. Am. Chem. Soc., 102: 2033-2038 (1980).
67. C. E. Bigge and M. P. Mertes, J. Org. Chem., 46: 1994-1997 (1981).
68. E. De Clercq, J. Balzarini, C. T.-C. Chang, C. F. Bigge, P. Kalaritis, and M. P. Mertes, Biochem. Biophys. Res. Commun., 97: 1068-1075 (1980).
69. R. E. Cline, R. M. Fink, and K. Fink, J. Am. Chem. Soc., 81: 2521-2527 (1959).
70. K. H. Scheit, Chem. Ber., 99: 3884-3891 (1966).
71. V. W. Armstrong and F. Eckstein, Nucleic Acids Res., Spec. Publ. Publ. 1, Information Retrieval Ltd., London, 1975, pp. s97-s100.
72. D. V. Santi and T. T. Sakai, Biochem. Biophys. Res. Commun., 42: 813-817 (1971).
73. A. Kampf, R. L. Barfknecht, P. J. Shaffer, S. Osaki, and M. P. Mertes, J. Med. Chem., 19: 903-908 (1976).
74. Y. Wataya, D. V. Santi, and C. Hansch, J. Med. Chem., 20: 1469-1473 (1977).
75. J. S. Park, C. T.-C. Chang, C. L. Schmidt, Y. Golander, E. De Clercq, J. Descamps, and M. P. Mertes, J. Med. Chem., 23: 661-665 (1980).
76. M. P. Mertes and M. T. Shipchandler, J. Heterocycl. Chem., 7: 751 (1970).
77. P. Langen, S. R. Waschke, K. Waschke, D. Barwolff, J. Reefschalger, P. Schultz, B. Preussel, and C. Lehmann, Acta Biol. Med. Ger., 35: 1625-1633 (1976).
78. E. De Clercq, J. Descamps, C. L. Schmidt, and M. P. Mertes, Biochem. Pharmacol., 28: 3249-3254 (1979).
]79. E. De Clercq, J. Descamps, P. F. Torrence, E. Krajewska, and D. Shugar, in Current Chemotherapy (W. Siegenthaler and R. Luthy, eds.), American Society of Microbiology, Washington, D.C., 1978, pp. 352-354.
80. S. Waschke, J. Reefschlager, D. Barwolff, and P. Langen, Nature, 255: 629-630 (1975).
81. T. J. Bardos, M. P. Kotick, and C. Szantay, Tetrahedron Lett., 1759-1764 (1966).
82. M. P. Kotick, C. Szantay, and T. J. Bardos, J. Org. Chem., 34: 3806-3813 (1969).

83. G. L. Szekeres and T. J. Bardos, J. Med. Chem., 13: 708-712 (1970).
84. T. J. Bardos, J. Aradi, Y. K. Ho, and T. I. Kalman, Ann. N.Y. Acad. Sci., 255: 522-531 (1975).
85. T. J. Bardos and T. K. Ho, in Chemistry and Biology of Nucleosides and Nucleotides (R. E. Harmon, R. K. Robins, and L. B. Townsend, eds.), Academic Press, New York, 1978, pp. 55-68.
86. P. Chandra, B. Kornhuber, and V. Ebener, in Modern Trends in Human Leukemia III (R. Weth, R. C. Gallo, P.-H. Hofschneider, and K. Mannweiler, eds.), Springer-Verlag, Berlin, 1979, pp. 145-155.
87. K. Baranski, T. J. Bardos, A. Bloch, and T. I. Kalman, Biochem. Pharmacol., 18: 347-358 (1969).
88. S. H. Schwartz, T. J. Bardso, G. H. Burgess, and E. Klein, J. Med. (Basel), 1: 174-179 (1970).
89. T. I. Kalman and T. J. Bardos, Mol. Pharmacol., 6: 621-630 (1970).
90. T. Nagamachi, P. F. Torrence, J. A. Waters, and B. Witkop, J. Chem. Soc., Chem. Commun., 1025-1026 (1972).
91. T. Nagamachi, J.-L. Fourrey, P. F. Torrence, J. A. Waters, and B. Witkop, J. Med. Chem., 17: 403-406 (1974).
92. P. F. Torrence, J. A. Waters, and B. Witkop, in Nucleic Acid Chemistry, Vol. 1 (L. B. Townsend and R. S. Tipson, eds.), Wiley, New York, 1978, pp. 367-370.
93. E. De Clercq, P. F. Torrence, J. A. Waters, and B. Witkop, Biochem. Pharmacol., 24: 2171-2175 (1975).
94. E. De Clercq, M. Luczak, D. Shugar, P. F. Torrence, J. A. Waters, and B. Witkop, Proc. Soc. Exp. Biol. Med., 151: 487-490 (1976).
95. P. F. Torrence, E. De Clercq, J. Descamps, G.-F. Huang, and B. Witkop, in Frontiers in Bioorganic Chemistry (Y. A. Ovchinnikov and M. N. Kolosov, eds.), Elsevier/North-Holland, Amsterdam, 1979, pp. 59-85.
96. S. Choi, T. I. Kalman, and T. J. Bardos, J. Med. Chem., 22: 618-621 (1979).
97. I. Wempen, I. L. Doerr, L. Kaplan, and J. J. Fox, J. Am. Chem. Soc., 82: 1624-1629 (1960).
98. K. A. Watanabe and J. J. Fox, J. Heterocycl. Chem., 6: 109-112 (1969).
99. M. Prystas and F. Sorm, Collect. Czech. Chem. Commun., 30: 1900-1912 (1965).
100. D. Kluepfel, Y. K. S. Murthy, and G. Sartori, Farm. Ed. Sci., 20: 757-763 (1965).
101. G.-F. Huang and P. F. Torrence, J. Org. Chem., 42: 3821-3824 (1977).
102. S. J. Kuhn and G. A. Olah, J. Am. Chem. Soc., 83: 4564-4571 (1961).

103. G.-F. Huang and P. F. Torrence, J. Carbohyd. Nucleosides Nucleotides, 5: 317-327 (1978).
104. E. De Clercq, J. Descamps, G.-F. Huang, and P. F. Torrence, Mol. Pharmacol., 14: 422-430 (1978).
105. W. Washtien, A. Matsuda, Y. Wataya, and D. V. Santi, Biochem. Pharmacol., 27: 2663-2666 (1978).
106. A. Matsuda, Y. Wataya, and D. V. Santi, Biochem. Biophys. Res. Commun., 84: 654-659 (1978).
107. M. P. Mertes, C. T.-C. Chang, E. De Clercq, G.-F. Huang, and P. F. Torrence, Biochem. Biophys. Res. Commun., 84: 1054-1059 (1978).
108. T. I. Kalman and J. C. Yalowich, in Drug Action and Design: Mechanism-Based Enzyme Inhibitors (T. I. Kalman, ed.), Elsevier/North-Holland, Amsterdam, 1980, pp. 75-91.
109. Y. Wataya, A. Matsuda, and D. V. Santi, J. Biol. Chem., 255: 5538-5544 (1980).
110. L. Maggiroa, C. T.-C. Chang, P. F. Torrence, and M. P. Mertes, J. Am. Chem. Soc., 103: 3192-3198 (1981).
111. C. B. Brouillete, C. T.-C. Chang, and M. P. Mertes, J. Med. Chem., 22: 1541-1544 (1979).
112. R. L. Barfknecht, R. A. Huet-Rose, A. Kampf, and M. P. Mertes, J. Am. Chem. Soc., 98: 5041-5043 (1976).
113. W. H. Prusoff and B. Goz, in Antineoplastic and Immunosuppressive Agents (A. C. Sartorelli and D. G. Johns, eds.), Springer-Verlag. New York, 1975, pp. 272-347.
114. W. H. Prusoff, M. S. Chen, P. H. Fischer, T. S. Lin, and G. T. Shiau, in Antibiotics, Vol. 2 (F. E. Hahn, ed.), Springer-Verlag, Berlin, 1979, pp. 236-261.
115. W. H. Prusoff, M. S. Chen, P. H. Fischer, T.-S. Lin, G. T. Shiau, R. F. Schinazi, and J. Walker, Pharmacol. Ther., 7: 1-34 (1979).
116. W. H. Prusoff, Biochim. Biophys. Acta, 32: 295-296 (1959).
117. E. C. Herrmann, Jr., Proc. Soc. Exp. Biol. N.Y., 107: 142-145 (1961).
118. H. E. Kaufman, A. B. Nesburn, and D. E. Maloney, Arch. Ophthalmol., 67: 583-591 (1962).
119. H. E. Kaufman, E. Martola, and C. Dohlman, Arch. Ophthalmol., 68: 235-239 (1962).
120. D. M. Gordon and D. A. Karnofsky, Am. J. Ophthalmol., 55: 229-234 (1963).
121. T. S. Lin, J. P. Neenan, Y. C. Cheng, W. H. Prusoff, and D. C. Ward, J. Med. Chem., 19: 495-498 (1976).
122. T. S. Lin and W. H. Prusoff, J. Med. Chem., 21: 106-109 (1978).
123. W. S. Mungall, G. L. Greene, G. A. Heavner, and R. Letsinger, J. Org. Chem., 40: 1659-1662 (1975).

124. R. L. Letsinger, J. S. Wilkes, and L. B. Dumas, J. Am. Chem. Soc., 94: 292-293 (1972).
125. M. D. Bick and R. Davidson, Proc. Natl. Acad. Sci. USA, 71: 2082-2086 (1974).
126. L. Rossler, G. J. Meyer, and G. Stocklin, J. Labelled Comp. Radiopharm., 13: 271 (1977).
127. R. C. Bleackley, A. S. Jones, and R. T. Walker, Nucleic Acids Res., 2: 683-690 (1975).
128. T. Ueda, H. Inoue, and A. Matsuda, Ann. N.Y. Acad. Sci., 255: 121-130 (1975).
129. P. F. Torrence, B. Bhooshan, J. Descamps, and E. De Clercq, J. Med. Chem., 20: 974-976 (1977).
130. A. Hampton, F. Kappler, and R. R. Chawla, J. Med. Chem., 22: 621-631 (1979).
131. W. A. Sheppard, in The Chemistry of the Cyano Group (Z. Rappoport, ed.), Interscience, New York, pp. 209-237, 1970.
132. C. T.-C. Chang, M. W. Edwards, P. F. Torrence, and M. P. Mertes, J. Med. Chem., 22: 1137-1139 (1979).
133. E. De Clercq, E. Krajewska, J. Descamps, and P. F. Torrence, Mol. Pharmacol., 13: 980-984 (1977).
134. D. Shugar, in Virus-Cell Interactions and Viral Antimetabolites (D. Shugar, ed.), Academic Press, New York, 1972, pp. 193-207.
135. D. Shugar, FEBS Lett. Suppl., 40: S48-S62.
136. M. Swierskowski and S. Shugar, J. Med. Chem., 12: 533-534 (1969).
137. H. Sternglanz and C. E. Bugg, Biochim. Biophys. Acta, 378: 1-11 (1975).
138. T. Kulikowski and D. Shugar, Nucleic Acids Res. Spec. Publ., 4: 7-10 (1978).
139. E. R. Kaufman and R. L. Davidson, Proc. Natl. Acad. Sci. USA, 75: 4982-4986 (1978).
140. K. K. Guari and G. Malorny, Arch. Exp. Pathol., 257: 21-22 (1967).
141. Y.-C. Cheng, B. A. Domin, R. A. Sharma, and M. Bobek, Antimicrob. Agents Chemother., 10: 119-122 (1976).
142. E. De Clercq, J. Descamps, and D. Shugar, Antimicrob. Agents Chemother., 13: 545-547 (1978).
143. E. De Clercq, Arch. Int. Physiol. Biochim., 87: 353-395 (1979).
144. E. De Clercq, J. Descamps, C. L. Schmidt, and M. P. Mertes, Biochem. Pharmacol., 28: 3259-3254 (1979).
145. C. L. Schmidt, C. T.-C. Chang, E. De Clercq, J. Descamps, and M. P. Mertes, J. Med. Chem., 23: 252-256 (1980).
146. V. S. Gupta, G. L. Bubbar, J. B. Meldrum, and R. J. Saunders, J. Med. Chem., 18: 973-976 (1975).
147. G. T. Shiau, R. F. Schinazi, M. S. Chen, and W. H. Prusoff, J. Med. Chem., 23: 127-133 (1980).
148. T. Y. Shen, J. F. McPherson, and B. O. Linn, J. Med. Chem., 9: 366-369 (1966).

149. P. F. Torrence, J. W. Spencer, A. M. Bobst, J. Descamps, and E. De Clercq, J. Med. Chem., 21: 228-231 (1978).
150. G.-F. Huang, M. Okada, E. De Clercq, and P. F. Torrence, J. Med. Chem., 24: 390-393 (1981).
151. L. A. Babiuk, B. Meldrum, V. S. Gupta, and B. T. Rouse, Antimicrob. Agents Chemother., 8: 643-650 (1975).
152. E. De Clercq, J. Descamps, P. J. Barr, A. S. Jones, P. Serafinowski, R. T. Walker, G.-F. Huang, P. F. Torrence, C. L. Schmidt, M. P. Mertes, T. Kulikowski, and D. Shugar, in Antimetabolites in Biochemistry, Biology and Medicine (J. Skoda and P. Langen, eds.), Pergamon Press, Oxford, 1979, pp. 275-285.
153. E. De Clercq, J. Descamps, P. De Somer, P. J. Barr, A. S. Jones, and R. T. Walker, Proc. Natl. Acad. Sci. USA, 76: 2947-2591 (1979).
154. E. De Clercq, J. Descamps, G. Verhelst, R. T. Walker, A. S. Jones, P. F. Torrence, and D. Shugar, J. Infect. Dis., 141: 563-574 (1980).
155. H. S. Allaudeen, J. W. Kozarich, J. R. Bertino, and E. De Clercq, Proc. Natl. Acad. Sci. USA, 78: 2698-2702 (1981).
156. T.-S. Chan, Proc. Natl. Acad. Sci, USA, 74: 1734-1738 (1977).
157. H. A. Rolton and H. M. Keir, Biochem. J., 143: 403-409 (1974).
158. G. M. Cooper, Proc. Natl. Acad. Sci. USA, 70: 3788-3792 (1973).
159. T. W. North and S. S. Cohen, Pharmacol. Ther., 4: 81-108 (1979).
160. R. A. Buchanan and F. Hess, Pharmacol. Ther., 8: 143-171 (1980).
161. G. A. Le Page, in Handbook of Experimental Pharmacology (A. C. Sartorelli and D. G. Johns, eds.), Springer-Verlag, New York, 1975, pp. 426-433.
162. C. E. Cass, in Antibiotics, Vol. II: Mechanism of Action of Antieukaryotic and Antiviral Compounds (F. E. Hahn, ed.), Springer-Verlag, New York, 1979, pp. 85-109.
163. S. S. Cohen, Med. Biol., 54: 299-326 (1976).
164. S. S. Cohen, in Nucleoside Analogues. Chemistry, Biology and Medical Applications (R. T. Walker, E. De Clercq, and F. Eckstein, eds.), Plenum Press, New York, 1979, pp. 225-245.
165. S. S. Cohen, Cancer, 40: 509-518 (1977).
166. W. W. Lee, A. Benitez, L. Goodman, and B. R. Baker, J. Am. Chem. Soc., 82: 2648-2649 (1960).
167. E. J. Reist, A. Benitez, L. Goodman, B. R. Baker, and W. W. Lee, J. Org. Chem., 27: 3274-3279 (1962).
168. C. P. J. Glaudemans and H. G. Fletcher, Jr., J. Org. Chem., 29: 3286-3290 (1964).
169. C. P. J. Glaudemans and H. G. Fletcher, Jr., J. Org. Chem., 28: 3004-3006 (1963).
170. M. Ikehara, M. Kaneko, and Y. Ogiso, Tetrahedron Lett., pp. 4673-4679 (1970).
171. M. Ikehara and Y. Ogiso, Tetrahedron, 28: 3695-3704 (1972).
172. R. Ranganathan, Tetrahedron Lett., 1185-1188 (1975).

173. K. Kadir, G. Mackenzie, and G. Shaw, J. Chem. Soc. Perkin Trans. I, 2304-2309 (1980).
174. G. P. Bodley, J. Gottlieb, K. B. McCredie, and E. J. Freireich, in Adenine Arabinoside: An Antirival Agent (D. Pavan-Langston, R. A. Buchanan, and C. A. Alford, Jr., eds.), Raven Press, New York, 1975, p. 281.
175. R. J. Whitley, S.-J. Soong, R. Dolin, G. J. Galasso, L. T. Chien, C. A. Alford, and the Collaborative Study Group, N. Engl. J. Med., 297: 289-294 (1977).
176. T. C. Merigan, First Int. Congr. Interferon Res., Washington, D.C., November 1980.
177. R. J. Whitley, A. J. Nahmias, S.-J. Soong, G. J. Galasso, C. L. Fleming, and C. A. Alford, Pediatrics, 66: 495-501 (1980).
178. M. S. Hirsch and M. N. Swartz, N. Engl. J. Med., 302: 903-907 (1980).
179. W. E. G. Muller, R. K. Zahn, K. Bittlingmaier, and D. Flake, Ann. N.Y. Acad. Sci., 284: 34-48 (1977).
180. M. S. Hershfield, J. Biol. Chem., 254: 22-25 (1979).
181. R. Vince and S. Daluge, J. Med. Chem., 20: 612-613 (1977).
182. J. A. Montgomery and K. Hewson, J. Med. Chem., 12: 498-504 (1969).
183. R. W. Brockman, F. M. Schabel, Jr., and J. A. Montgomery, Biochem. Pharmacol., 26: 2193-2196 (1977).
184. F. M. Schabel, Jr., in Nucleoside Analogues: Chemistry, Biology and Medical Applications (R. T. Walker, E. De Clercq, and F. Eckstein, eds.), Plenum Press, New York, 1979, pp. 363-394.
185. L. L. Bennett, Jr., W. M. Shannon, P. W. Allan, and G. Arnett, Ann. N.Y. Acad. Sci., 255: 342-358 (1975).
186. R. W. Sidwell, R. L. Tolman, J. H. Hoffman, G. P. Khare, L. B. Allen, and R. K. Robins, Intersci. Conf. Antimicrob. Agents Chemother., 12: 43 (1972).
187. S. Hanessian, J. Med. Chem., 16: 290-292 (1973).
188. W. W. Lee, L. V. Fisher, and L. Goodman, J. Heterocycl. Chem., 8: 179-180 (1971).
189. T. A. Khwaja, R. Harris, and R. K. Robins, Tetrahedron Lett., 4681-4684 (1972).
190. R. W. Sidwell, L. B. Allen, J. H. Huffman, T. A. Khwaja, R. L. Tolman, and R. K. Robins, Chemotherapy, 19: 325-340 (1975).
191. C. Lopez and A. Giner-Sorolla, Ann. N.Y. Acad. Sci., 284: 351-357 (1977).
192. M. Bobek, Y. C. Cheng, and A. Bloch, J. Med. Chem., 21: 597-598 (1978).
193. G. B. Elion, J. L. Rideout, P. De Miranda, P. Collins, and D. J. Bauer, Ann. N.Y. Acad. Sci., 255: 468-480 (1975).
194. W. A. Creasey, in Handbook of Experimental Pharmacology, Vol. 38, Pt. II (A. C. Sartorelli and D. G. Johns, eds.), Springer-Verlag, New York, 1974, pp. 232-256.

195. W. B. Pratt, Fundamentals of Chemotherapy, Oxford University Press, Oxford, 1973, pp. 304-305.
196. D. A. Stevens, G. W. Jordan, T. F. Waddell, and T. C. Merigan, N. Engl. J. Med., 289: 873-877 (1973).
197. J. Furth and S. Cohen, Cancer Res., 28: 2061-2067 (1968).
198. F. Graham and G. Whitmore, Cancer Res., 30: 2636-2644 (1970).
199. D. W. Kufe, P. P. Major, E. M. Egan, and G. P. Beardsley, J. Biol. Chem., 255: 8997-9000 (1980).
200. M. W. Myers-Robfogel and A. A. Spataro, Cancer Res., 40: 1940-1943 (1980).
201. A. R. Hanze, J. Am. Chem. Soc., 89: 6720-6725 (1960).
202. G. W. Camiener, Biochem. Pharmacol., 17: 1981-1991 (1968).
203. V. E. Marquez, P. S. Lin, J. A. Kelley, J. S. Driscoll, and J. J. McCormack, J. Med. Chem., 23: 715-717 (1980).
204. P. S. Lin, V. E. Marquez, J. A. Kelley, and J. S. Driscoll, J. Org. Chem., 45: 5225-5227 (1980).
205. M. Bobek, Y. C. Cheng, and A. Bloch, J. Med. Chem., 21: 597-598 (1978).
206. K. Kikugawa and M. Ichino, J. Org. Chem., 37: 284-288 (1972).
207. A. F. Russell, M. Prystasz, E. K. Hamamura, J. P. H. Verheyden, and J. G. Moffatt, J. Org. Chem., 39: 2182-2186 (1974).
208. B. Shimizu and F. Shimizu, Chem. Pharm. Bull., 18: 1060-1062 (1970).
209. J. J. Fox, W. Miller, and I. Wempen, J. Med. Chem., 9: 101-105 (1966).
210. J. H. Bunchenal, V. E. Currie, M. D. Dowling, J. J. Fox, and I. H. Krakoff, Ann. N.Y. Acad. Sci., 255: 202-212 (1975).
211. R. A. Sanchez and L. E. Orgel, J. Mol. Biol., 47: 531-543 (1970).
212. G. Ramani, J. Am. Chem. Soc., 98: 7381-7390 (1976).
213. G. R. Higgins, N. Movassaghi, A. Pyesmany, R. Baehner, R. Chard, and D. Hammond, Proc. Am. Assoc. Cancer Res., 20: 341 (1979).
214. P. Alberto, M. Rozencweig, D. Gangji, A. Brugarolas, F. Cavalli, P. Siegenthaler, H. H. Hansen, and R. Sylvester, Eur. J. Cancer, 14: 195-201 (1978).
215. K. A. Watanabe, A. Reichman, K. Hirota, C. Lopez, and J. J. Fox, J. Med. Chem., 22: 21-24 (1979).
216. C. Lopez, K. A. Watanabe, and J. J. Fox, Antimicrob. Agents Chemother., 17: 803-806 (1980).
217. J. A. Beisler, M. M. Abbasi, and J. S. Driscoll, J. Med. Chem., 22: 1230-1231 (1979).
218. A. M. Mian, R. A. Long, L. B. Allen, R. W. Sidwell, R. K. Robins, and T. A. Khwaja, J. Med. Chem., 22: 514-518 (1979).
219. Y. F. Shealy,and C. A. O'Dell, J. Heterocycl. Chem., 13: 1353-1354 (1976).
220. H. E. Renis, Cancer Res., 30: 189-194 (1970).
221. H. E. Renis, G. E. Underwood, and J. H. Hunter, Antimicrob. Agents Chemother., 1967: 675-679 (1968).

222. H. E. Prince, E. Grunberg, M. Buck, and R. Cleeland, Proc. Soc. Exp. Biol. Med., 130: 1080-1086 (1969).
223. G. A. Gentry and J. F. Aswell, Virology, 65: 294-296 (1975).
224. R. L. Miller, J. P. Iltis, and F. Rapp, J. Virol., 23: 679-684 (1977).
225. G. A. Gentry, G. P. Allen, J. McGowan, J. Aswell, and D. Campbell, in Oncogenesis and Herpesvirus III (G. de-Thé, W. Henle, and F. Rapp, eds.), Pt. 1, Int. Agency Res. Cancer, Lyon, France, 1978, pp. 1007-1012.
226. T. Ooka and A. Calendar, Virology, 104: 219-223 (1980).
227. E. Werner, G. Müller, R. K. Zahn, J. Arendes, and D. Falke, J. Gen. Virol., 43: 261-271 (1979).
228. J. F. Aswell and G. A. Gentry, Ann. N.Y. Acad. Sci., 284: 342-350 (1977).
229. J. F. Aswell, F. P. Allen, A. T. Jamieson, D. E. Campbell, and G. A. Gentry, Antimicrob. Agents Chemother., 12: 243-254 (1977).
230. A. Matsukage, T. Takahashi, C. Nakayama, and M. Sanegoshi, J. Biochem., 83: 1511-1515 (1978).
231. E. De Clercq, E. Krajewska, J. Descamps, and P. F. Torrence, Mol. Pharmacol., 13: 980-984 (1977).
232. T. Kulikowski, Z. Zawadzki, D. Shugar, J. Descamps, and E. De Clercq, J. Med. Chem., 22: 647-652 (1972).
233. T. Kulikowski, Z. Zawadzki, D. Shugar, J. Descamps, and E. De Clercq, J. Med. Chem., 22: 647-652 (1972).
234. C. Nakayama, H. Machida, and M. Saneyoshi, J. Carbohyd. Nucleosides Nucleotides, 6: 295-308 (1979).
235. P. F. Torrence, G.-F. Huang, M. W. Edwards, B. Bhooshan, J. Descamps, and E. De Clercq, J. Med. Chem., 22: 316-319 (1979).
236. E. De Clercq, P. F. Torrence, J. A. Waters, and B. Witkop, Biochem. Pharmacol., 24: 2171-2175 (1975).
237. T. Ueda, S. Watanabe, and A. Matsuda, J. Carbohyd. Nucleosides Nucleotides, 5: 523-535 (1978).
238. H. Machida, A. Kininaka, H. Yoshino, K. Iheda, and Y. Mizuno, Antimicrob. Agents Chemother., 17: 1030-1031 (1980).
239. R. F. Schinazi, M. S. Chen, and W. H. Prusoff, J. Med. Chem., 22: 1273-1277 (1979).
240. G. E. Underwood, in Third International Congress of Chemotherapy, Vol. 1 (H. P. Kuemmerle and P. Preziosi, eds.), Hafner, New York, 1964, pp. 858-860.
241. B. Rada and J. Doskocil, Pharmacol. Ther., 9: 171-217 (1980).
242. P. Calabresi, Ann. N.Y. Acad. Sci., 130: 198-208 (1965).
243. V. Myska, J. Elis, J. Plevova, and H. Raskova, Lancet, 1: 1230-1231 (1967).
244. S. M. H. Jaffari and A. Hussain, Ind. J. Med. Res., 57: 808-814 (1969).

245. W. Saenger and D. Suck, Nature, 242: 610-612 (1973).
246. W. Saenger, D. Suck, M. Knappenberg, and J. Dirkx, Biopolymers, 18: 2015-2037 (1979).
247. S. Rodaway and A. Marcus, J. Biol. Chem., 255: 8402-8404 (1980).
248. D. D. Von Hoff and M. Slavik, Adv. Pharmacol. Ther., 14: 285-326 (1977).
249. D. D. Von Hoff, M. Slavik, and F. M. Muggia, Ann. Intern. Med., 85: 237-245 (1976).
250. J. Vesely and A. Cihak, Pharmacol. Ther. A, 2: 813-840 (1978).
251. A. Piskala and F. Sorm, Collect. Czech. Chem. Commun., 29: 2060-2076 (1964).
252. L. J. Hanka, J. S. Evans, D. J. Mason, and A. Dietz, Antimicrob. Agents Chemother., 619-624 (1966).
253. A. Piskala, P. Riedler, and F. Sorm, Nucleic Acids Res., Spec. Publ., 1: S17-S20 (1975).
254. M. W. Winkley and R. K. Robins, J. Org. Chem., 35: 491-495 (1970).
255. U. Niedballa and H. Vorgrüggen, J. Org. Chem., 39: 3672-3674 (1974).
256. G. A. Omura, Proc. Am. Assoc. Cancer Res., 18: 25 (1977).
257. R. J. Suhadolnik, Prog. Nucleic Acid Res. Mol. Biol., 22: 193-291 (1979).
258. R. I. Glazer and K. D. Hartman, Mol. Pharmacol., 17: 250-255 (1980).
259. P. A. Jones and S. M. Taylor, Cell, 20: 85-93 (1980).
260. P. Pithova, A. Piskala, J. Pitha, and F. Sorm, Collect. Czech. Chem. Commun., 30: 2801-2811 (1965).
261. J. A. Beisler, J. Med. Chem., 21: 204-208 (1978).
262. Z. H. Israili, W. R. Vogler, E. S. Mingioli, J. L. Pirkle, R. W. Smithwick, and J. H. Goldstein, Cancer Res., 36: 1453-1461 (1976).
263. J. A. Beisler, M. M. Abbasi, and J. S. Driscoll, Cancer Treat. Rep., 60: 1671-1674 (1976).
264. J. A. Beisler, M. M. Abbasi, J. A. Kelley, and J. S. Driscoll, J. Carbohydr. Nucleosides, Nucleotides, 4: 281-299 (1977).
265. J. A. Beisler, M. M. Abbasi, J. A. Kelley, and J. S. Driscoll, J. Med. Chem., 20: 806-812 (1977).
266. J. T. Witkowski, R. K. Robins, R. W. Sidwell, and L. N. Simon, J. Med. Chem., 15: 1150-1154 (1972).
267. R. W. Sidwell, J. H. Huffman, G. P. Khare, L. B. Allen, J. T. Witkowski, L. N. and R. K. Robins, Science, 177: 705-706 (1972).
268. R. W. Sidwell, R. K. Robins, and I. W. Hillyard, Pharmacol. Ther., 6: 123-146 (1979).
269. J. G. Bekesi, J. P. Roboz, E. Zimmerman, and J. F. Holland, Cancer Res., 36: 631-639 (1976).

270. L. W. Klassen, G. W. Williams, J. L. Reinersten, W. L. Gerber, and A. D. Steinberg, Arthritis Rheum., 22: 145-154 (1979).
271. J. B. McCormick, P. A. Webb, and K. M. Johnson, in Ribavirin a Broad Spectrum Antiviral Agent (R. A. Smith and W. Kirkpatrick, eds.), Academic Press, New York, 1980, pp. 213-214.
272. R. A. Smith, in Ribavirin, a Broad Spectrum Antiviral Agent (R. A. Smith and W. Kirkpatrick, eds.), Academic Press, New York, 1980, pp. 99-118.
273. P. Prusiner and M. Sundaralingam, Nature New Biol., 244: 116-117 (1973).
274. D. G. Streeter, J. T. Witkowski, G. P. Khare, R. W. Sidwell, R. J. Bauer, R. K. Robins, and L. N. Simon, Proc. Natl. Acad. Sci. USA, 70: 1174-1178 (1973).
275. C. M. Smith, L. J. Fontenelle, H. Unger, L. W. Brox, and J. F. Henderson, Biochem. Pharmacol., 23: 2727-2735 (1974).
276. J. C. Drach, J. W. Barnett, M. A. Thomas, S. H. Smith, and C. Shipman, Jr., in Ribavirin, a Broad Spectrum Antiviral Agent (R. A. Smith and W. Kirkpatrick, eds.), Academic Press, New York, 1980, pp. 119-128.
277. J. S. Oxford, J. Antimicrob. Chemother., 1: 7-23 (1976).
278. B. Eriksson, E. Helgstrand, N. G. Johannson, A. Larsson, A. Misiorng, J. O. Noren, L. Philipson, K. Stenberg, G. Stening, S. Stridh, and B. Oberg, Antimicrob. Agents Chemother., 11: 946-951 (1977).
279. S. Harris and R. K. Robins, in Ribavirin, a Broad Spectrum Antiviral Agent (R. A. Smith and W. Kirkpatrick, eds.), Academic Press, New York, 1980, pp. 1-21.
280. A. K. Drabikowska, L. Dudycz, and D. Shugar, J. Med. Chem., 22: 653-657 (1979).
281. E. De Clercq, M. Luczsk, J. C. Reepmeyer, K. L. Kirk, and L. A. Cohen, Life Sci., 17: 187-194 (1976).
282. J. Goddard, in Ribavirin, a Broad Spectrum Antiviral Agent (R. A. Smith and W. Kirkpatrick, eds.), Academic Press, New York, 1980, pp. 231-233.
283. E. De Clercq, J. Descamps, P. De Somer, and A. Holy, Science, 200: 563-565 (1978).
284. H. J. Schaeffer, L. Beauchamp, P. de Miranda, G. B. Elion, D. J. Bauer, and P. Collins, Nature, 272: 583-585 (1978).
285. G. B. Elion, P. A. Furman, J. A. Fyfe, P. de Miranda, L. Beauchamp, and J. J. Schaeffer, Proc. Natl. Acad. Sci. USA, 74: 5716-5720 (1978).
286. T. W. North and S. S. Cohen, Proc. Natl. Acad. Sci. USA, 75: 4684-4688 (1978).
287. J. A. Fyfe, P. M. Keller, P. A. Furman, R. L. Miller, and G. B. Elion, J. Biol. Chem., 253: 8721-8727 (1978).

288. P. A. Furman, H. H. St. Clair, J. A. Fyfe, J. L. Rideout, P. M. Keller, and G. B. Elion, J. Virol., 32: 72-77 (1979).
289. P. A. Furman, P. V. McGuirt, P. M. Keller, J. A. Fyfe, and G. B. Elion, Virology, 102: 420-430 (1980).
290. J. R. Barrio, J. D. Bryant, and G. E. Keyser, J. Med. Chem., 23: 572-574 (1980).
291. E. De Clercq and A. Holy, J. Med. Chem., 22: 510-513 (1979).
292. E. Klein, G. H. Burgess, A. Bloch, H. Milgrom, and O. A. Holtermann, Ann. N.Y. Acad. Sci., 255: 216-224 (1975).
293. J. J. Jaffe, Ann. N.Y. Acad. Sci., 255: 306-316 (1975).
294. H. Kasai, Z. Ohashi, F. Harada, S. Nishimura, W. J. Oppenheimer, P. F. Crain, J. G. Liehr, D. L. vonMinden, and J. A. McCloskey, Biochemistry, 14: 4198-4208 (1975).
295. S. Yokoyama, T. Miyazawa, Y. Tituka, Z. Yamaizumi, H. Kasai, and S. Nishimura, Nature, 282: 107-109 (1979).
296. A. L. McNamara and D. W. E. Smith, J. Biol. Chem., 253: 5964-5970 (1978).
297. P. E. Olsen and E. E. Penhoet, Biochemistry, 15: 4649-4654 (1976).
298. W. T. Brisco, A. C. Griffen, C. McBride, and J. M. Bowen, Cancer Res., 35: 2586-2593 (1975).
299. J. R. Katze, Biochem. Biophys. Res. Commun., 84: 527-535 (1978).
300. J. R. Katze and W. R. Farkas, Proc. Natl. Acad. Sci. USA, 76: 3271-3275 (1975).
301. N. Shindo-Okada, N. Okada, T. Ohgi, T. Goto, and S. Nishimura, Biochemistry, 19: 395-400 (1980).
302. N. Okada, N. Noguchi, S. Nishimura, T. Ohgi, T. Goto, P. F. Crain, and J. A. McCloskey, Nucleic Acids Res., 5: 2289-2295 (1978).
303. W. Okada, N. Shindo-Okada, S. Sato, Y. H. Itoh, K.-I. Oda, and S. Nishimura, Proc. Natl. Acad. Sci. USA, 75: 4247-4251 (1978).
304. J. R. Katze, Nucleic Acids Res., 5: 2513-2524 (1978).
305. R.-M. Landin, M. Boisnard, and G. Petrissant, Nucleic Acids Res., 7: 1635-1648 (1979).
306. C. D. Jackson, C. C. Irving, and B. H. Sells, Biochim. Biophys. Acta, 217: 64-71 (1970).
307. W. R. Farkas, J. Biol. Chem., 255: 6832-6835 (1980).
308. B. A. Roe, A. F. Stankiewicz, H. L. Rizi, C. Weisz, M. N. Dilauro, D. Pike, C. V. Chen, and E. Y. Chen, Nucleic Acids Res., 6: 673-688 (1979).
309. M. Marini and J. F. Mushinsky, Biochim. Biophys. Acta, 562: 252-270 (1979).
310. J. R. Katze and W. T. Beck, Biochem. Biophys. Res. Commun., 96: 313-319 (1980).
311. A. J. Shatkin, Cell, 9: 645-653 (1976).

312. F. M. Rottman, in Biochemistry of Nucleic Acids (B. F. C. Clark, ed.), 17: 45-73 (1978).
313. A. K. Banerjee, Microbiol. Rev., 44: 175-205 (1980).
314. C. H. Kim and R. H. Sarma, J. Am. Chem. Soc., 100: 1571-1590 (1978).
315. M. Bouloy, S. J. Plotch, and R. M. Krug, Proc. Natl. Acad. Sci. USA, 75: 4886-4890 (1978).
316. S. J. Plotch, M. Bouloy, and R. M. Krug, Proc. Natl. Acad. Sci. USA, 76: 1618-1622 (1979).
317. R. T. Borchardt, J. Med. Chem., 23: 347-357 (1980).
318. P. K. Chiang, G. L. Cantoni, J. P. Bader, W. M. Shannon, H. J. Thomas, and J. A. Montgomery, Biochem. Biophys. Res. Commun., 82: 417-423 (1978).
319. R. J. Rousseau, L. B. Townsend, and R. K. Robins, Biochemistry, 5: 756-760 (1966).
320. J. A. May and L. B. Townsend, J. Chem. Soc. Perkin Trans. I, 125-129 (1975).
321. J. A. Montgomery, A. T. Shortnacy, and S. D. Clayton, J. Heterocyc. Chem., 14: 195-197 (1977).
322. N. M. Kredich, J. Biol. Chem., 255: 7380-7385 (1980).
323. M. S. Hershfield, J. Biol. Chem., 254: 22-25 (1979).
324. M. Robert-Gero and E. Lederer, in Frontiers in Bioorganic Chemistry and Molecular Biology (Y. A. Ovchinnikov and M. N. Kolosov, eds.), Elsevier/North-Holland, Amsterdam, 1979, pp. 113-128.
325. M. Pankaskie and M. M. Abdel-Monem, J. Med. Chem., 23: 121-127 (1980).
326. F. Hirata and J. Axelrod, Science, 209: 1082-1090 (1980).
327. A. C. Schroeder, T. J. Bardos, and Y.-C. Cheng, J. Med. Chem., 24: 109-112 (1981).
328. I. M. Kerr and R. E. Brown, Proc. Natl. Acad. Sci. USA, 75: 256-260 (1978).
329. C. Baglioni, Cell, 17: 255-264 (1979).
330. P. F. Torrence, Mol. Aspects Med., 5: 129-171 (1982).

6

SYNTHESIS AND CHARACTERIZATION OF NITROSOUREAS

DONALD J. REED

Oregon State University
Corvallis, Oregon

I. INTRODUCTION

An effective chemist in drug development must have some understanding of the interplay between the design and synthesis of drugs, biological test systems, human toxicity, pharmacodynamics of parent drug and its metabolites, modes of drug action, and clinical efficacy of single drugs and drug combinations. This is particularly true for the nitrosoureas, which are an extremely interesting class of drugs for cancer chemotherapy due to their unique chemical and biological characteristics. Many new nitrosourea congeners are being synthesized and tested in laboratories around the world. The basis for these efforts and some of the factors to be considered in the design, synthesis, and testing of new congeners are the subject of this chapter. Because of the unique properties of certain nitrosoureas, they may remain important research tools for cell research long beyond any clinical usefulness.

II. HISTORICAL BACKGROUND

The Cancer Chemotherapy National Service Center screening program provided the interest and resources for antitumor activitiy. 1-Methyl-3-nitro-1-nitrosoguanidine was found to increase the life span of mice implanted intraperitoneally with leukemia L1210 cells. Investigators at the Southern Research Institute observed that 1-methyl-1-nitrosourea was an even more effective agent against L1210 cells [1]. They subsequently initiated a program which has resulted in the synthesis and testing of hundreds of N-nitrosoureas. The congeners of major importance are those containing a 2-chloroethyl moiety on the nitrogen atom attached to the nitroso group. Three drugs emerged and underwent intense testing: 1,3-bis(2-chloroethyl)-1-nitrosourea (BCNU), 1-(2-chloroethyl)-3-cyclohexyl-1-nitrosourea (CCNU), and 1-(2-chloroethyl)-3-(trans-4-methylcyclohexyl)-1-nitrosourea (methyl CCNU). Because of the ability of these lipophilic drugs to cross the blood-brain barrier and to be effective against solid tumors (including brain tumors), as well as leukemias, great interest developed in their clinical efficacy. A large body of literature exists from 20 years of study of these and of other nitrosoureas. The National Cancer Institute considers nitrosoureas to be one of the most important classes of antitumor agents developed by the Cancer Chemotherapy Program [2].

III. SYNTHESIS

Conventional synthesis of nitrosoureas utilizes the reaction of an amine with an organic isocyanate to yield a parent urea [1] (Fig. 6.1). The urea is nitrosated under conditions that ultimately favor the formation of the 1-nitroso rather than the 3-nitroso isomer. A bulky R group on the N-3 amine nitrogen often assures a predominance of the 1-nitroso isomer.

$$RNCO + H_2NR' \rightarrow RNHCONHR' \rightarrow RN(NO)CONHR' + RNHCON(NO)R'$$

1-Nitroso 3-Nitroso

FIGURE 6.1 Steps in the synthesis of nitrosoureas.

A. Synthesis Procedures

Unsymmetrical rather than symmetrical 1,3-disubstituted ureas comprise the majority of the parent ureas employed for nitrosourea syntheses. Commercial availability of 2-chloroethylisocyanate has provided a convenient precursor which requires only redistillation prior to use. Whereas a large variety of amines are commercially available, the synthesis of many nitrosoureas involves either custom synthesis of a particular amine or resolution of either urea or nitrosourea isomers. For example, May et al. [3] prepared 1-(2-chloroethyl)-3-(trans-4-hydroxycyclohexyl)-1-nitrosourea (trans-4-hydroxy-CCNU (Table 6.1) and the corresponding cis-4-hydroxy-CCNU by reaction of 2-chloroethylisocyanate with 4-hydroxycyclohexylamine followed by nitrosation and separation of the cis- and trans-4-hydroxy CCNUs from their 3-nitroso isomers by preparative high-pressure liquid chromatography (HPLC). In contrast, Johnston et al. [4] prepared large quantities of pure trans-4-aminocyclohexanol by the hydrolysis of fractionated cis, trans-N-(4-hydroxycyclohexyl)acetamide. Failure to obtain pure cis-acetamide by fractionation required preparation of pure cis-4-aminocyclohexanol via catalytic hydrogenation of 2-oxa-3-azabicyclo[2.2.2]oct-5-ene hydrochloride [4]. Synthesis of nitrosoureas containing a monohydroxylated methylcyclohexyl moiety required the catalytic reduction of the appropriate aromatic amine. Pure cis-3-hydroxy-trans-4-methyl CCNU (Table 6.2) and trans-3-hydroxy-trans-4-methyl CCNU were prepared by catalytic hydrogenation of 5-acetamido-o-cresol followed by hydrolysis to yield cis, trans-3-hydroxy-cis, trans-4-methylcyclohexylamine which was converted to cis, trans-3-hydroxy-cis, trans-4-methyl CCNU. Pure isomers were isolated by preparative HPLC and their structures determined by mass spectrometry (MS) and detailed nuclear magnetic resonance (NMR) analysis with $Eu(fod)_3$ shift reagent [5].

The general lack of therapeutic efficacy of the 3-isomers of nitrosoureas has led to considerable effort to establish the most appropriate nitrosation conditions for individual ureas. Nitrosating agents have been discussed in some detail and they include anhydrous sodium nitrite, dinitrogen trioxide, dinitrogen tetraoxide, and transnitrosation from a nitrosourea [6]. Unsymmetrical ureas that contain two protons on both carbons alpha to the urea nitrogen atoms generally yield a mixture of nitroso isomers, with the exception that a methyl substitutent directs exclusive nitrosation to the nitrogen attached to the methyl group [6]. For further discussion of the nitrosation step, see Johnston et al. [7].

TABLE 6.1 Nitrosoureas in Commercial Use and Certain of Their Metabolites

Code	Compound	R- = NH-C(=O)-N(NO)-CH_2-CH_2-C1*	Reference
BCNU NSC 409962	1-3-Bis(2-chloroethyl)-1-nitrosourea	R-CH_2-CH_2-C1	7
CCNU NSC 79037	1-(2-Chloroethyl)-3-cyclohexyl-1-nitrosourea		7
trans-2-Hydroxy CCNU NSC 253947	1-(2-Cyloroethyl)-3-trans-2-hydroxycyclohexyl)-1-nitrosourea	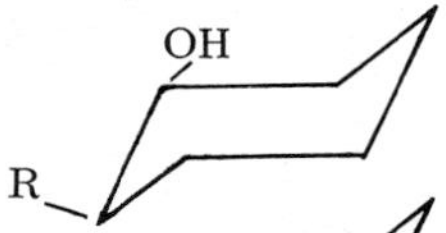	3
cis-3-Hydroxy CCNU NSC 253945	1-(2-Chloroethyl)-3-(cis-3-hydroxycyclohexyl)-1-nitrosourea	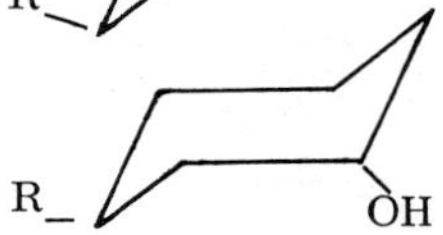	3
cis-4-Hydroxy CCNU NSC 239724	1-(2-Chloroethyl)-3-cis-4-hydroxycyclohexyl)-1-nitrosourea	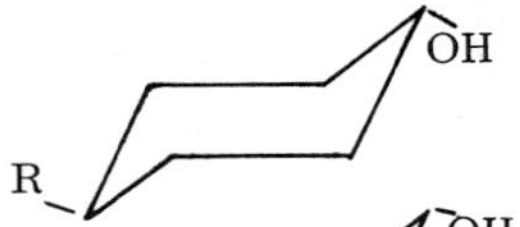	3
trans-4-Hydroxy CCNU NSC 239717	1-(2-Chloroethyl)-3-(trans-4-hydroxycyclohexyl)-1-nitrosourea	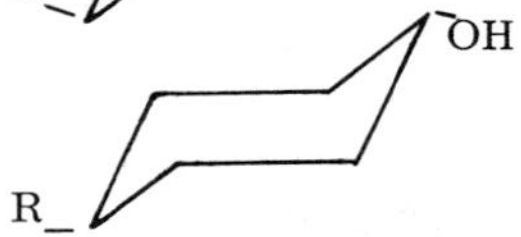	3

TABLE 6.2 Methyl CCNU Congeners and Certain Metabolites

Code	Compound	R = NH-C(=O)-N(NO)-CH_2CH_2-Cl	Reference
Me CCNU NSC 95441	1-(2-Chloroethyl)-3-(*trans*-4-methylcyclohexyl)-1-nitrosourea	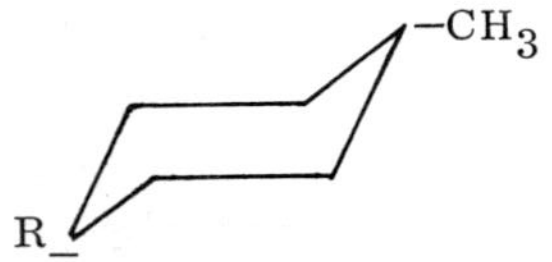 R, $-CH_3$	7
cis-4-Hydroxy-*trans*-4-methyl CCNU	1-(2-Chloroethyl)-3-(*cis*-4-hydroxy-*trans*-4-methylcyclohexyl)-1-nitrosourea	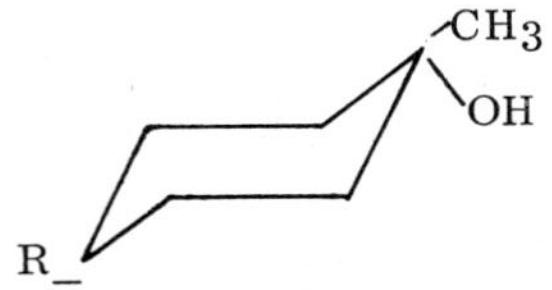 R, CH_3, OH	5
trans-4-Hydroxy-*cis*-4-methyl CCNU	1-(2-Chloroethyl)-3-(*trans*-4-hydroxy-*cis*-4-methylcyclohexyl)-1-nitrosourea	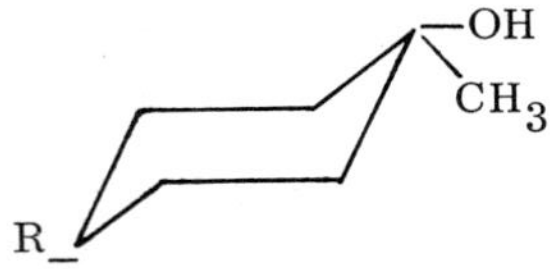 R, $-OH$, CH_3	5
cis-3-Hydroxy-*trans*-4-methyl CCNU	1-(2-Chloroethyl)-3-(*cis*-3-hydroxy-*trans*-4-methylcyclohexyl)-1-nitrosourea	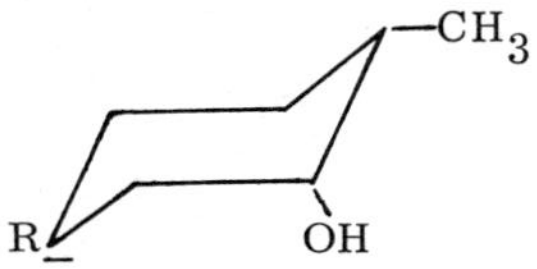 R, $-CH_3$, OH	5

TABLE 6.2 (Continued)

Code	Compound	R = NH-C(=O)-N(NO)-CH_2CH_2-Cl	Reference
trans-3-Hydroxy-*trans*-4-methyl CCNU	1-(2-Chloroethyl)-3-(*trans*-3-hydroxy)-*trans*-4-methyl-cyclohexyl)-1-nitrosourea	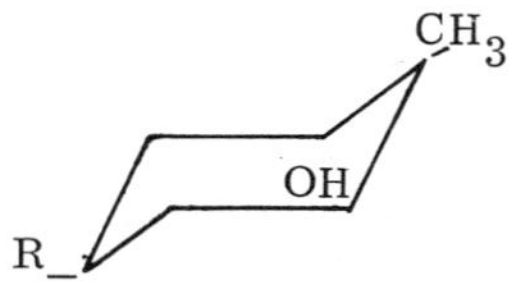 R, OH, CH_3	5
trans-4-Hydroxymethyl CCNU	1-(2-Chloroethyl)-3-(*trans*-4-hydroxymethylcyclohexyl)-1-nitrosourea	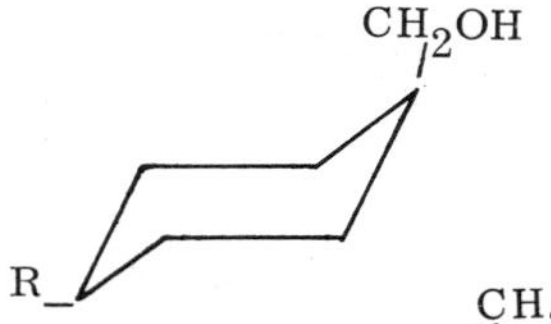 R, CH_2OH	5
α-Hydroxymethyl CCNU	1-(1-Hydroxy-2-chloroethyl)-3-(*trans*-4-methylcyclohexyl)-1-nitrosourea	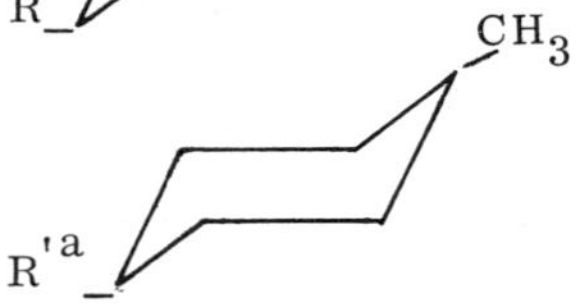 R'[a], CH_3	5

[a] R', NH-C(=O)-N(NO)-CH(OH)-CH_2-Cl.

B. Analytical Techniques

The prominent infrared absorption bands in the carbonyl stretching region (1620-1750 cm^{-1}) characterize the nitrosoureas. Nitrosation of urea functions was found to cause consistently a shift toward higher wave numbers in the carbonyl region [1]. Nitroso isomer identification has been established by proton magnetic resonance (PMR) spectroscopy by demonstrating a spectral symmetry of the $ClCH_2CH_2N(NO)$ group (A_2B_2 system) [7, 8]. Mass spectral fragmentation patterns have been shown to be very useful in establishing nitroso isomer identification [3, 5]. Ultraviolet (UV) absorbance at about 230 nm provides a means of detection and quantitation of nitrosoureas. Quantitation by HPLC at nanomole levels is made possible with sensitive UV flow detectors [3, 5]. An elegant analytical method based on stable isotope dilution analysis and mass spectrometry has been described for BCNU [9].

IV. CHEMICAL DEGRADATION

The chemistry of the nitrosoureas is complex and new degradation products continue to be identified. New pathways continue to be proposed to illustrate the chemical steps that may occur in the formation of these degradation products. Some products are very reactive intermediates that are essential for the biological effects of the nitrosoureas by mechanisms that remain poorly understood.

A. Degradation Pathways and Reactive Intermediates

Decomposition of nitrosoureas in aqueous solution is spontaneous and dependent on pH, buffer, and temperature. Typical decomposition rates afford a range of half-lives from 46 min for chlorozotocin [6] to 70 min for methyl CCNU [10]. Isocyanate formation during nitrosourea degradation was established in early studies [11]. Alkylating species were observed indirectly with the nitrobenzylpyridine assay method [12]. Vinyl carbonium ions were suggested as the alkylating species from BCNU [13]. However, Reed and co-workers [10] examined in detail the decomposition of CCNU and methyl CCNU at pH 7.4 in phosphate buffer and found the major alkylating species to be capable of 2-chloroethylation. 2-Chloroethanol is a major decomposition product with small amounts of acetaldehyde, vinyl chloride, and ethylene. At the same time, Colvin et al. [14] concluded that BCNU decomposition produced primarily a chloroethylcarbonium ion intermediate as the alkylating species. Dependence on pH was later noted for the difference in degradation products with low pH, producing acetaldehyde, whereas neutral pH produces greatly enhanced quantities of 2-chloroethanol [15].

Recent studies illustrate the complexity of the degradation events of the 2-chloroethylnitrosoureas. Lown and Chauhan [16] described the synthesis of three 2-(alkylimino)-3-nitrosooxazolidines that correspond to degradation intermediates of BCNU, CCNU, and methyl CCNU. These intermediates are proposed to be formed via a minor pathway (Fig. 6.2) of degradation, yet may account in part for the 2-hydroxyethylated nucleoside products reported by other workers.

The appropriateness of chloride ion as a leaving group for 2-chloroethylnitrosoureas has been discussed in terms of an effective chemical compromise in reactivity. Chloride leaving group ability is low enough to not favor competing pathways of nitrosourea degradation involving oxadiazoline, imino-N-nitrosooxazolidinones, or hybrid migrations which can limit 2-chloroethyl alkylations (Fig. 6.2). Yet, after chloroethylation, labilization of the chloride and production of interstrand cross-links can occur. It appears that the probability of cross-linking events is maximized with chloroethylation compared to other haloethylation [18]. Interestingly, FCCNU, which contains a decafluorocyclohexyl ring, rapidly converts to the corresponding 1(1_H_-decaflurocyclohexyl)-3-nitrosoimidazolidin-2-one by chloride being a leaving group [19]. CCNU did not form a detectable quantity of the imidazolidine derivative, which suggests that a

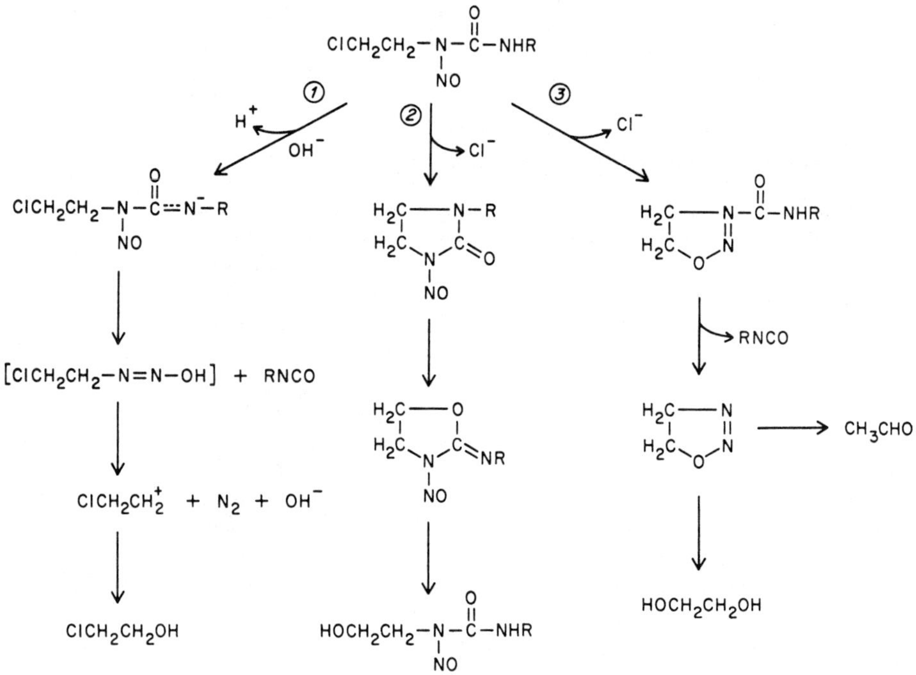

FIGURE 6.2 Possible routes of nitrosourea degradation, including the Formation of 2-(Alkylimino)-3-nitroso oxazolidine and 4,5-Dihydro-1-2,2-oxadiazole intermediates. (From Refs. 16 and 17.)

decafluorocyclohexyl moiety enhances the nucleophilicity of the N-3 nitrogen atom to facilitate the cyclization and the loss of chloride ion [19].

Brundrett [20] has found evidence for the intermediacy of 4,5-dihydro-1,2,3-oxadiazole in BCNU decomposition. Formation of ethylene glycol as a degradation product of BCNU was noted. They concluded that its formation is best explained by an oxidiazole intermediate. Again this intermediate is thought to play only a minor role in the decomposition of BCNU at physiological pH and to have little or no antitumor activity [20].

V. METABOLISM

The short half-lives of the nitrosoureas in buffer at physiological pH and in vivo as plasma half-lives led to an initial assumption that these drugs would have little opportunity to undergo metabolism in vivo (for a review, see Ref. 21). Not only was this assumption erroneous, it is now generally accepted that the biological activity of CCNU is expressed through its metabolites; these are formed by an extremely rapid monohydroxylation of the cyclohexyl ring by cytochrome P-450-dependent enzymes. Evidence is accumulating to suggest that in vivo denitrosation is important to the pharmacodynamics of certain nitrosoureas.

A. Cytochrome P-450 Monooxygenase-Dependent Hydroxylation

During the past 15 years cytochrome P-450-dependent enzymes have been established as the major enzymes responsible for the biotransformation of lipophilic drugs. Lipophilic nitrosoureas, including CCNU and methyl CCNU, undergo cytochrome P-450-dependent monooxygenation at cyclohexyl ring carbon atoms (Tables 6.1 and 6.2). Methyl CCNU is also hydroxylated in the 2-chloroethyl side chain (Table 6.2). Cytochrome P-450 present in rat liver microsomes prepared from liver of phenobarbital-induced rats catalyzes rapid monooxygenation of CCNU to yield 5-hydroxy CCNU metabolites [3,21-25]. Within 2 min after intravenous administration of CCNU to rats, a majority of the CCNU in the liver is metabolized and hydroxy CCNU metabolites are detectable in all organs examined [24]. Methyl CCNU displays a slower rate of monooxygenation than CCNU and has a more complex metabolic pattern than CCNU [5]. The presence of a _trans_-4-methyl group decreases the rate of monooxygenation of methyl CCNU 25% compared to CCNU [5]. The methyl group is hydroxylated to some extent and a small amount of _trans_-4-hydroxy-_cis_-4-methyl CCNU formation occurs possibly via a free-radical intermediate which facilitates some methyl group "flip" [26].

Efforts have been made toward metabolism-directed design of new nitrosourea congeners. An attempt was made to direct the metabolic formation of specific hydroxy CCNU metabolites with specific deuterium labeling of the cyclohexyl ring [27]. Whereas a metabolic shift is achieved, the fraction of the metabolite desired, _trans_-2-hydroxy CCNU, remains too small compared to total metabolite formation for a noticeable change in therapeutic effect.

More recently, fluorinated congeners of CCNU were synthesized and tested in hopes that such congeners would be more effective antitumor agents than CCNU due to possible blocking of ring hydroxylation and changes in physiochemical characteristics [19]. The 3-(1H-decafluorocyclohexyl) analog of CCNU (FCCNU) was found to be more toxic and possess less antitumor activity than CCNU. This congener favors chemical decomposition via a 3-nitrosoimidazolidin-2-one intermediate. A mixture of this intermediate and a 1-(nonafluorocyclohexyl) derivative appears to be responsible for the observed toxicity of FCCNU [19].

B. Nitrosourea Denitrosation

The lack of antitumor activity of methylurea as well as other ureas demonstrates the requirement of the N-nitroso moiety [28]. Chemically, the nitroso moiety of methyl CCNU can be quantitatively removed with the formation of methyl CCU by hydrogenation in ethanol in the presence of 5% rhodium on charcoal at 25°C and 1 atm [5]. Biologically, BCNU undergoes denitrosation, which is catalyzed by liver microsomes in the presence of NADPH [29]. Recent evidence has demonstrated that nitric oxide is formed as a product of denitrosation under anaerobic conditions [30]. Cytochrome P-450 can form a nitroso complex during denitrosation of CCNU with an absorption maximum at 445 nm [24]. Certain nitrosoureas can undergo denitrosation in vivo with loss of antitumor activity, especially after induction of the liver endoplasmic reticulum with phenobarbital. Phenobarbital pretreatment of rats bearing intracerebral 9L tumors eliminates the antitumor activity of BCNU and decreases the efficacy of PCNU [1-(2-chloroethyl)-3-(2,6-dioxo-3-piperidyl)-1-nitrosourea] and CCNU [31]. Decreased systemic toxicity to the host rats is observed, which agrees with a microsomal-catalyzed rate of BCNU disappearance that doubles by phenobarbital pretreatment [31].

Denitrosation is a parameter that may have great importance in the design and efficacy of new nitrosourea drugs. Every nitrosourea examined thus far can undergo anaerobic denitrosation catalyzed by liver microsomes in the presence of NADPH [30]. The rates of denitrosation reveal a sufficient variation between the nitrosoureas tested to indicate that a low denitrosation rate may modify the therapeutic index of a congener.

VI. MODE OF ACTION

Many nitrosoureas are remarkable in their ability to achieve complete cures of various tumors in test animals. Except for one factor, these drugs undoubtedly would be equally impressive in achieving cures of many neoplasms in humans. This factor, toxicity to normal cells as well as malignant cells, is extremely severe with the nitrosoureas. A wide range of toxicities is exhibited when nitrosoureas are administered to either test animals or humans. These include bone marrow suppression (myelosuppression or myelotoxicity), alopecia (loss of hair), interference with spermatogenesis, and of particular importance to patients, nausea and vomiting. Since rapidly proliferating cells or tissue have growth characteristics similar to tumor cells, they are the most susceptible to these cytotoxic effects. Alteration of genetic material is expressed not only by tytotoxicity, but also by the ability of the nitrosoureas to be mutagenic and somewhat carcinogenic. These effects have been reviewed [32]. Cytotoxicity is so severe with the 2-chloroethylnitrosoureas that cancer cell kill plays a greater role than transformation of normal cells to malignancy and tumor formation.

Much of the effort on development of new nitrosoureas has been directed toward decreasing the dose-limiting bone marrow suppression. Chlorozotocin is an example of a drug that was designed to maintain therapeutic efficacy while attempting to minimize host toxicity [33]. Sections VI.A and VI.B should provide some views as to why chlorozotocin does not achieve this goal to the extent desired.

A. Alkylation

Nonenzymic degradation of 2-chloroethylnitrosoureas, which may be protein mediated under certain conditions [34], is responsible for the generation of a common but penultimate alkylating intermediate, 2-chloroethyldiazene hydroxide (Fig. 6.2). This hypothetical intermediate (also known as a diazohydroxide) is very unstable and yet appears to have an important role in the selective alkylation events of DNA. This role has been discussed in detail for the corresponding diazene hydroxides derived from degradation of methyl- and ethylnitrosourea [35, 36]. Formation of either 2-chloroethanol or 1-bromo-2-chloroethane in the presence of bromide ion during CCNU degradation is strong evidence for an intermediate capable of 2-chloroethylation of biological molecules [10]. Evidence against a classical SN_1 reaction mechanism for BCNU alkylation has been reported by Brundrett et al. [37] from studies with deuterated BCNU. They propose that a reaction which has a 2-chloroethylcarbonium ion intermediate would yield products predominantly from rearranged 1-chloroethylcarbonium ion and cyclic chloronium ions. The major product, 2-chloroethanol, was mostly unrearranged (90%) [37]. Since SN_2 reactions of the diazene hydroxide are of low activation energy, little selectivity is proposed for the concerted loss of N_2 and alkylation of either sulfur, oxygen, or nitrogen atoms [37]. Differences in oxygen atom alkylation by ethyl- and methylnitrosoureas would suggest that alkylation site affinity for the diazene hydroxide cannot be ruled out entirely [36].

Ludlum and co-workers have studied extensively alkylation modifications of DNA and RNA bases by nitrosoureas. Structures of the modified bases are shown in Fig. 6.3. Properties of these derivatives are reviewed [38].

The modified bases have been categoriezed into two classes: those derived from a single substitution at a nucleophilic site and those involving a two-step modification. The haloethyl, hydroxyethyl, and aminoethyl modified bases are placed in the first group [38]. The formation of

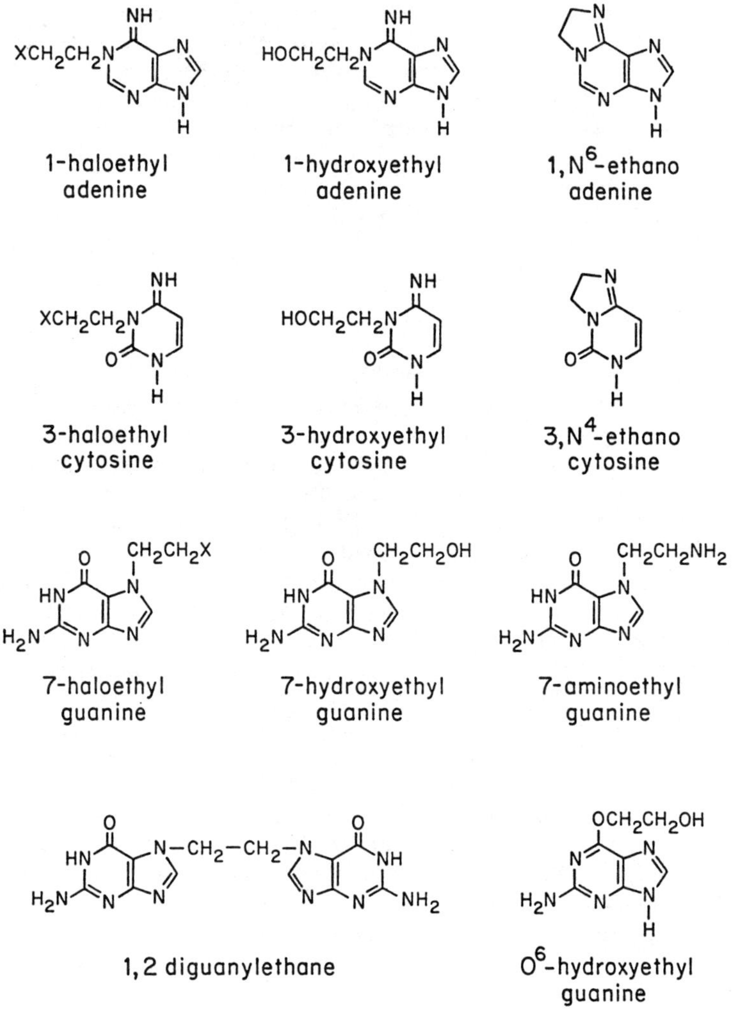

1-haloethyl adenine

1-hydroxyethyl adenine

1,N^6-ethano adenine

3-haloethyl cytosine

3-hydroxyethyl cytosine

3,N^4-ethano cytosine

7-haloethyl guanine

7-hydroxyethyl guanine

7-aminoethyl guanine

1,2 diguanylethane

O^6-hydroxyethyl guanine

FIGURE 6.3 Structures of alkylated bases derived from 2-haloethylnitrosourea alkylation events as identified by Ludlum and Tong. (From Ref. 38.]

diguanylethane represents a DNA cross-linking event which probably is intrastrand in nature but interstrand cross-linking cannot be ruled out at this time [39]. Some of the unique cytotoxic properties of the nitrosoureas may relate to interstrand DNA cross-linking processes which were first observed with purified DNA by physical studies by Kohn [18] and Lown and co-workers [40]. We are still unable to describe these events chemically and therefore we cannot fully assess their impact on loss of cellular function, including cellular repair processes. Studies on DNA cross-linking have been reviewed [41]. Efforts to quantitate alkylation of DNA in intact cells and bone marrow has led workers to conclude that differences in DNA alkylation may relate to differences of bone marrow toxicity of nitrosoureas [42]. These workers conclude that decreased myelotoxicity of an individual nitrosourea compared to other nitrosoureas may relate to localization of DNA modification within chromatin rather than alteration of rate and extent of DNA repair. In this regard, Tew [43] has observed that within the nuclear matrix there exist transcriptionally active regions of chromatin that are preferentially modified by nitrosoureas. This rather speculative hypothesis of nitrosourea cytotoxicity is greatly limited by our meager knowledge of the structure of chromatin and the molecular events necessary for nuclear DNA function.

B. Carbamylation

Carbamylation (also known as carbamoylation) events can occur after nitrosourea degradation to yield an organic isocyanate and a diazene hydroxide (Fig. 6.2). The organic moiety of the isocyanate may contain a functional group such as a hydroxyl group leading to a possible intramolecular carbamylation reaction to form a cyclic urethane. Extensive in vitro intramolecular carbamylation is known to occur with chlorozotocin [44] but whether exclusive intramolecular carbamylation takes precedence in vivo over intermolecular carbamylation is not known. The extent of intermolecular carbamylation in vitro has been assayed by the carbamylation of [^{14}C]-lysine and quantitation of products by chromatography [45]. This assay has been utilized extensively on the basis that the isocyanate would attack in a random manner any amino, hydroxyl, or thiol functional group. Thus classification of nitrosoureas based on their comparative carbamylation of lysine in vitro has been utilized extensively to rank them on their in vivo or intracellular carbamylating ability. It is now apparent that such a comparison is not an adequate estimate of protein modification because many organic isocyanates are excellent pseudosubstrates which are capable of irreversible inactivation of a specific enzyme at its catalytic site.

Originally, Brown and Wold [46,47] found that butyl isocyanate and octyl isocyanate were active-site-directed inactivators of elastase and chymotrypsin, respectively. Babson et al. [48] observed that active-site specific inactivation of chymotrypsin occurred by cyclohexyl isocyanate released during degradation of CCNU. A 70-fold excess of lysine over chymotrypsin concentration is necessary to detect any effect on the stoichiometric inactivation of chymotrypsin [48]. Subsequently, Frischer and Ahmad [49] observed that only glutathione reductase out of 19 erythrocyte enzymes assayed is inactivated in vivo during chemotherapy of patients with BCNU. Further studies by Babson and Reed [50] have shown that inactivation of glutathione reductase occurs only when the enzyme is in a reduced state (i.e., NADPH reduction) and two thiol groups are present at the active site. The inactivation of catalytic activity appears to occur as a thiocarbamate adduct forms between the isocyanate and possibly the distal thiol group at the active site [50].

The importance of these observations is that certain enzymes and proteins have either a catalytic or functional site at a region of hydrophobicity that is capable of high affinity binding of organic isocyanate with R groups of proper size and character. Thus a very high probability exists for a successful collision between a particular isocyanate and protein functional group. Active-site-directed interactions of this type take precedence over undirected reactions between other functional groups lacking the associated hydrophobic region for initial binding of the R group of the isocyanate. Such pockets or crevices in proteins have a very important role in the overall specificity and affinity of enzymes and other proteins (i.e., receptor proteins) for substrates and/or pseudosubstrates. The ability of cyclohexylisocyanate to prevent stoichiometrically the polymerization of brain tubulin is another example of highly specific irreversible binding of isocyanate to a protein [51].

Evidence for in vivo carbamylation of proteins by nitrosoureas includes not only organ and tissue distribution of radiolabel following administration of nitrosoureas radiolabeled in the isocyanate precursor moiety, but also from the nature of the urinary metabolites. Kohlhepp et al. [52] observed that major urinary metabolites of CCNU have molecular weights of 629, 413, 329, and 243 and they represent 5%, 20%, 20%, and 5%, respectively, of total excreted ^{14}C following administration of ^{14}C ring-labeled CCNU. They concluded that the higher molecular-weight metabolites are conjugates of peptides derived from active-site-directed inactivation of specific enzymes. Lysine does not contribute significantly to the composition of the urinary metabolites. Major amino acids present in the peptides were cysteine, serine, glutamic acid, alanine, glycine, and aspartic acid [52].

What role does carbamylation have in the overall biological effects of the nitrosourea? First, it must be accepted that any attempt to correlate carbamylation activity measured by an in vitro assay of lysine carbamylation to an in vivo structure-activity study is based on a weak premise. Only after much more is understood about selective protein carbamylation in vivo can appropriate correlations be made between carbamylation and cytotoxicity for the many nitrosoureas being evaluated for antineoplastic activity.

Kann [53] has suggested that carbamylation of a yet undetermined enzyme(s) is the basis for radiation synergism by a nonalkylating nitrosourea, BCyNU. Kann [53] has examined several nonalkylating nitrosoureas for antitumor activity (Table 6.3). Carbamylation effects may cause inhibition of macromolecular synthesis [54], selective metabolic effects on de novo purine synthesis [75], inhibition of RNA processing [55], inhibition of tubulin polymerization [51], inhibition of DNA repair [56], and inhibition of transglutaminase [76,77,78].

An example of the complexity of carbamylation events is the comparison between chlorozotocin and ACNA (Tables 6.4 and 6.5), neither of which is capable of in vitro carbamylation of lysine [42]. Chlorozotocin has curative antitumor activity for murine L1210 leukemia at doses that are not myelosuppressive [57]. ACNU, however, is a potent bone marrow toxin that also has curative antitumor activity for murine L1210 leukemia [58]. These differences in bone marrow toxicity may be related to a difference between chlorozotocin and ACNU in rates of intramolecular carbamylation. ACNU is a potent inactivator of glutathione reductase via carbamylation, while chlorozotocin is without effect on this enzyme [50]. Thus ACNU may carbamylate certain proteins quite effectively even though it is efficient at intramolecular carbamylation. Babson and Reed [50] have found a good correlation between the ability of ACNU and CCNU to inactivate glutathione reductase and myelosuppression, whereas chlorozotocin and GANU are not able to inactivate glutathione reduction and are not myelosuppressive. These agents may have different tissue-specific binding sites for alkylation within the substructure of chromatin. Green et al. [42] have concluded that differential toxicity of chlorozotocin and GANU (Table 6.4) for bone marrow and tumor cells, as compared to ACNU and CCNU, may be mediated in part by the observed qualitative differences in subnucleosomal alkylation sites. However, the selective cytotoxicity of haloethylnitrosoureas to Walker 256 rat carcinoma cell lines has been attributed to the carbamylation rather than to alkylation effects possibly at the preferential target—the nuclear matrix [79]. One must conclude that selective alkylation and carbamylation events that modify macromolecules are both important in correlation of structure-activity relationships and that in vitro assays are unable to measure the selectivity of such specific macromolecular modifications.

VII. DESIGN BASIS FOR NEW CONGENERS

The ability of the nitrosoureas to cross the blood-brain barrier, whereas many antitumor drugs fail to do so, has resulted in much interest in the lipophilic character of the nitrosoureas. Based on a cancer quantitative structure-activity relationship (QSAR), some guidelines for the design of new nitrosoureas have been advanced. After an extensive study of a QSAR for 90 nitrosoureas against L1210 leukemia in mice, it was concluded that the lipophilic character of the nitrosoureas is the most important parameter

TABLE 6.3 Nonalkylating Nitrosoureas

Code	Compound	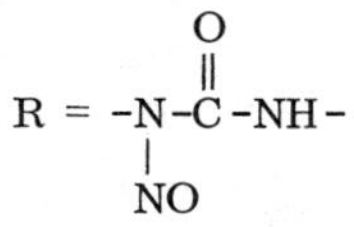 R = -N(NO)-C(=O)-NH-	Reference
BCyNU NSC-80590	1,3-Bis(cyclohexyl)-1-nitrosourea	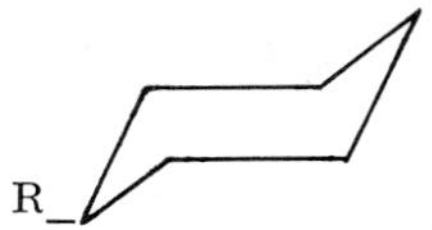 R–cyclohexyl	53
trans-4-Hydroxy BCyNU NSC-305715	1,3-Bis(*trans*-4-hydroxycyclohexyl)-1-nitrosourea	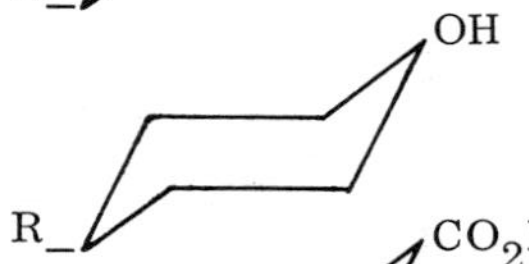 R–cyclohexyl–OH	53
cis-4-Carboxyl BCyNU NSC-305716	1,3-Bis(*cis*-4-carboxylcyclohexyl)-1-nitrosourea	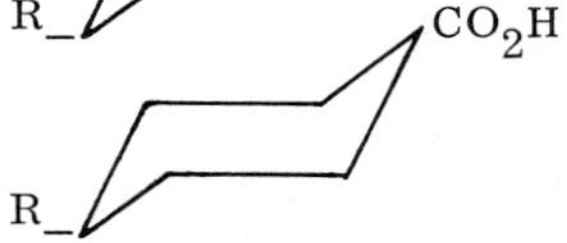 R–cyclohexyl–CO_2H	53

TABLE 6.4 Nitrosoureas Developed for Greater Water Solubility and Reduced Myelosuppression

Code	Compound	$R- = NH-\underset{\displaystyle \|}{C}-\underset{\displaystyle |}{N}-CH_2-CH_2-Cl$ O NO	Reference
Chlorozotocin NSC 178248	1-(2-Chloroethyl)-3-(D-2-glucopyranosyl)-1-nitrosourea	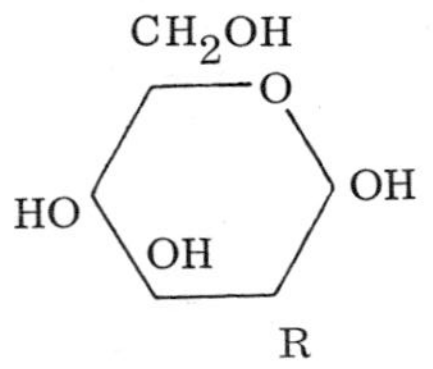 CH_2OH, O, HO, OH, OH, R	32
cis-Acid NSC 153174	1-(2-Chloroethyl)-3-(4-cis-carboxycyclohexyl)-1-nitrosourea	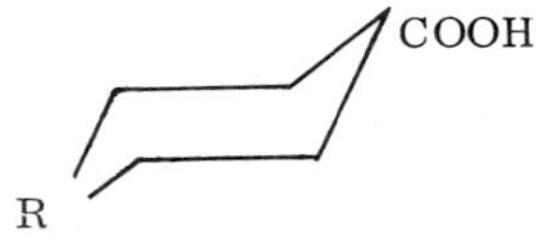 COOH, R	69
MCNU	1-(2-Chloroethyl)-3-(methyl-α-D-glucopyranose-6-yl)-1-nitrosourea	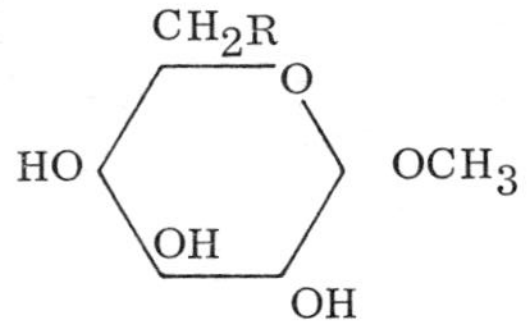 CH_2R, O, HO, OCH_3, OH, OH	70

TABLE 6.4 (Continued)

Code	Compound	R- = NH-C(=O)-N(NO)-CH_2-CH_2-Cl	Reference
TA-077	1-(2-Chloroethyl)-3-isobutyl-3-(β-maltosyl)-1-nitrosourea	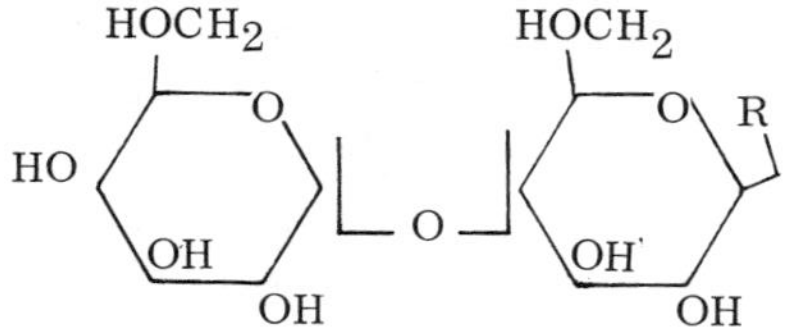 $HOCH_2$, HO, OH, OH, O, $HOCH_2$, O, R, OH, OH	71
GANU NSC D 254157	1-(2-Chloroethyl)-3-(β-D-glucopyranosyl)-1-nitrosourea	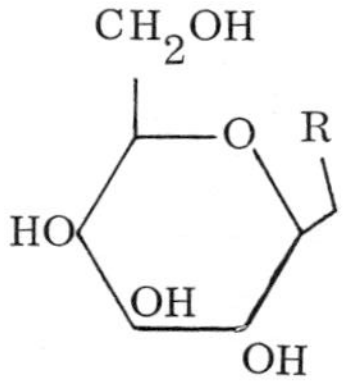 CH_2OH, O, R, HO, OH, OH	8

TABLE 6.5 New Nitrosourea Congeners in Clinical Trials

Code	Compound	R– = NH–C(=O)–N(NO)–CH_2–CH_2–Cl	Reference
HECNU NSC 294895	1-(2-Chloroethyl)-3-(2-hydroxy-ethyl-1-nitrosourea	R–CH_2–CH_2OH	63
CNCC 1.C.1.G.1325	N,N'-Bis(N-(2-chloroethyl)-N-nitrosocarbonyl]cystamine	S–CH_2–CH_2–R | S–CH_2–CH_2–R	72
RPCNU 1.C.1.G.1163	1-(2-Chloroethyl)-3-(2,3,4-triacetyl-1-ribopyranosyl)-1-nitrosourea	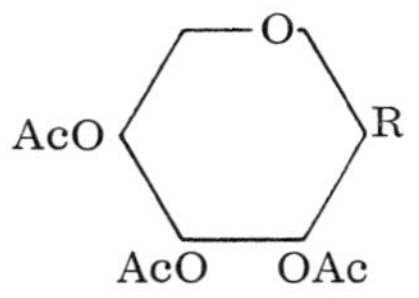 O, R, AcO, AcO, OAc	73
RFCNU 1.C.1.G.1105	1-(2-Chloroethyl)-3-[2,3-isopropylidene 5-(nitro-4-benzoyl)-1-ribofuranosyl]-1-nitrosourea	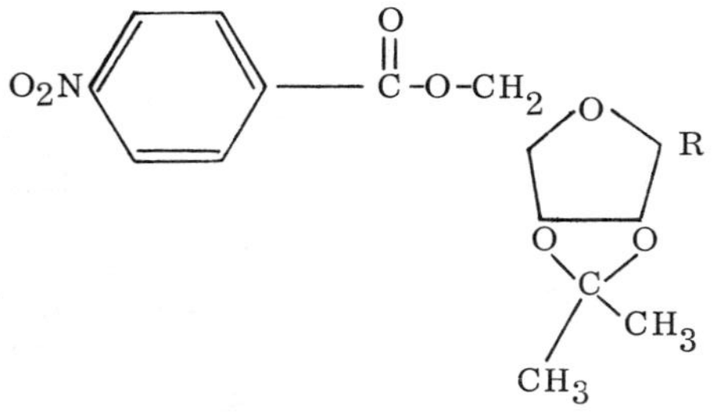 O_2N, C(=O)–O–CH_2, O, R, O, O, C, CH_3, CH_3	73

TABLE 6.5 (Continued)

Code	Compound	R– = NH–C(=O)–N(NO)–CH_2–CH_2–Cl	Reference
ACNU	1-(2-Chloroethyl)-3-(4-amino-2-methylpyrimidine-5-yl)methyl-1-nitrosourea	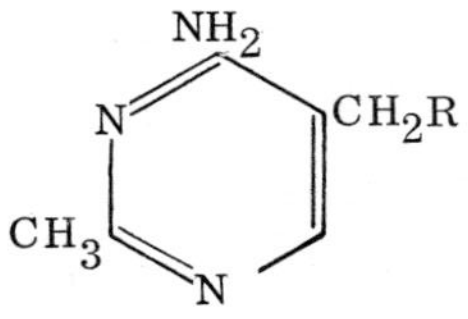 NH_2, CH_2R, CH_3, N, N (pyrimidine ring)	74

determining their antitumor activity [59]. P-values were measured for 43 nitrosoureas and efforts to make nitrosourea congeners somewhat more hydrophilic became a central point in the study (Table 6.4). Justified concern was expressed about the limitation of functional groups such as COOH, which are almost completely ionized at physiological pH, pH 7.4, to confer greater hydrophilicity when un-ionized functional groups showed a better correlation. Making the R group more polar yet un-ionized with a disaccharide was suggested [59]. Interestingly, at about the same time, this approach was being tested with three nitrosoureas containing either a β-maltosyl, β-lactosyl, or β-cellubiosyl R group [60]. Testing of these congeners against various types of tumors is in progress.

Increasing evidence supports the concept that carbamylation capability remains an important factor in the design of new nitrosourea congeners. DNA alkylation events have a greater chance for cell killing when the rate of DNA repair is decreased. Day et al. [61] have identified a group of 8 (among 39) human tumor cell strains that are deficient in DNA repair ability. This deficiency is being studied in regard to susceptibility to DNA cross-links caused by CNU, BCNU, and CCNU [61, 62]. Eisenbrand et al. [63] have designed and synthesized a congener series of 1,1'-polymethylene bis-3-(2-chloroethyl)-3-nitrosoureas as transport forms of polymethylene diisocyanates. These compounds may cause some interesting cross-linking reactions primarily with proteins. Studies with these and other new nitrosoureas has led Eisenbrand and co-workers [64] to conclude that the nonalkylating part of the 2-chloroethylnitrosourea is important for the biological effects of these drugs. Various new nitrosoureas in clinical trial are shown in Table 6.5.

Certain nitrosoureas have been shown to cause a prolonged in vivo depression of cytochrome P-450 content and cytochrome P-450-dependent enzyme activities of liver microsomes when measured in vivo [65, 66]. A single nonlethal dose of CCNU in vivo decreased liver cytochrome P-450 content and drug metabolism of rat liver microsomes by 40-70% for up to 6 weeks. This unique suppression is without parallel by any other drug and cannot be explained except for possible persistent alkylation and/or carbamylation effects by the degradation intermediates of the nitrosoureas. This effect could well be the basis for a new congener series that could modulate the activity of these and other drugs that are substrates for the cytochrome P-450 enzymes.

Fourteen (2-chloroethyl)nitrosourea congeners of L-amino acid amides have been synthesized and found to be highly active against L1210 cells in mice [80]. A congener of sarcosinamide exhibited especially high antitumor activity, liver acute toxicity and extremely long half-life [80]. Lin et al. [67] have combined two active agents for antitumor activity, thiocolchicine and nitrosourea, into a single analog for potential improved biological and pharmacological properties. Colvin and Brundrett [68] have found that chloroethylnitrosocarbamate, $Cl\text{-}CH_2\text{-}CH_2\text{-}N(NO)\text{-}C(=O)\text{-}O\text{-}CH_3$ and chloroethylnitrosoacetamide, $Cl\ CH_2\ CH_2\text{-}N(NO)\text{-}C(=O)\text{-}CH_3$ are about 500 times more potent DNA cross-linking agents than the chloroethylnitrosoureas when exposed to cells in vitro. However, these compounds are rapidly destroyed by a plasma esterase. These observations are potentially important for congener design studies.

VIII. CONCLUSIONS

Nitrosourea cytotoxicity remains a very complex effect with unique characteristics. Much more needs to be understood at the molecular level to provide even rudimentary explanation of the chemical modifications caused by the alkylations and carbamylating events of the nitrosoureas. If potent toxicity of the nitrosoureas could be ameliorated without sacrificing tumor cell cytotoxicity, the clinical impact of these drugs would be enormous. Design and testing of new congeners on a rational basis should continue to be a worthwhile activity in the years ahead.

ACKNOWLEDGMENTS

The author wishes to acknowledge support by Grant CH-199 from the American Cancer Society and the National Cancer Institute Grant CA-25561.

REFERENCES*

1. T. P. Johnston, G. S. McCaleb, and J. A. Montgomery, J. Med. Chem., 6: 669 (1963).
2. S. K. Carter, F. M. Schabel, Jr., L. E. Broder, and T. P. Johnston, Adv. Cancer Res., 16: 273 (1972).
3. H. E. May, R. Boose, and D. J. Reed, Biochemistry, 14: 4723 (1975).
4. T. P. Johnston, G. S. McCaleb, and J. A. Montgomery, J. Med. Chem., 18: 634 (1975).

---

*The following books are the result of recent international symposia on the nitrosoureas: Nitrosoureas: Current Status and New Developments, edited by A. W. Prestayko, S. T. Crooke, L. H. Baker, S. K. Carter, and P. S. Schein, Academic Press, New York, 1981, 416 pp.; and Nitrosoureas in Cancer Treatment, edited by B. Serrou, P. S. Schein, and J.-L. Imbach, Elsevier, New York, 1981, 310 pp.

5. H. E. May, S. J. Kohlhepp, R. B. Boose, and D. J. Reed, Cancer Res., 39: 762 (1979).
6. J. A. Montgomery, Cancer Treat. Rep., 60: 651 (1976).
7. T. P. Johnston, G. S. McCaleb, P. S. Opliger, and J. A. Montgomery, J. Med. Chem., 9: 892 (1966).
8. T. Machinami, S. Nishiyama, K. Kikuchi, and T. Suami, Bull. Chem. Soc. Jpn., 48: 3763 (1975).
9. R. J. Weinkam, J. H. C. Wen, D. E. Furst, and V. A. Levin, Clin. Chem., 24: 45 (1978).
10. D. J. Reed, H. E. May, R. B. Boose, K. M. Gregory, and M. A. Beilstein, Cancer Res., 35: 568 (1975).
11. E. R. Garrett, S. Goto, and J. F. Stubbins, J. Pharm. Sci., 54: 119 (1965).
12. G. P. Wheeler and S. Chumley, J. Med. Chem., 10: 259 (1967).
13. J. A. Montgomery, R. James, G. S. McCaleb, and T. P. Johnston, J. Med. Chem., 10: 668 (1967).
14. M. Colvin, J. W. Cowens, R. B. Brundrett, B. S. Kramer, and D. B. Ludlum, Biochem. Biophys. Res. Commun., 60: 515 (1974).
15. J. A. Montgomery, R. James, G. S. McCaleb, M. C. Kirk, T. P. Johnston, J. Med. Chem., 18: 568 (1975).
16. J. W. Lown and S. M. S. Chauhan, J. Med. Chem., 24: 270 (1981).
17. J. W. Lown, A. V. Joshua, and L. W. McLaughlin, J. Med. Chem., 23: 798 (1980).
18. K. W. Kohn, Cancer Res., 37: 1450 (1977).
19. A. B. Foster, M. Jarman, P. L. Coe, J. Sleigh, and J. C. Tatlow, J. Med. Chem., 23: 1226 (1980).
20. R. B. Brundrett, J. Med. Chem., 23: 1245 (1980).
21. D. J. Reed, in Nitrosoureas Current Status and New Developments (A. W. Prestayko, S. T. Crooke, L. H. Baker, S. K. Carter, and P. S. Schein, eds.), Academic Press, New York, 1981, p. 51.
22. H. E. May, R. Boose, and D. J. Reed, Biochem. Biophys. Res. Commun., 57: 426 (1974).
23. D. J. Reed and H. E. May, Life Sci., 16: 1263 (1975).
24. D. J. Reed and H. E. May, in Microsomes and Drug Oxidations (V. Ullrich, I. Roots, A. Hildebrandt, R. W. Estabrook, and A. H. Conney, eds.), Pergamon Press, Elmsford, N.Y., 1977, p. 680.
25. J. Hilton and M. D. Walker, Biochem. Pharamacol., 24: 2153 (1975).
26. D. W. Potter and D. J. Reed, in Microsomes, Drug Oxidations, and Chemical Carcinogenesis (M. A. Coon et al., eds.), Academic Press, New York, 1980, p. 371.
27. P. B. Farmer, A. B. Foster, M. Jarman, M. R. Oddy, and D. J. Reed, J. Med. Chem., 21: 514 (1978).
28. H. E. Skipper, F. M. Schabel, Jr., M. W. Trader, and J. R. Thomson, Cancer Res., 21: 1154 (1961).
29. D. L. Hill, M. C. Kirk, and R. F. Struck, Cancer Res., 35: 296 (1975).

30. D. W. Potter and D. J. Reed, Pharmacologist, 23: 168 (1981).
31. V. A. Levin, J. Stearns, A. Byrd, A. Finn, and R. J. Weinkam, J. Pharmacol. Exp. Ther., 208: 1 (1979).
32. D. B. Ludlum, in Cancer, A Comprehensive Treatise (F. F. Becker, ed.), Vol. 5, Plenum Press, New York, 1977, p. 285.
33. T. Anderson, M. G. McMenamin, and P. S. Schein, Cancer Res., 35: 761 (1975).
34. R. J. Weinkam, T.-Y. J. Liu, and H.-S. Lin, Chem.-Biol. Interact., 31: 167 (1980).
35. D. E. Jensen and D. J. Reed, Biochemistry, 17: 5098 (1978).
36. D. E. Jensen, Biochemistry, 17: 5108 (1978).
37. R. B. Brundrett, J. W. Cowens, M. Colvin, and I. Jardine, J. Med. Chem., 19: 958 (1976).
38. D. B. Ludlum and W. P. Tong, in Nitrosoureas in Cancer Treatment (B. Serrou, P. S. Schein, and J.-L. Imbach, eds.), Elsevier, New York, 1981, p. 21.
39. W. P. Tong and D. B. Ludlum, Cancer Res., 41: 380 (1981).
40. J. W. Lown, L. W. McLaughlin, and Y.-M. Chang, Bioorg. Chem., 7: 97 (1978).
41. K. W. Kohn, L. C. Erickson, and G. Laurent, in Nitrosoureas in Cancer Treatment (B. Serrou, P. S. Schein, and J.-L. Imbach, eds.), Elsevier, New York, 1981, p. 33.
42. D. Green, J. D. Ahlgreen, and P. S. Schein, in Nitrosoureas in Cancer Treatment (B. Serrou, P. S. Schein, and J.-L. Imbach, eds.), Elsevier, New York, 1981, p. 49.
43. K. D. Tew, in Nitrosoureas in Cancer Treatment (B. Serrou, P. S. Schein, and J.-L. Imbach, eds.), Elsevier, New York, 1981, p. 61.
44. T. P. Johnston, G. S. McCaleb, and J. A. Montgomery, J. Med. Chem., 18: 104 (1975).
45. G. P. Wheeler, B. J. Bowdon, J. A. Grimsley, and H. H. Lloyd, Cancer Res., 34: 194 (1974).
46. W. E. Brown and F. Wold, Biochemistry, 12: 828 (1973).
47. W. E. Brown and F. Wold, Biochemistry, 12: 835 (1973).
48. J. R. Babson, D. J. Reed, and M. A. Sinkey, Biochemistry, 16: 1584 (1977).
49. H. Frischer and T. Ahmad, J. Lab. Clin. Med., 89: 1080 (1977).
50. J. R. Babson and D. J. Reed, Biochem. Biophys. Res. Commun., 83: 754 (1978).
51. A. E. Brodie, J. R. Babson, and D. J. Reed, Biochem. Pharmacol., 29: 652 (1980).
52. S. J. Kohlhepp, H. E. May, and D. J. Reed, Drug Metab. Dispos., 9: 135 (1981).
53. H. E. Kann, Jr., in Nitrosoureas: Current Status and New Developments (A. W. Prestayko, S. T. Crooke, L. H. Baker, S. K. Carter, and P. S. Schein, eds.), Academic Press, New York, 1981, p. 95.
54. H. E. Kann, Jr., K. W. Kohn, and J. M. Lyles, Cancer Res., 34: 398 (1974).

55. H. E. Kann, Jr., K. W. Kohn, L. Widerlite, and D. Gullion, Cancer Res., 34: 1982 (1974).
56. H. E. Kann, Jr., M. A. Schott, and A. Petkas, Cancer Res., 40: 50 (1980).
57. L. C. Panasci, D. Green, R. Nagourney, P. Fox, and P. S. Schein, Cancer Res., 37: 2615 (1977).
58. R. A. Nagourney, P. A. Fox, and P. S. Schein, Cancer Res., 38: 65 (1978).
59. C. Hansch, A. Leo, C. Schmidt, P. Y. C. Jow, and J. A. Montgomery, J. Med. Chem., 23: 1095 (1980).
60. T. Suami, T. Machinami, and T. Hisamatsu, J. Med. Chem., 22: 247 (1979).
61. R. S. Day III, C. H. J. Ziolkowski, D. A. Scudiero, S. A. Meyer, A. S. Lubiniecki, A. J. Girardi, S. M. Galloway, and G. D. Bynum, Nature, 288: 724 (1980).
62. L. C. Erickson, G. Laurent, N. A. Sharkey, and K. W. Kohn, Nature, 288: 727 (1980).
63. G. Eisenbrand, H. H. Fiebig, and W. J. Zeller, Z. Krebsforsch., 86: 279 (1976).
64. G. Eisenbrand, M. Habs, W. J. Zeller, H. Fiebig, M. Berger, O. Zelesny, and D. Schmähl, in Nitrosoureas in Cancer Treatment (B. Serrou, P. S. Schein, and J.-L. Imbach, eds.), Elsevier, New York, 1981, p. 175.
65. D. J. Reed and H. E. May, Biochimie, 60: 989 (1978).
66. C. L. Littrst, Biochem. Pharmacol., 30: 1014 (1981).
67. T.-S. Lin, G. T. Shiau, W. H. Prusoff, and R. E. Harmon, J. Med. Chem., 23: 1440 (1980).
68. M. Colvin and R. Brundrett, in Nitrosoureas: Current Status and New Development (A. W. Prestayko, S. T. Crooke, L. H. Baker, S. K. Carter, and P. S. Schein, eds.), Academic Press, New York, 1981, p. 43.
69. T. P. Johnston, G. S. McCaleb, S. D. Clayton, J. L. Frye, C. A. Krauth, and J. A. Montgomery, J. Med. Chem., 20: 279 (1977).
70. S. Sekido, K. Ninomiya, and M. Iwasaki, Cancer Treat. Rep., 63: 961 (1979).
71. K. Tsujihara et al., Proc. Jpn. Cancer Assoc., 39th Annu. Meet., Tokyo, 660, Abstr. (1980) [Ref. 5 in M. Ogawa's article in Nitrosoureas in Cancer Treatment (B. Serrou, P. S. Schein, J.-L. Imbach, eds.), Elsevier, New York, 1981, p. 249].
72. J.-L. Imbach, J. Martinez, J. Oiry, Ch. Bourut, E. Chenu, R. Maral, and G. Mathe, in Nitrosoureas in Cancer Treatment (B. Serrou, P. S. Schein, and J.-L. Imbach, eds.), Elsevier, New York, 1981, p. 123.
73. J. L. Montero and J.-L. Imbach, C.R. Acad. Sci., 279C: 809 (1974).
74. M. Arakawa, F. Shimizu, and N. Okada, Gann, 65: 191 (1974).

75. D. P. Groth, J. M. D'Angelo, W. R. Vogler, E. S. Mingioli and B. Betz, Cancer Res., 31: 332 (1971).
76. A. Tarantino, P. Thompson, and K. Laki, Cancer Biochem. Biophys., 4: 33 (1979).
77. J. Hunyadi, G. Szegedi, T. Szabo, A. Ahmed and K. Laki, Cancer Res., 41: 1677 (1981).
78. L. Fesus, A. Falus, A. Erdei and K. Laki, J. Cell Biol., 89: 706 (1981).
79. K. D. Tew and A. L. Wang, Molec. Pharmacol., 21: 729 (1982).
80. T. Suami, T. Kato, H. Takino and T. Hisamatsu, J. Med. Chem., 25: 829 (1982).

7

METAL COMPLEXES AS ANTITUMOR AGENTS

DAVID H. PETERING, WILLIAM E. ANTHOLINE,* and LEON A. SARYAN

University of Wisconsin-Milwaukee
Milwaukee, Wisconsin

*Present affiliation: The Medical College of Wisconsin, Milwaukee, Wisconsin

I. INTRODUCTION

Many reviews have been written in the past decade which summarize the current information about the chemical, biochemical, and biological properties of metal-containing antitumor agents. However, few efforts have been made to integrate and interpret this information on the objective basis of the biological chemistry which the complexes may undergo as they enter and move about within organisms. Therefore, we have focused on the use and application of inorganic chemistry to study how cytotoxic complexes and ligands may react in biological systems. Of necessity, as well as design, the choice of material is selective and illustrative. The intent is to provide the reader with detailed insight into the bioinorganic chemistry of several metal complexes and through this to show how one can couple a basic interest in inorganic chemistry to the study of the mechanism of action of metal complexes and metal-binding drugs.

II. HISTORY

Two decades ago Arthur Furst set forth the hypothesis that many antitumor agents interact with biological systems through the formation of metal chelates between functional groups of the drugs and essential transition metals of the organisms [1]. The hypothesis was based solely on the plausible formation of five- and six-membered chelate rings between drug and metal ion. It was made without regard for the basic question of the probability of formation of such structures in biological systems, which contain a variety of metal-binding molecules that naturally can compete with the drug for the metal ion.

In the same period, French and Freedlander prepared a number of bis(thiosemicarbazones) as potential antitumor agents, which were designed expressly to bind transition metals [2,3]. H.G. Petering and co-workers subsequently provided the first definitive information about a metal complex with significant antitumor activity when they showed that 3-ethoxy-2-oxobutyraldehyde bis(thiosemicarbazone) must be activated through formation of its copper complex [4].

Nevertheless, it was not until the discovery of the remarkable chemotherapeutic effectiveness of cis-dichlorodiammine platinum(II) by Rosenberg that attention was drawn to the real and potential importance of metal complexes as a general, unexplored class of antitumor agents [5]. However, the field remains in its infancy. Despite the more recent findings of antitumor activity of α-N-heterocyclic carboxaldehyde thiosemicarbazone metal complexes, Ga^{3+} salts, and some rhodium carboxylate dimers [6, 7], it was still a surprise to the pharmacological and medical communities to discover that bleomycin, an established, clinically used antibiotic, probably reacts with cells in the form of a metal complex [8].

Therefore, this chapter begins with a general introduction to the interaction of ligands and metal complexes with biological systems. A conceptual picture is drawn in which illustrative examples from bis(thiosemicarbazone) studies are included.

III. REACTIONS OF LIGANDS AND METAL COMPLEXES WITH BIOLOGICAL SYSTEMS—A CONCEPTUAL INTRODUCTION

Biological systems contain a variety of transition metals in differing concentration and location amid a large concentration of competing ligands, including proteins, nucleic acids, and smaller metabolites [9]. Such metals as Fe, Cu, and Zn, although present in trace amounts, serve as cofactors in many enzymes, as constituents of other macromolecular structures, and in general, play important roles in many metabolic pathways. Clearly, there are homeostatic mechanisms to govern the movements and distribution of transition metal ions in organisms. Even in the best studied example of iron, however, there remain many unanswered questions. It is also evident that when the metabolism of essential transition metals goes awry, as in the case of copper in Wilson's disease, such metals become highly toxic, Thus ligands that can bind to essential metals or mobilize them from their normal metabolic pathways can disrupt cellular function. Similarly, once new complexes are formed between exogenous ligands and metal ions in the organism, new reactions of the bound metal may occur outside its normal range of activities. Therefore, the first conceptual problem is whether an antitumor agent with metal-binding capacity can bind to metals in the living system with sufficient thermodynamic or kinetic stability to permit formation of new metal complexes on a reasonable biological time scale.

The imposition of nonphysiological heavy metal complexes upon organisms brings together potentially reactive metal sites with systems that contain an array of possible reactants. At this point, the problem in analyzing how complexes of essential and nonessential heavy metals interact with cells and fluids is conceptually the same: Given the chemical properties of the metal complex, what reactions occur in the interaction of the complex with the myriad of biomolecules confronting it? This is a problem that requires an understanding of the inorganic chemistry of the complex as well as an appreciation of the organism as a complicated multiphase, metal-ligand mixture with which external ligands and complexes may react.

Finally, to describe the mechanism of action of a drug, the chemical reactions taking place in cells must be causally related to the biological response to the drug, namely, cytotoxicity in the case of an antitumor agent. Except in general terms, however, it is often difficult to establish a satisfying cause-and-effect relationship between biochemical and cellular responses.

IV. BIS(THIOSEMICARBAZONATO)Cu(II) COMPLEXES

To illustrate the conceptual picture we have set forth, the bioinorganic pharmacology of bis(thiosemicarbazone) antitumor agents will be discussed. French and Freedlander [2, 3] synthesized a variety of bis(thiosemicarbazones) as potential chelating agents for essential transition metals (Fig. 7.1). Some had antitumor activity. H. G. Petering and others carried out extensive antitumor studies on this series of compounds and some of its metal complexes [4, 6, 10-12]. In particular, 3-ethoxy-2-oxobutyraldehyde bis(thiosemicarbazone), H_2KTS, has excellent, broad-spectrum activity in animals but has not been examined in humans beyond phase I testing.

The major conceptual questions at that point were whether H_2KTS does bind metals in animals and whether such reactions participate in the antitumor activity or toxicity of the drug. In antitumor studies both CuKTS and ZnKTS are active forms of the drug [11]. Using diets deficient in zinc or copper, it was found that the ligand required nutrient copper, but not zinc, for activity. Hence the formation of CuKTS is inferred as a necessary activation step [13].

This interpretation is reinforced by studies in cell culture [14]. In a standard assay of cytotoxicity, H_2KTS is inactive against cells maintained in "metal-free" media and is only activated by Cu^{2+} among nutritionally essential metal ions. The apparent activity of ZnKTS is rationalized with the aid of measurements of equilibrium binding of Zn^{2+} and Cu^{2+} to H_2KTS in aqueous solution and in plasma [15, 16]. The latter was chosen as a representative mixture of biological chelating agents for Zn and Cu. The apparent log stability constant of ZnKTS at pH 7.4 is 5.9, whereas that for CuKTS is 18.4. Not surprisingly, ZnKTS dissociates in plasma, for Zn-amino acid complexes have larger stability constants. Similarly, the sta-

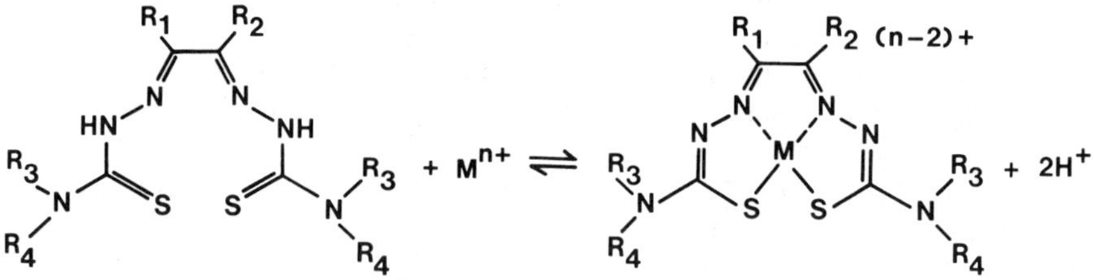

FIGURE 7.1 Metal chelation by bis(thiosemicarbazone) ligand.

bility of CuKTS in plasma is reasonable in light of its large stability constant. Thus ZnKTS readily dissociates in organisms liberating H_2KTS which chelates "available" copper to form the active complex.

What is the source of copper which activates H_2KTS? The question of ligand activation by thermodynamically and kinetically "available" essential metals is important but relatively unexplored. The problem is considered again in the sections on monothiosemicarbazones and bleomycin. In general, there is little nonmacromolecular-bound transition metals in cells. This is clearly seen in molecular weight profiles of bound forms of Cu and Zn in liver cytoplasm [17]. Similarly, in plasma, iron is bound almost entirely to transferrin, 80% of the copper to ceruloplasmin, and about 70% of the zinc to α_2-macroglobulin [18, 19]. Most of the remainder of the zinc is bound to albumin, and only a small fraction to amino acids [19].

Once it is established that CuKTS is the active form of the drug, how does it react with and attack cells? Experiments directed toward these questions should examine the problem broadly with complementary chemical and cellular studies. Since ligands and metal complexes are usually not antimetabolites or structural relatives of active, well-understood complexes, it is difficult to predict how they might react in vivo. Thus it is useful to survey the physiochemical properties of the complexes, which may reasonably suggest how these species behave in cells. For typical copper complexes, one considers the thermodynamics and kinetics of several types of reactions:

$$Cu^{2+} + H_2KTS \rightleftharpoons CuKTS + 2H^+ \quad \text{Complex formation} \tag{1}$$

$$Cu(II)KTS + Red \rightleftharpoons Cu(I)KTS^{1-} + Ox \quad \text{Redox reaction} \tag{2}$$

$$Cu(II)KTS + L \rightleftharpoons Cu(II)L^{2+} + KTS^{2-} \quad \text{Ligand substitution} \tag{3}$$

$$Cu(II)KTS + B: \rightleftharpoons CuKTS \cdot B \quad \text{Adduct formation} \tag{4}$$

$$Cu(II)KTS + X \rightleftharpoons CuKTS\text{-}X \quad \text{Ligand modification} \tag{5}$$

Furthermore, it is instructive to compare the properties of complexes which differ in biological activity in an effort to correlate changes in activity with systematic variation in physiochemical characteristics of the compounds. In fact, peripheral R-group substitution can markedly alter the in vitro cytotoxicity of bis(thiosemicarbazonato) metal complexes as shown in Fig. 7.1 and Table 7.1. Thus comparisons of the chemical, cellular, and biological behavior of active and inactive complexes can be made.

TABLE 7.1 Comparative Cytotoxicity of Copper and Zinc Bis(Thiosemicarbazones)

Numbering for figure 7.2	R_1	R_2	R_3	R_4	Relative in vitro cytotoxicity	
					Cu complex	Zn complex
1	$CH(OET)CH_3$	H	H	H	(+)	(-)
2	$CH(OET)CH_3$	H	CH_3	H	(+)	(-)
3	$CH(OET)CH_3$	H	CH_3	CH_3	(-)	(+)
4	CH_3	H	H	H	(+)	(-)
5	CH_3	H	CH_3	H	(+)	(-)
6	CH_3	H	CH_3	CH_3	(-)	(+)
7	H	H	H	H	(-)	
8	2-Formylpyridine thiosemicarbazone				(+)	

Source: Ref. 14.

Examination of reaction 3 suggests that ligand substitution or addition processes will be thermodynamically or kinetically unfavorable in vivo [16, 20,21]. However, CuKTS can be slowly reduced and dissociated as follows [20,21]:

$$Cu(II)KTS + 2RSH \qquad Cu(I)SR + RSSR + H_2KTS \tag{6}$$

It was hypothesized, therefore, that CuKTS reacts with thiols of tumor cells. A thorough investigation of the reaction of the complex with Ehrlich ascites cells confirmed in detail the occurrence of reaction 6 in cells [22, 23].

Reaction 6 is important in the mechanism of action of CuKTS. This is shown by the parallel behavior of copper complexes of ligands 1-6 in Table 7.1 in reactions with thiols and cells [23]. Figure 7.2 shows the linear free energy correlation between the relative pseudo-first-order rate constants of reaction of these complexes with dithiothreitol and with cells as a function of their reduction potentials. The close similarity of the complexes among the two reactions provides mechanistic support for reaction 6 and focuses on the subtle changes in ligand structure which affect activity. With these results, a unified picture emerges which links the chemical, biochemical, and cellular information about CuKTS, in which complexes with sufficient reactivity towards sulfhydryl groups are also generally active against cells.

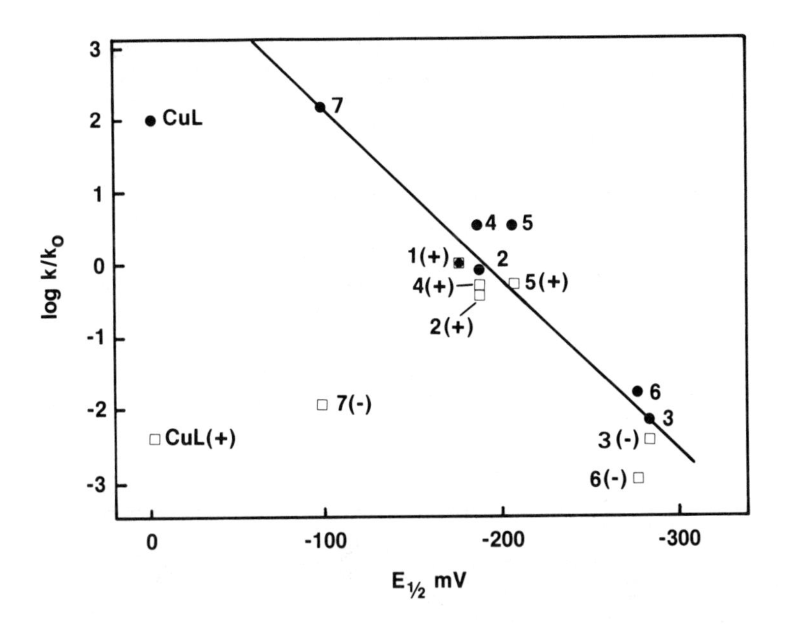

FIGURE 7.2 Linear free energy correlations relating pseudo-first-order rate constants for reaction 6 and the reactions of copper complexes with Ehrlich cells. k_0 is the rate for CuKTS. Numbering is given in Table 7.1. (●) reaction 6, with dithiothreitol as the thiol reagent (□) reaction with cells. In vitro cytotoxicities of complexes are given in parentheses. (From Refs. 14, 21, and 23.)

The finding that zinc activates compounds 3 and 6 in Table 7.1 is intriguing. The pattern of activity is correlated with the apparent stability constants of the complexes. As with the copper complexes, the addition of the second methyl group to the N-4 nitrogen of the thiosemicarbazone moiety markedly enhances the electron donating character of that nitrogen. Thus the log apparent stability constants for the zinc complexes of ligands 1-3 are 5.9, 6.4, and 9.7, respectively, at pH 7.4 [15,24]. It has been estimated that in plasma zinc complexes with log K_{app} constants greater than 8 are necessary if the complex is to remain significantly associated when present in 10 μM concentration [24]. Thus activity is correlated with thermodynamic stability of the complex. Although little has been done to explore the antitumor activity of bis(thiosemicarbazonato) zinc complexes, $ZnKTSM_2$ does inhibit tumor growth and on a cellular level disrupts both DNA synthesis and oxidative phosphorylation [24,25]. It is interesting to observe that even complexes of zinc, the least toxic of the major trace metals, Fe, Cu, and Zn, can be cytotoxic, when administered as a stable complex.

The last, most elusive task is to relate the biochemical reactions of a drug with their consequent biological effects. Basically, H_2KTS and CuKTS are known to inhibit DNA synthesis and stimulate cell respiration [22,23,26, 27]. The experimental problem is to establish kinetically and quantitatively the relationship between these effects and cell death. Although incomplete, the following results illustrate one approach to this question. At the core of the work is the exposure of Ehrlich cells in vitro to CuKTS to obtain the cellular data, followed by inoculation of similarly exposed cells, washed free of unbound drug, into mice to assess cytotoxicity. The results are collated in Figure 7.3. Inhibition of DNA synthesis but not cellular respiration correlates with the stoichiometry of cytotoxicity (Fig. 7.3a). Data on the cytotoxicity of lower concentrations of CuKTS are needed to test this relationship further. Furthermore, the time required to inhibit DNA synthesis is similar to the exposure time of cells necessary to produce a cytotoxic response. The apparent much slower inhibition of O_2 uptake by cells may

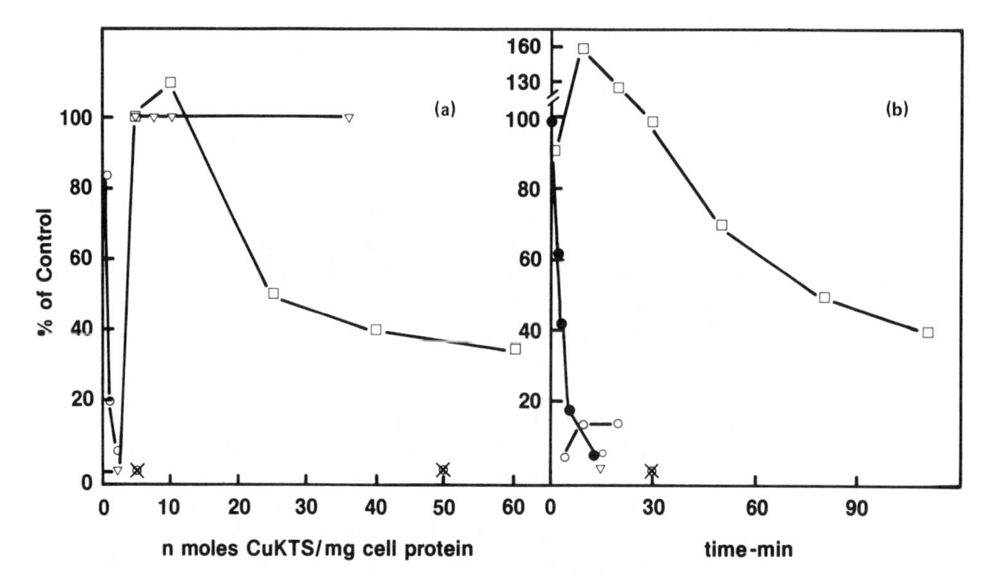

FIGURE 7.3. Concentration and time dependence of effects of CuKTS upon Ehrlich cells relative to untreated controls. Panel a: (○) thymidine incorporation into DNA, (⊠) cell survival in animals after in vitro incubation with CuKTS, (□) cell respiration after 2 hr in the presence of CuKTS, (▽) Cu from CuKTS not specifically bound to Zn,Cu binding protein. (From Ref. 28.) Panel b: symbols as in A. (○) 1 nmol of CuKTS per milligram of cell protein, (⊠) 5 nmol/mg, (□) 50 nmol/mg, (▽) 0.4 nmol/mg, (●) 7.6 nmol/mg CuKTS for reaction rate of complex with Ehrlich cells. (From Refs. 22, 23, and 27 and unpublished information.)

be a combination of opposing reactions, the Cu-catalyzed reduction of O_2 by thiols enhancing O_2 consumption, and the inhibition of mitochondrial respiration (Fig. 7.3b). The rate of reaction of CuKTS with the cells is on the same time scale as that for the inhibition of DNA synthesis and the rapid enhancement of oxygen uptake.

What, then, may be the molecular relationship between the generalized chemical reaction of CuKTS in equation 6 and the inhibition of DNA synthesis? In reaction 6, copper is released to cellular thiols, disulfides are formed, and copper can act as a redox catalyst for the reduction of O_2 to radical species by sulfhydryl groups. Any of these effects may be envisioned to disrupt cellular activities. Interestingly, at or near drug concentrations which significantly inhibit DNA synthesis and produce cytotoxicity, Cu from CuKTS binds predominantly if not exclusively to a low-molecular-weight protein called Zn, Cu binding protein (BP), which has metallothionein-like properties [17, 28]. In the process, the zinc bound to BP is replaced by copper from CuKTS. The presence of this protein in large quantity in Ehrlich cells and the finding of Zn-metallothionein in rapidly regenerating rat liver has led researchers to suggest that such a protein may be required for rapid cell division [29, 30]. If so, the displacement of zinc by copper may interfere with the role of the former in promoting cell division.

V. α-N-HETEROCYCLIC CARBOXALDEHYDE THIOSEMICARBAZONES

A. Introduction

α-N-Heterocyclic carboxaldehyde thiosemicarbazones were explored first as antitumor agents by Brockman and French and co-workers [31-33]. Although none of the compounds have shown significant antitumor activity in humans [34], their excellent effects in animals together with the extensive studies of the properties of these drugs make them important models in this area of metal-containing antitumor agents.

Like the bis(thiosemicarbazones), these monothiosemicarbazones were designed as potential biological metal-chelating agents (Fig. 7.4).

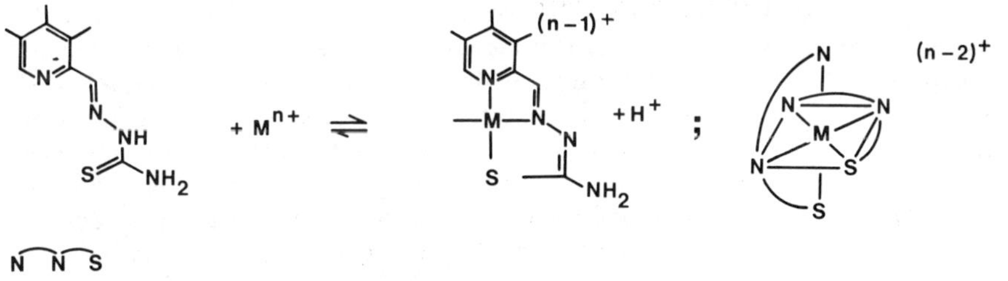

FIGURE 7.4 Metal chelating by α-N-heterocyclic carboxaldehyde thiosemicarbazone ligand to produce 1:1 and 2:1 ligand-to-metal complexes.

Until recently the screening and mechanistic studies of this series of compounds have centered upon the metal-free ligand [35, 36]. Among the key observations made in that work were that monothiosemicarbazones sequester large quantities of iron from animals and humans [34, 37, 38], and that a particularly sensitive site of inhibition by these compounds is ribonucleoside diphosphate reductase (RDR), the key enzyme in the conversion of ribonucleotides to deoxyribonucleotides [39, 40]. Because early RDR preparations were activated by Fe II, it was attractive to hypothesize that metal interactions were important to the mechanism of inhibition of this enzyme [41]. The initial view was that the drug formed a mixed-ligand complex with iron, bound in a coordinatively unsaturated way to the enzyme.

$$E\cdot Fe + \overset{\frown\frown}{N\ \ N\ \ S} \rightleftharpoons E\cdot Fe\begin{matrix} /N \\ -N \\ \backslash S \end{matrix} \qquad (7)$$

Although other workers found that RDR need not be activated by extra Fe II, this reaction remained of interest because the native mammalian enzyme does contain bound iron [42]. These early observations and hypotheses then raised the following questions: Is the free ligand or a metal complex the reactive form of the drug (for at least iron complexes of drug exist in organisms along with the ligand)? If a metal complex is important, which metal(s) are involved, and how is it mobilized from the host? Finally, what are the detailed mechanisms of reaction of ligands or complexes which lead to cytotoxicity?

To consider the nature of the cytotoxic forms of monothiosemicarbazones, it is necessary to react drug and cells under metal-free conditions which minimize interconversion of ligand and its metal complexes [43]. In one approach, cells and drug are incubated in Eagle's minimal essential medium (MEM), which contains little contaminant iron, copper, or zinc. Then, cells are washed free of drug and injected into animals or placed in cell culture to assess long-term viability of the treated cells. In this procedure, little drug can interact with the metal content of the host organism or the culture medium. In Table 7.2 a representative set of results for 1-formylisoquinoline thiosemicarbazone and its iron and copper complexes is given. Even at huge concentrations, short exposure of cells to the ligand has no deleterious effect on their survival. However, both iron and copper complexes significantly inhibit cell proliferation in mice, although Cu(IQ-1) is much more active under these conditions. A recent study using Chinese hamster ovary (CHO) cells provides similar results [44]. There has been only one brief report of the antitumor activity of an iron complex in animals [45]. In that work, bis(1-formylisoquinoline thiosemicarbazonato) Fe(II) was 40 times more active than the free ligand against mouse ascites sarcoma 180.

The question of the possible formation and stability of metal complexes in vivo has been examined with the measurement of stability constants

TABLE 7.2 Cytotoxicity and Cellular Effects of 1-Formylisoquinoline Thiosemicarbazone and Its Iron and Copper Complexes

Drug	Cytotoxicity[a]		50% inhibition of DNA synthesis (nmol/mg)	Cellular uptake
	Concentration (nmol/mg)	T/C		
IQ-1	500	1.1	0.35	–
Fe(IQ-1)$_2$	360	1.6	0.09	70% (100 nmol/mg)
Cu(IQ-1)	48	2.8	0.6	82% (36 nmol/mg)

[a]Cells incubated with drug, washed free of drug after 1 hr and injected with mice. T/C is ratio of the life span of animals with drug-treated cells to those with control cells.
Source: Ref. 43.

for Fe, Cu, and Zn monothiosemicarbazones (Table 7.3). With the exception of 2-formylpyridine thiosemicarbazonato Zn(II), the other complexes have large stability constants and might form and remain associated in the presence of typical competing biological ligands.

TABLE 7.3 Stability Constants of Metal Complexes of α-N-Heterocyclic Carboxaldehyde Thiosemicarbazones

Complex	Log stability constants		
	K_1	β_2	K_{app} (pH 7.4)
$Fe(III)L_2^+$[a]	–[b]	26.5	–
$Fe(II)L_2$[a, c]	–[b]	23.0	15.8
$Cu(II)L^+$[d, e]	16.9		13.3
$Zn(II)^+$[d]	9.2		5.6

[a]Unpublished information.
[b]$K_2 > K_1$.
[c]Ref. 46.
[d]Ref. 47.
[e]The log adduct stability constant of $Cu(II)L^+$ with ethylenediamine is 5.5.

B. Iron Complexes

Structural studies on the iron 2-formylpyridine monothiosemicarbazone complex have been initiated. According to electron paramagnetic resonance (EPR) measurements, $Fe(III)L_2$ is low spin [46]. Similarly, $Fe(II)L_2$ is expected to be diamagnetic. For such complexes, in which there is a spin-state change of the iron upon complexation, K_2 is greater than K_1 (Table 7.3) [46]. Thus FeL species are not favored under conditions of limiting concentration of thiosemicarbazone. Unpublished studies of the iron complexes show that they react very slowly in ligand substitution processes. Thus there are reasonable alternatives to reaction 7 (step a of reaction 8):

$$E\cdot Fe(II) + NNS \underset{}{\overset{a}{\rightleftharpoons}} E\cdot Fe(NNS) \xrightarrow[(NNS)]{b} E\cdot Fe(NNS)_2 \overset{c}{\rightleftharpoons} E + Fe(NNS)_2 \quad (8)$$

The formation of $Fe(NNS)_2$ is likely to be favored. The ligand, therefore, may remove iron from the enzyme (c) or possibly react with the enzyme as an octahedral complex (b). That the latter is the case is supported by the finding that preformed FeL_2 inhibits RDR, to which no exogenous Fe^{2+} has been added, several times better than the ligand itself [43].

Given the activity of intact Fe(II) complexes, how might they form in vivo? Two sources are prime candidates for iron donors, ferritin, the liver storage form of iron, and transferrin, the plasma transfer protein for iron. The reaction of HL with ferritin iron occurs over several days [46]. Similarly, HL is unreactive with transferrin even in the presence of nitrilotriacetate (NTA) [48]. However, the following reaction has much more favorable kinetics and is a plausible model for the mechanism of iron mobilization by HL [48].

$$Tr\cdot Fe(III)\cdot HCO_3 + 2HL \xrightarrow[NTA]{RSH} Tr + HCO_3^- + Fe(II)L_2 + 2H^+ \quad (9)$$

In reaction 9, NTA is thought to compete with HCO_3^- for binding to the protein. In so doing it labilizes the iron, making it susceptible to reduction by thiols or ascorbate. The Fe(II)-protein species is unstable and breaks down in the presence of HL to yield $Fe(II)L_2$. The substitution reaction of HL with transferrin and NTA does not take place because the apparent stability of $Fe(III)L_2$ is not large enough to extract the iron from the protein in the absence of reduction (Table 7.3).

The nature of the detailed interactions of iron monothiosemicarbazones with tumor cells has not been worked out. The complexes are readily taken up by Ehrlich cells and rapidly inhibit DNA synthesis at less than 0.1 nmol of drug per milligram of cell protein for several different chelates (Table 7.2). However, sustained cytotoxicity requires exposure to much larger concentrations of these materials.

C. Copper Complexes

A much clearer picture of the reaction of 2-formylpyridine thiosemicarbazonato copper(II) (CuL) in biological systems has been developed. Since the ligand is tridentate, the copper complex contains an in-plane coordination site for a solvent molecule, anion, or Lewis base. EPR measurements of CuL^+ in plasma, culture media, or cells show shifts in the hyperfine structure and g consistent with adduct formation [46,49]. Hence adduct species of these copper complexes may be expected in organisms. CuL is rapidly and irreversibly taken up by cells [49]. Although the complex bears a 1+ charge, adducts between the complex and amino acids probably form and may facilitate uptake. Once inside, CuL is thought to bind to thiols such as glutathione, for the frozen EPR spectrum of the complex in cells closely resembles that of CuL in the presence of glutathione (GSH) [6, 49,50].

Absorbance and EPR spectra of CuL in cells taken over time show that there is a very slow destruction of the complex which has a first-order decay of 4.5×10^{-5} sec^{-1} when 0.1 mM CuL is incubated with 1-15 mg of cell protein per milliliter [49]. This is a steady state; however, thiols are lost from the cell and oxygen is being consumed during this period. Apparently, CuL acts as a redox catalyst for the reaction of thiols with oxygen.

In solution, the reaction of CuL with glutathione has qualitatively similar properties [49]. Reduction occurs anaerobically with a rate constant of 6.25 M^{-1}/sec. In the presence of O_2, the reaction proceeds to a steady state in which oxygen continues to be reduced. The initial rate data for the aerobic reaction yield a smaller constant, 1.95 M^{-1}/sec, indicative of the involvement of O_2 in the reaction of CuL with thiols. Assays of oxygen radical production with the spin trap 5,5-dimethyl-1-pyrroline-N-oxide shows that large amounts of $O_2^{\cdot -}$ and $\cdot$OH are generated during the reaction [49].

The linkage between biochemical and cellular effects of CuL has yet to be made. Biochemically, it behaves much like CuKTS. Yet, unlike CuKTS, the levels of CuL which inhibit DNA synthesis and cause cytotoxicity are quite different. Clearly, more study is necessary to understand the importance of various biochemical properties of copper complexes for cytotoxicity.

D. Structure-Activity Relationships

Considerable effort has focused on empirical structure-function relationships involving chemical, enzymatic and antitumor properties [51]. Considering, in particular, chemical linear free energy correlations for 5-substituted-2-formylpyridine thiosemicarbazones, Knight et al. concluded that the stability constants and adduct formation constants with ethylenediamine have small ρ-values in linear free energy correlations and hence are not very sensitive to large changes in the substituent in the 5-position of the pyridine ring [51]. In contrast, reduction potentials for both copper and iron complexes are significantly altered by changes in substituent. Given the apparent role of reaction 2 in the cytotoxic interaction of CuL with Ehrlich cells, ring substitutions may therefore have a large effect on the antitumor activity of Cu and perhaps Fe monothiosemicarbazones.

VI. METAL BLEOMYCINS

The other principal members of the class of essential metal complexes with antitumor activity are derived from the antibiotic bleomycin (Fig. 7.5). The history of investigation of this clinically useful glycopeptide shows the conceptual novelty of the consideration of essential metal-ligand interactions in organisms. Bleomycin (Blm) was originally isolated from Streptomyces verticillus as CuBlm and shown to have significant antitumor properties in animals as a copper complex [52, 53]. Nevertheless, the drug was studied clinically, pharmacologically, and mechanistically for a number of years solely as the metal-free material [54]. The only role for metals such as CuII, ZnII, and CoII in these studies was as inhibitors of a DNA-strand scission reaction involving the drug [55]. In 1975, however, Ishida et al. showed that FeII stimulated this reaction [56]. Shortly, thereafter, attention was directed again to the role of CuII in the activities of Blm [50, 57, 58]. It was the excellent studies of Horwitz and colleagues, carefully documenting the requirement of FeII for the strand scission reaction,

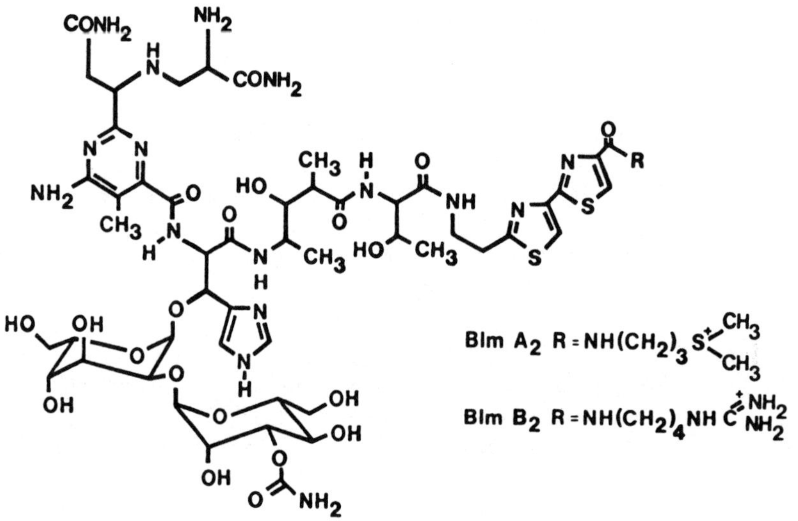

FIGURE 7.5 Structure of bleomycin. Major isomers are Blm-A_2 and Blm-B_2. (From Ref. 77.)

which stimulated a great surge of interest in the chemistry of metal bleomycins, particularly Fe(II)Blm [59, 60). Subsequent studies have shown Blm to be a fascinating, versatile ligand for transition metal ions and have begun to elucidate the reaction of Fe(II)Blm with DNA. Following our guidelines set forth above for obtaining biologically relevant information about metal complexes, this section will focus on the implication of chemical studies on metal bleomycins for their possible biological activity. Because of the tremendous current interest in metal bleomycins, the reader has available a wealth of recent reviews on this subject. Two monographs, as well as a comprehensive review of the chemistry of metal bleomycins by Dabrowiak, are particularly useful [54, 61, 62].

A. Biological Studies

The complexity of the question of the nature of the reactions of Blm and metal bleomycins with biological systems is apparent from the following results from antitumor and cytotoxicity studies of such materials. According to Rao et al. [63], metal-free Blm as well as the Cu(II), Zn(II), and Fe(III) Blm complexes all inhibit the growth of Ehrlich ascites tumor in mice. The order of activity on a molar basis is Cu(II)Blm > Blm > Zn(II)Blm > Fe(III)Blm >> Co(II)Blm ~ untreated control. In cell culture, a 60-min incubation of cells with drugs under "metal-free" conditions to minimize formation or interconversion of complexes shows a similar order of activity against Ehrlich cells, with Fe(III)Blm less cytotoxic than Blm, Cu(II)Blm, or Zn(II)Blm. Thus, in contrast to the results with thiosemicarbazones, the bleomycin ligand is active under metal-free incubation conditions in cell culture experiments. Second, several metal complexes are also active, but Fe(III)Blm, closely related to the putative active form of Blm, Fe(II)Blm, is less active than the others. Thus the question is raised: Are bleomycin and its metal complexes distinct pharmacological agents in vivo or do they converge to a single proximate agent? To address this question, it is important to understand the stability and reactivity of the various metal complexes.

B. Chemical Properties of Metal Bleomycins

Sugiura has published a series of equilibrium constants for different metal bleomycins determined by computer analysis of pH titration data [64]. More detailed studies of the pH-dependent dissociation of Cu(II)Blm using EPR, fluorescence, and absorbance measurements, however, do not agree with his findings [65]. In the latter work, log apparent stability constants measured at lower pH values can be extrapolated to 18.0 at pH 7 [65-67]. Besides high thermodynamic stability, ligand exchange reactions of Cu(II)Blm appear to be very slow (Table 7.4). Finally, the complex reacts very slowly with a selection of sulfhydryl reagents without significant catalysis of oxygen reduction by thiols (Table 7.4). Thus chemical studies predict that Cu(II)Blm will be rather stable and unreactive in biological systems.

TABLE 7.4 Kinetics of Some Reactions of Cu(II)Blm

$$Cu(II)Blm + L \overset{k}{\rightleftharpoons} Cu(II)L + Blm$$

L = EDTA[a] $k = 3 \times 10^{-6}\ M^{-1}/sec$ at pH 7.4

$$Cu(II)Blm + 2RSH \overset{k}{\rightleftharpoons} Cu(I)SR + (1/2)RSSR + H_2Blm$$

RSH:	
glutathione	$k = 1.2 \times 10^{-2}\ M^{-1}/sec$
cysteine	$= 1.2 \times 10^{-1}\ M^{-1}/sec$
2-mercaptoethanol	$= 9.5 \times 10^{-3}\ M^{-1}/sec$

[a]Extrapolated from pseudo-first-order data at lower pH. EDTA, ethylenediaminetetraacetic acid.
Source: Refs. 65-67.

Nevertheless, Takahashi et al. present data showing that thiols in homogenates of tumor cells reductively dissociate Cu(II)Blm and maintain the copper in its Cu(I) state even after Sephadex chromatography [58]. In terms of the relative unreactivity of Cu(II)Blm with model thiols, this result is surprising and deserves further study. Although interpreted as a way to release Blm so that it can react with FeII in cells, this reaction would also release copper inside of cells as does CuKTS. Thus this feature of the reaction may, itself, initiate a cytotoxic response.

The apparent stability constants of Zn(II)- and Fe(II,III)Blms have not yet been determined but are much smaller than that for Cu(II)Blm, for CuII stoichiometrically displaces these metals from their complexes with Blm. Qualitatively, zinc competes well with FeII for binding to Blm [67]. The major question is whether Zn(II)Blm or the Fe(II,III) can form by the reaction of BLM with these metals in the organism and whether such complexes can exist without exchanging metals with cellular ligands of higher stability with the metals.

This question has two parts, one relating to the stability of the bleomycin complexes, the other to the availability of transition metals in the organism for reaction with Blm. The information available about the first aspect is summarized below. No studies have been carried out to resolve the second part; however, if the plasma distribution of zinc, copper, and iron is any indication, the order of availability to external ligands is Zn >> Cu > Fe. A significant amount of zinc is bound to exchangeable sites—amino acids and albumin; a smaller fraction of the copper is in such form; but virtually all of the iron is tightly bound to transferrin [18, 19]. Thus, whether there is iron in cells available for chelation must be carefully documented.

The pH-dependent dissociations of Fe(III)- and Fe(II)Blm have been studied [68, 69]. Figure 7.6 shows that Fe(III)Blm dissociates in two steps, as does CuBlm [68, 69]. The first is described as [68]

$$\text{Fe(III)Blm} + \text{H}^+ \overset{K = 10^{4.3}}{\rightleftharpoons} \text{Fe(III)BlmH}^+ \qquad (10)$$

Low spin: g = 2.45, 2.18, 1.89 High spin: g = 9.4, 4.3

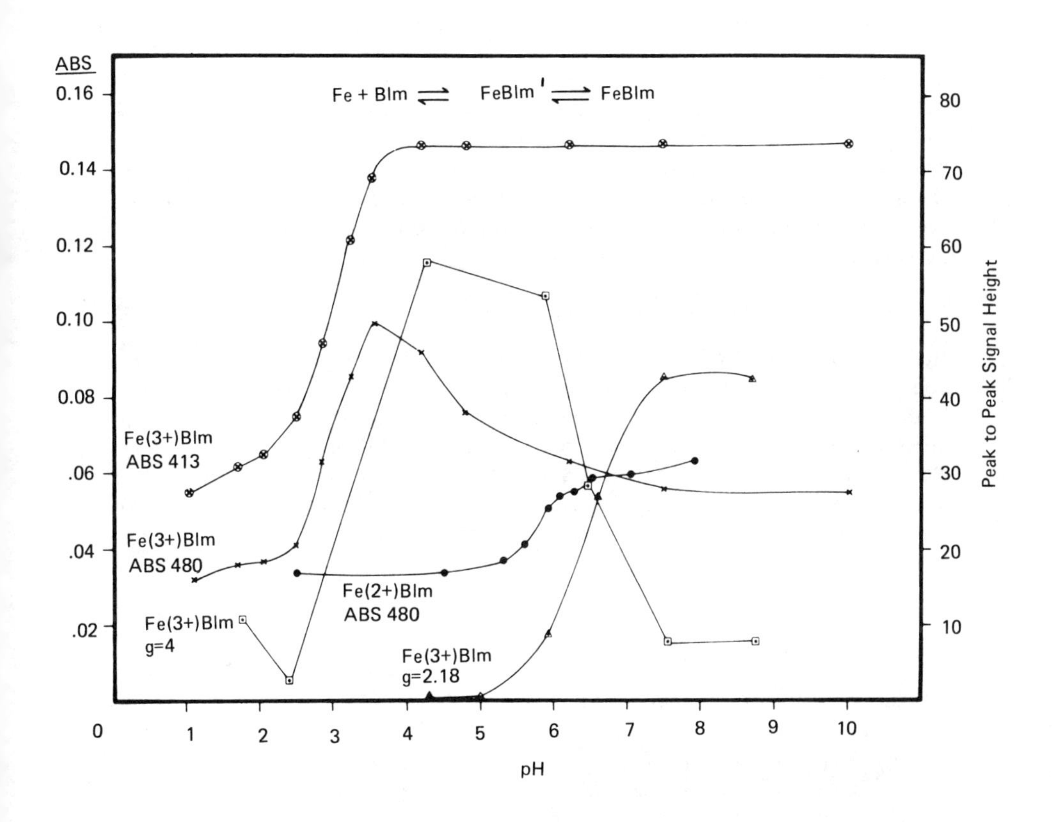

FIGURE 7.6 The pH dependence of the absorbance at 413 nm and 480 nm for Fe(3+)Blm and at 480 nm for Fe(2+)Blm (left ordinate) in addition to the pH dependence versus the peak-to-peak signal height (right ordinate) for high-spin Fe(3+)Blm at g = 4 and low-spin Fe(3+)Blm at g = 2.18. All solutions are made up in a 0.1 M NaCl. The concentration of both Fe(3+)Blm and Fe(2+)Blm is approximately 0.2 mM. (From Ref. 69, reproduced with permission of Biochem. Biophys. Res. Commun.)

The second is curve fit to the following process;

$$Fe(III)BlmH^{+} + 2.5H^{+} \underset{}{\overset{K = 10^{2.7}}{\rightleftharpoons}} Fe(III) + H_{3.5}Blm \qquad (11)$$

Figure 7.6 also shows a titration event for Fe(II)Blm, described previously by Sausville et al. [60]. A single proton is involved:

$$Fe(II)Blm + H^{+} \overset{K = 10^{5.7}}{\rightleftharpoons} Fe(II)BlmH^{+} \qquad (12)$$

That the protonation produces an intermediate Fe(II)Blm species is inferred from a ^{13}C nuclear magnetic resonance (NMR) relaxation study of Fe(II)Blm at pH 5.3 [69, 70]. It was concluded that Fe(II)Blm is only bound to the primary and secondary amine groups, consistent with the partial dissociation of the ligand structures from the metal at this pH. It is noted that whether or not the iron bleomycins are stable in biological systems, equations 10 and 12 indicate that part of the structure is bound weakly to the metal and suggest that adduct species may form in which part of the ligand structure is displaced by Lewis bases.

C. Structures of Metal Bleomycins

Because of the size of Blm and diversity of its functional groups, it has not been easy to define the coordination sites in Blm for various metal ions. The cornerstone for studies in this area is the x-ray structure of the copper complex of a biosynthetic intermediate (P-3A) of CuBlm (Figure 7.7) [71]. The copper binds to five nitrogen atoms from primary and secondary amines, pyrimidine, peptide bond, and imidazole. All of these groups are located in the left half of the structure of Blm.

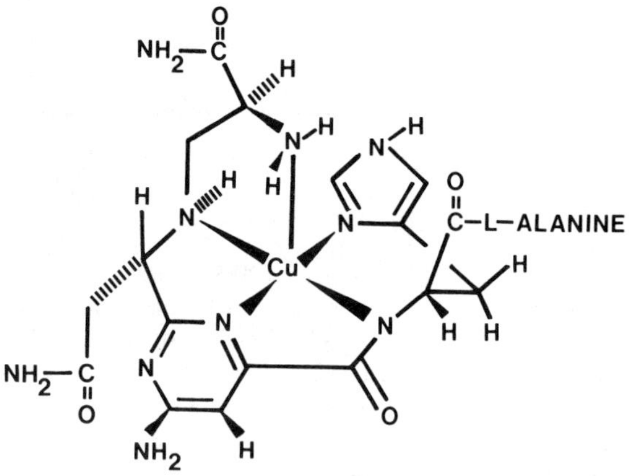

FIGURE 7.7 Structure of Cu(P-3A), a biosynthetic intermediate of CuBlm. (Reproduced with permission of J. Inorg. Biochem.)

The extension of these results to other complexes has been made principally by NMR studies. Qualitatively, in diamagnetic complexes such as Zn(II)Blm and Fe(II)Blm·CO, large changes in chemical shift of resonances in Blm have been identified with sites of metal binding [72-75]. In general, such changes are confined to the left half of the molecule, leading to the idea that there is a common region for metal binding in bleomycin. However, there is controversy as to which groups may be directly bound to zinc, in part because there are six groups associated with large shifts: primary and secondary amines, pyrimidine, imidazole, the mannose carbonyl function, and the valerate residue [76].

The structure proposed by Oppenheimer for Fe(II)Blm·CO based on ^1H NMR of the complex contains the primary amine as an in-plane ligand and the carbamoyl nitrogen as the axial ligand trans to CO. The axial amide is not attractive either as a ligand for iron or as the trans axial ligand to stabilize the binding of CO to the complex. In contrast, Sugiura presents EPR evidence from the comparison of Fe(II)Blm·NO· and NO· complexes of modified iron bleomycins that the primary amine acts as the fifth axial ligand in Fe(II)Blm (Fig. 7.5). Similar comparisons lead to the same model for Fe(III)Blm.

Glickson and co-workers have assigned the contact shifted NMR resonances in Fe(II)Blm, a high-spin, paramagnetic complex [78]. They argue that ligands may include the valerate hydroxyl or carbonyl, α-amine, imidazole, pyrimidine, and/or carbamoyl oxygen, which differ in part from those for the Fe(II)Blm·CO complex. It is unlikely that the binding of CO to the complex causes a major reorganization of the metal ligand structure. Although the precise structures of the site of iron bleomycins have not been determined, the binding of Fe(II)Blm to CO, NO·, and O_2 and Fe(III)Blm to a variety of Lewis bases having N, O, and S donor atoms suggests that these are naturally 5-coordinate complexes, which form adduct species [68, 77, 79]. In this respect, they seem comparable to iron in myoglobin and hemoglobin [68].

There are other subtleties to metal-bleomycin adduct formation which suggest that under some conditions intermolecular and possibly intramolecular metal-bithiazole interactions occur [80-83]. In the presence of Fe(II) Blm or Fe(II)Blm·NO, which are paramagnetic and have extensively broadened ligand resonances, the ^1H NMR spectrum of excess added Blm contains broadened bithiazole resonances [80]. All of the others remain sharp. Addition of thiol reverses the broadening of bithiazole. The results are consistent with the ability of bithiazole sulfur or nitrogen atoms to bind to iron. According to similar NMR studies adduct formation between Cu(II)Blm or Co(II)Blm and another molecule of Blm occurs, which appears to involve interaction of the extra bithiazole with the metal centers [81, 82]. Another recent proton nuclear relaxation study of Mn(II)Blm also suggests that the bithiazole but not the imidazole group is bound to manganese [83].

D. Redox Chemistry of FeBlm

Interest naturally centers around the strand scission of DNA by Fe(II)Blm and O_2. Burger et al. have studied the kinetics of oxidation of Fe(II)Blm by O_2 [84]. An intermediate thought to be a dioxygen adduct is detected in stopped-flow absorbance studies:

$$\text{Fe(III)Blm} + O_2 \underset{}{\overset{k_1}{\rightleftharpoons}} \text{Fe(II)Blm}\cdot O_2 \xrightarrow{k_2} \text{Fe(III)Blm}' \qquad (13)$$

g = 2.26, 2.18, 1.94 (Ref. 77, 84)

$$\xrightarrow{k_3} \text{Fe(III)Blm}$$

g = 2.45, 2.18, 1.89

In this reaction sequence the probable intermediate, Fe(II)Blm·O_2, reacts to yield Fe(III)Blm', a paramagnetic species having EPR g values characteristic of low-spin Fe(III). In the presence of DNA this intermediate turns over at the same rate as reaction with DNA occurs [85]. Hence this species is probably the activated form of Fe(III)Blm which attacks DNA. Reminiscent of the work with cytochrome P-450, an intermediate with these same g values can also be generated from the reaction of Fe(III)Blm with H_2O_2 under anaerobic conditions [85]. Peisach and co-workers have suggested that the product of this reaction is a two-electron reduced form of O_2 bound to low-spin ferric iron in bleomycin. Either Fe(III)-OH· or Fe(III)-O_2H would satisfy this description. Support for the presence of reduced O_2 in this intermediate comes from the demonstration of a broadening of its EPR line width when $^{17}O_2$ having a nuclear spin of 5/2 is used in place of $^{16}O_2$ to oxidize Fe(II)Blm [85]. To get to this state in equation 13, one can imagine that the Fe(II)Blm·O_2 adduct adds another molecule of Fe(II)Blm to form a binuclear complex and then undergoes an internal electron transfer to yield the product. However, the rate constant, k_2, in equation 13 has been measured as 0.33 sec^{-1}, which does not indicate that a bimolecular process is involved [84].

It will be noted that the g values of Fe(III)Blm' are contracted toward the spin-only value of 2.00 in comparison with Fe(III)Blm, the final, stable Fe(III) species. Apparently, the electronic orbital angular momentum is quenched in the intermediate. Adduct formation between Fe(III)Blm and cysteine or glutathione produces this same type of alteration in g values [79]. In fact, EPR spectra of a number of adducts of Fe(III)Blm with ligands containing Lewis base donor atoms O, N, and S show clearly that only sulfur-containing bases cause this shift in g values [77]. Thus the finding that the intermediate, Fe(III)Blm', species is an oxygen donor adduct is unexpected.

Consideration of how reaction 13 might occur in vivo centers on how he redox stable Fe(III)Blm can be reduced to Fe(II)Blm. The complex might act as catalyst of oxygen reduction by cellular reductants so that the small amounts of Blm that enter cells might exert significant effects [79, 86]. Antholine and Petering showed that Fe(III)Blm catalyzes the reduction of oxygen by thiols according to the following minimal mechanism [79]:

$$Fe(III)Blm^{+} + RSH \rightleftharpoons Fe(III)Blm\cdot SR + H^{+} \quad (14)$$

$$Fe(III)Blm\cdot SR \longrightarrow Fe(II)Blm + (1/2)RSSR \quad (15)$$

$$Fe(II)Blm + O_2 \xrightarrow{fast} Fe(III)Blm^{+} + \text{reduced } O_2 \quad (16)$$

This seqquence is formally equivalent to the catalytic cycle of oxygen reduction by thiols carried out by 2-formylpyridine thiosemicarbazonato Cu(II) [49]. A second, less biologically plausible, but still very interesting, catalytic cycle has been described by Bachur's group in which excess FeII is the reductant and Blm is considered to be the catalyst [87].

E. Reaction of FeBlm with DNA

The right side of the bleomycin molecule contains bithiazole and positively charged R groups. Fluorescence and NMR studies clearly show that they interact and bind to DNA with a binding constant and stoichiometry of 1.2×10^5 M^{-1} and 1 Blm/5-6 base pairs, respectively [88]. Binding and intercalation involve the bithiazole and positively charged R group [88, 89]. There is a clear preference for strand scission to occur on pyrimidine nucleosides on the 3' side of guanosine in single- and double-stranded DNA [90]. The reasons for this specificity have not been elucidated [91]. Thus it is now known that Cu(II)phleomycin, which differs only in its partially saturated bithiazole group, does not intercalate into DNA as does Cu(II)Blm [91]. Yet Fe(II)phleomycin cleaves DNA with the same specificity as Fe(III)Blm. Hence the role of intercalation of drug into DNA in the strand scission reaction is in question.

Using Fe(II)Blm·NO as a model for Fe(II)Blm·O_2, EPR studies show significant perturbations of the electronic structures of the complex when it interacts with DNA [69, 92]. The perturbation appears to be in the xy plane of the iron site. This is striking because the metal site is several bonds away from the region in Blm of principal binding to DNA. The difference in spectra can be used to monitor binding of the complex to DNA. The reaction has a definite stoichiometry of about 1 Fe(II)Blm·NO/10-30 base pairs of DNA [69]. A recent NMR study confirms the binding of Fe(II)Blm to DNA by its bithiazole and R groups [93]. Interestingly, however, the study reveals no significant structural effect on the iron binding site. In contrast to this, when Fe(II)Blm·CO binds to DNA, NMR shifts in the histidine imidazole protons are observed [80]. Assuming that an imidazole nitrogen is an in-plane ligand of Fe(II), this result is consistent with the interpretation of the change in EPR spectrum of Fe(II)Blm$\cdot$NO upon binding to DNA, in which xy plane perturbation of the iron site occurs [69].

The reaction of Blm + FeII, DNA, and O_2 has the following properties. The redox reaction occurs 60 times faster in the presence of DNA than in its absence [86]. Thus the kinetics of reaction also support a structural modification of the iron site in the Fe(II)Blm$\cdot$DNA complex. Furthermore, there is no spectral evidence for an intermediate dioxygen adduct in the reaction [86]. Both superoxide and hydroxyl radicals have been spin trapped [66, 77, 94]. However, the reaction seems to be insenstitive to the presence of superoxide dismutase and catalase to scavenge $O_2^{\cdot-}$ and H_2O_2 [56, 60]. Together with the ability of bleomycin to bind to DNA, this result has led to the view that the reduced oxygen species generated from Fe(II)Blm and O_2 reacts with DNA without diffusion from the site, presumably because it is bound directly to iron [85]. This hypothesis is consistent with the details of the oxidation of Fe(II)Blm by O_2 described above. Depending on the conditions, the products of strand scission include free bases and a material that can be converted to malondialdehyde [59, 60]. The nature of the reactions involved are being investigated [95].

Complicating this picture are data on the stoichiometry of the reaction. According to Fig. 7.8, 5±1 electrons or Fe(II)Blm sites react with O_2 and DNA to cleave one bond in DNA as measured by malondialdehyde formation. Within error, the data are independent of relative FeII, Blm, and DNA base concentration. According to these results, Blm can act as a ferroxidase in strand scission, as observed above in the redox process alone [87]. Other workers have not observed increases in bond cleavage above 1:1 ratios of Fe/Blm [8, 86]. Interestingly, the data require that multiple Fe(II) atoms diffuse into a given site of reaction. Yet, remarkably, the stoichiometry is relatively constant, even though the initial binding sites of Blm to the polymer may be widely separated and FeII may be in excess of Blm.

That multiple electrons are required in the reaction is consistent with both the relative unreactivity of the one-electron reduced form of O_2, superoxide ion, and the highly reactive nature of hydroxyl radical, possibly generated as a bound Fe(II)OH adduct as described above [85, 96]. Thus, using $OH^{\cdot}$ as the initial attacking species, Grollman and Takeshita envision strand scission to occur as shown in Fig. 7.9 [89]. The stoichiometry of this mechanism is 4 Fe(II)/2 O_2/bond cleaved and is consistent with data in Fig. 7.8 and some of the results for Fe(II)/O_2 ratios in strand scission [8]. However, recent work shows that the reaction sequence outlined in Fig. 7.9 is probably oversimplified [95].

F. Cellular Studies

Experiments suggesting that both Blm and Cu(II)Blm cleave DNA in cells have been published [58]. However, Nunn and Lunec's data show that both drugs can inhibit cell growth 99% without causing observable increases in strand

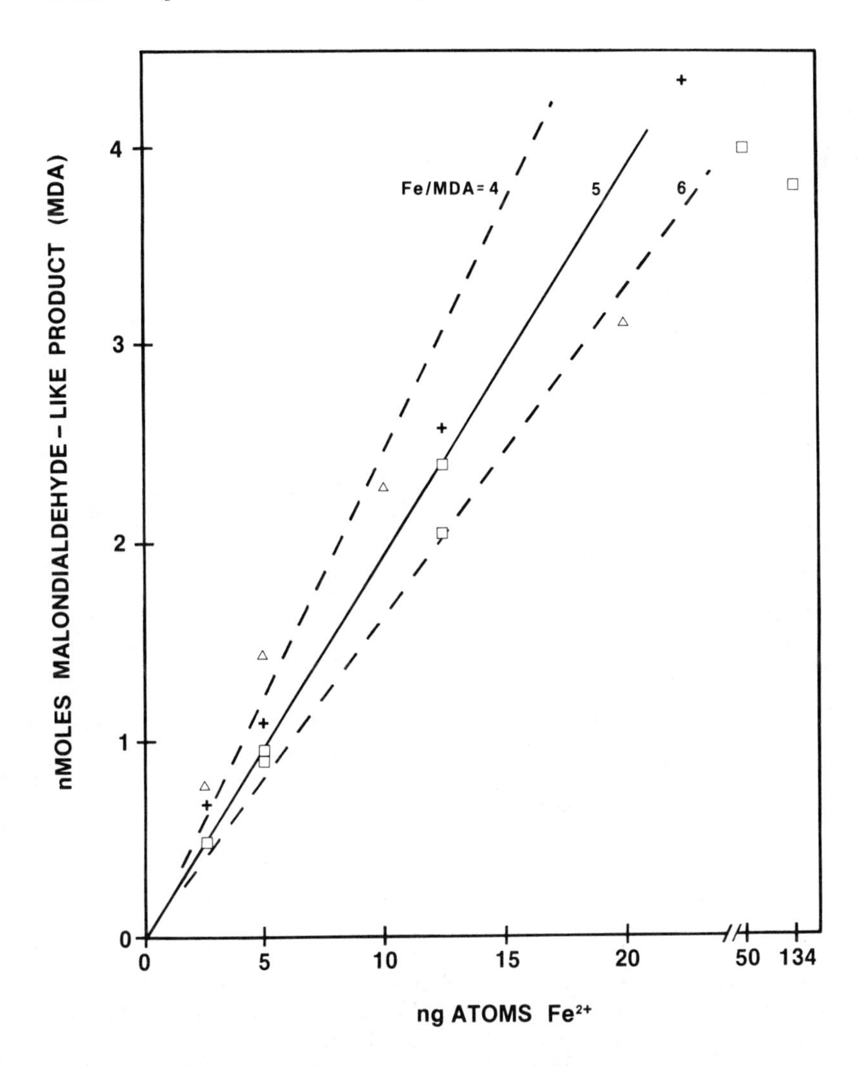

FIGURE 7.8 Stoichiometry of DNA strand cleavage by Fe^{2+} plus Blm [DNA] = 0.25 mM (50 nmol). (□) [Blm] = 0.025 mM (5 nmol) Fe^{2+} varied in 62 mM phosphate buffer, pH 7.0; (Δ) as in ( ) except 31 mM phosphate buffer, pH 7.0; (+) [Blm] = [Fe^{2+}] in 62 mM phosphate buffer, pH 7.0. (Unpublished information.)

scission [97]. Similarly, among antitumor drugs bleomycin does not stand out in the production of chromosome breaks [98]. Furthermore, bleomycin specifically stops the cell cycle in G_2, a process not readily related to strand scission [99]. It is important to point out that very little bleomycin,

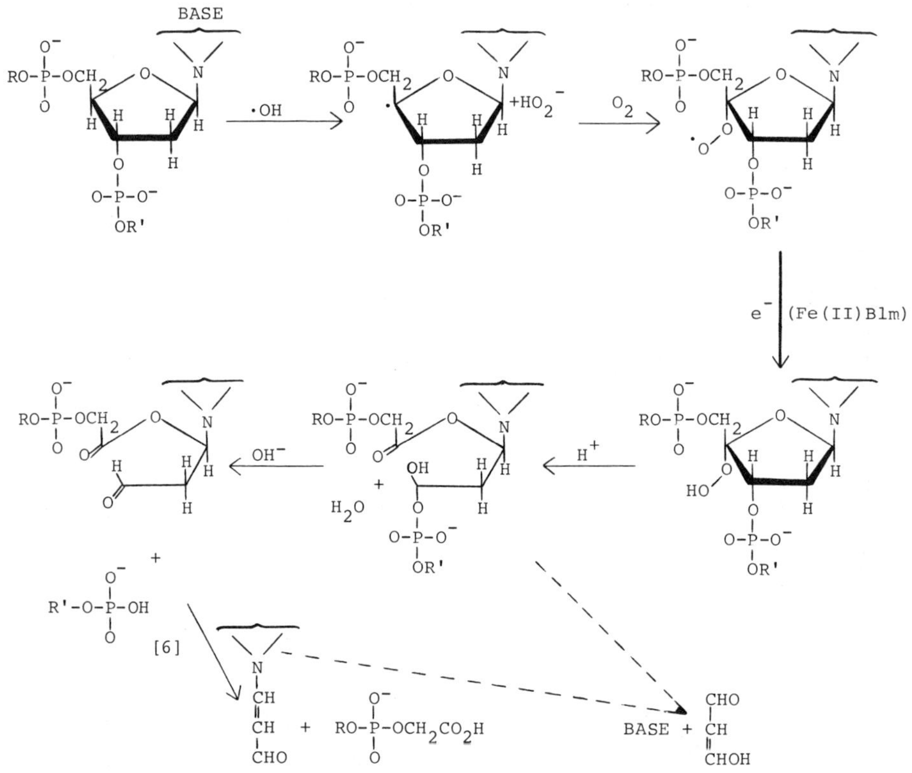

FIGURE 7.9 Mechanism of DNA strand cleavage by Fe(II)Blm. (Adapted from ref. 90.)

or its Cu or Co complexes, enters cells [67, 100-102], presumably because the ligand and complexes are charged polar molecules which may not easily penetrate the membrane lipid bilayer. Hence the relationship of the in vitro chemistry of bleomycin to the cellular response requires further study.

VII. CIS-DICHLORODIAMMINE PLATINUM(II)

The only metal complex that is currently used in the chemotherapy of human cancers is cis-dichlorodiammine platinum(II) [103, 104]. In contrast to the copper and iron complexes discussed in this chapter, this is a complex of a nonessential heavy metal. cis-Platinum has a broad spectrum of chemotherapeutic activity, and has been used successfully against tumors of the head and neck, testicular carcinoma, squamous cell carbinoma, malignant lymphoma, endometrial carcinoma, and ovarian adenocarcinoma.

Rosenberg and his colleagues were the first to observe that platinum compounds had biological activity. They found that bacterial division could be arrested by compounds formed from the dissolution of platinum wire electrodes in culture media containing NH_4Cl [105]. In 1969, Rosenberg's group reported that cis-platinum and some related species have a potent cytotoxic effect against a variety of experimental tumors [106, 107]. It was observed that the biological activity of square-planar platinum(II) complexes was restricted to neutral complexes in the cis configuration; trans complexes, such as trans-dichlorodiammine platinum (II), are either inactive against tumors, or active only at much higher concentrations than the corresponding cis analogs.

A number of symposia on cis-platinum have been held [108-111] and reviews covering the basic chemistry, biochemistry [103, 112-114], and clinical findings [5, 104] have recently appeared. This chapter will concentrate on the relationship of the chemical and biochemical properties of platinum complexes to their reactions in organisms.

A. Chemistry

The biochemistry of square-planar Pt(II) complexes appears to center on their properties in substitution reactions:

$$-\mathrm{Pt}-X + \underline{Y} \longrightarrow -\mathrm{Pt}-Y + X \qquad (17)$$

Under pseudo-first-order conditions for Y, a two-term rate constant is observed:

$$k = k_1 + k_2[Y] \qquad (18)$$

Three alternative pathways of reaction exist. Two are in k_1 and involve rate-determining dissociation of $X(k_1')$ or solvolysis of the complex (k_1'') followed by rapid addition or substitution of Y. The other involves direct

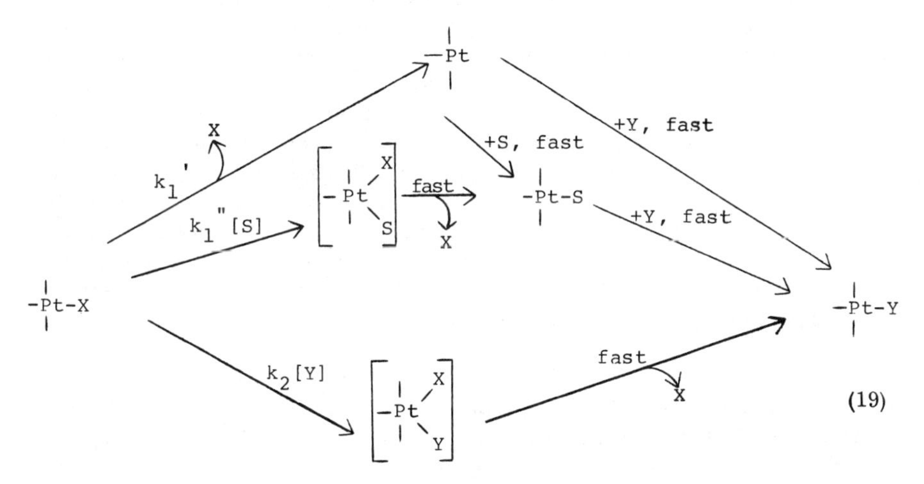

(19)

displacement of X by Y (k_2). In this mechanism,

$$k_1 = k_1' + k_1''[S] \tag{20}$$

and for the case of solvent in large excess of reactant complex, the expression is a constant. This type of platinum chemistry has been studied and reviewed in great detail [112, 115, 116]. The key observation is that platinum chloroammine complexes react slowly in substitution reactions but with varying rates depending on the nature of Y. Nucleophiles with sulfur in various oxidation states react more rapidly than those containing nitrogen, which in turn are more reactive than oxygen-containing compounds.

B. Biological Studies

The interaction of cis-$Pt(NH_3)_2Cl_2$ with organisms has been described in terms of a controlling role for Cl^- on its reactivity [112]. Since water molecules, but not hydroxyl groups, are displaced much more rapidly than chloride in substitution reactions* the degree of solvolysis of cis-platinum is an important determinant of reactivity of the platinum center. For example, under equilibrium conditions in plasma with $[Cl^-] \sim 0.1$ M, most of the platinum is in the form of $Pt(II)(NH_3)_2Cl_2$ (Fig. 7.10). However, in a tissue having a much lower $[Cl^-]$ (0.004 M), mono- and diaquo species comprise about 40% of the total concentration of platinum. As a consequence, the neutral parent complex is unreactive in plasma and can diffuse through membranes into cells where it hydrolyzes and reacts with cellular ligands, particularly nucleic acid bases in DNA. However, according to one study, nuclei may have a $[Cl^-]$ as high as 0.15 M [117], rather than the lower average value for tissue given above.

A more complete picture of the reactivity of cis-platinum must also include the kinetic properties of these reactions and the description of the competition reactions of multiple ligands in organisms with forms of the complex. According to Fig. 7.10, both reactions with water molecules (I→II, II → III) are slow reactions. Thus the distribution of platinum species is to some extent kinetically controlled. In addition, recent studies show that V can form dimer and trimer bridged hydroxo species [118]. Given the preference of platinum for soft ligands, Cl^- is probably the principal inorganic competitor of water and hydroxide for binding to the metal center. However, recent studies show that 50 nM phosphate greatly inhibits the binding of cis-$Pt(Cl)(H_2O)$ to DNA [119]. Thus, other, harder anions also seem to have important effects on the chemistry of the complex.

*For the reaction dien Pt-X + pyridine → dien Pt-pyridine + X, X = OH_2 reacts about 50 times more rapidly than X = Cl. (Ref. 115, Table 95.)

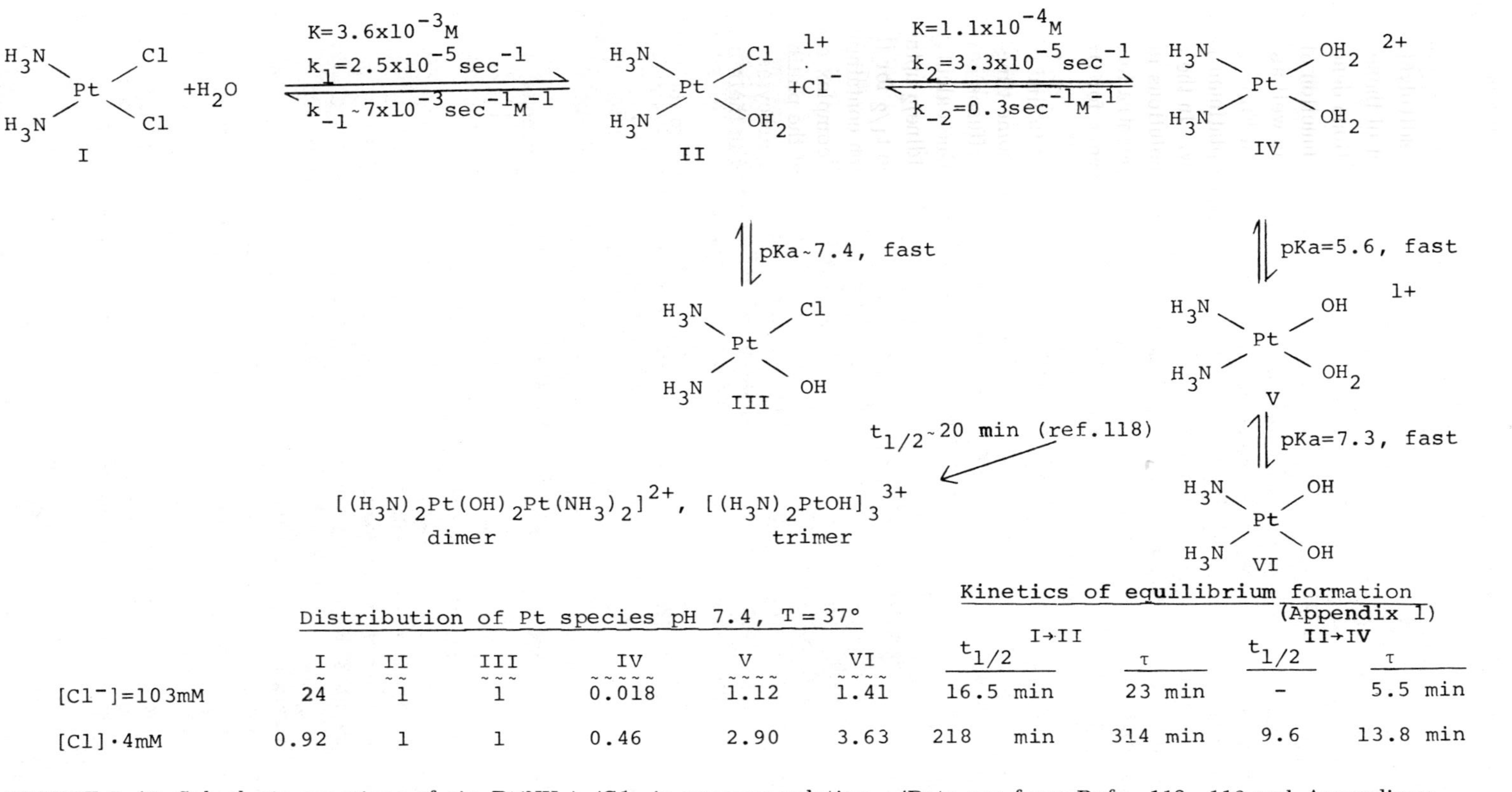

Distribution of Pt species pH 7.4, T = 37°

	I	II	III	IV	V	VI
$[Cl^-]$=103mM	24	1	1	0.018	1.12	1.41
[Cl]·4mM	0.92	1	1	0.46	2.90	3.63

Kinetics of equilibrium formation (Appendix I)

	I→II $t_{1/2}$	I→II τ	II→IV $t_{1/2}$	II→IV τ
$[Cl^-]$=103mM	16.5 min	23 min	-	5.5 min
[Cl]·4mM	218 min	314 min	9.6	13.8 min

FIGURE 7.10 Solvolysis reactions of cis-$Pt(NH_3)_2(Cl_2$ in aqueous solution. (Data are from Refs. 112, 118 and Appendixes 1 and 2.)

To find the half-time ($t_{1/2}$) for the establishment of the solvolysis equilibria, or the relaxation times (τ) for the reestablishment of these equilibria as other reactions occur to perturb them, the equations described in Appendixes 1 and 2 can be used. It is noted that $t_{1/2}$ is a function of the initial concentration of chloride and of the platinum complex as well as its equilibrium concentration. The calculated results are given in Fig. 7.10 for the condition of water and chloride in large excess of the platinum reactants and products. The approach to each equilibrium is slow. In the calculations, the difference in $t_{1/2}$ for high- and low-chloride solutions is largely accounted for by the difference in the equilibrium concentrations of the parent cis-platinum complex in these media. The $t_{1/2}$ and τ for II$\rightleftharpoons$IV are faster than the values for the first equilibrium.

It is for kinetic reasons, therefore, that one may expect to find that the neutral complex, cis-$Pt(NH_3)_2Cl_2$, exists in plasma for some time without significant dissociation. During this time it readily diffuses across plasma membranes into blood cells and tissues [120-122]. One calculation for the first-order diffusion rate constant of cis-Pt-Cl_2 (pyridine)$_2$ uptake into Ehrlich cells gives a value of about 2 min^{-1}* [123]. The $t_{1/2}$ for this process is much smaller than $t_{1/2}$ or τ for I$\rightleftharpoons$II in a solution containing 0.1 M chloride. However, it is also evident that the dichloro complex reacts with plasma proteins in blood (Fig. 7.11). Within 1 hr 40% of the platinum in blood is bound to protein. The same study showed that erythrocytes rapidly pick up platinum from plasma and bind it irreversibly in their intracellular space.

According to Appendix 3, one may envision contributions to the overall rate constant of reaction from rate-limiting solvolysis of cis-platinum and possibly from direct reaction of the dichloro species, depending on the relative magnitude of k_1 and k_3. Rate constants for direct substitution vary widely depending on the nature of the nucleophile [124].

Some results of a study showing the distribution of intravenous, injected $^{195}Pt(NH_3)_2Cl_2$ among tissues is illustrated in Fig. 7.12 [120]. The interesting features are first the rapid disappearance of platinum from blood into a variety of tissues prior to the initial 30-min point and, more important, the long-term stability of the metal in each tissue. In harmony with these observations, tumors do not preferentially accumulate cis-platinum. Contrasted with this pattern are data for another neutral complex, CuKTS [125]. Here, marked changes in tissue concentration occur for hours, including a slow increase in liver copper. That is, even though CuKTS is kinetically more reactive in model systems, it is cis-platinum which is rapidly and irreversibly accumulated by a variety of tissues.

---

*In the calculations, $\frac{d[Pt]}{dt}_{cell} = k[Pt]_{external\ medium}$ and 2.5 mg cell protein = 10^7 cells = 0.00075 ml of total aqueous cell volume.

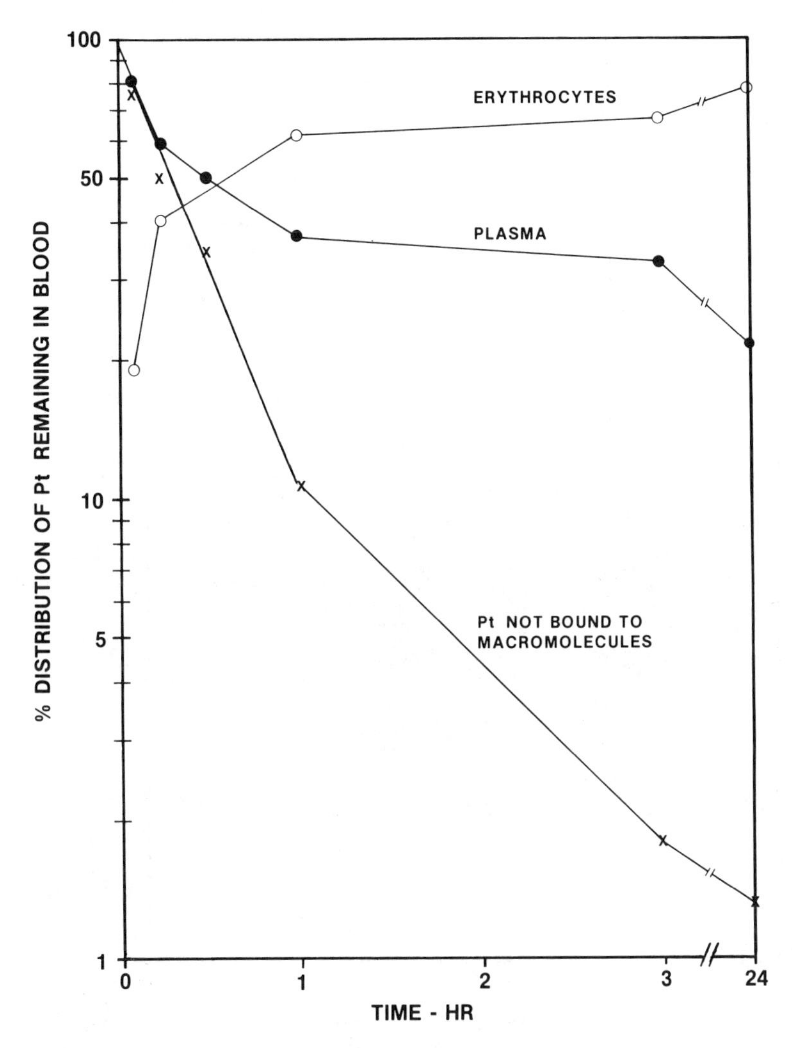

FIGURE 7.11 Kinetics of distribution of cis-platinum among components of blood. (From Ref. 121.)

How is the platinum sequestered in cells? Recently, Choie et al. studied the time-dependent changes in cis-platinum distribution among subcellular components of rat liver and kidney [122]. As shown in Fig. 7.13, most of the kidney platinum localized in the cytosol. More than half is rapidly bound to trichloroacetic acid-precipitable macromolecules. A fraction of the rest binds to membranes and organelles. A significant amount of

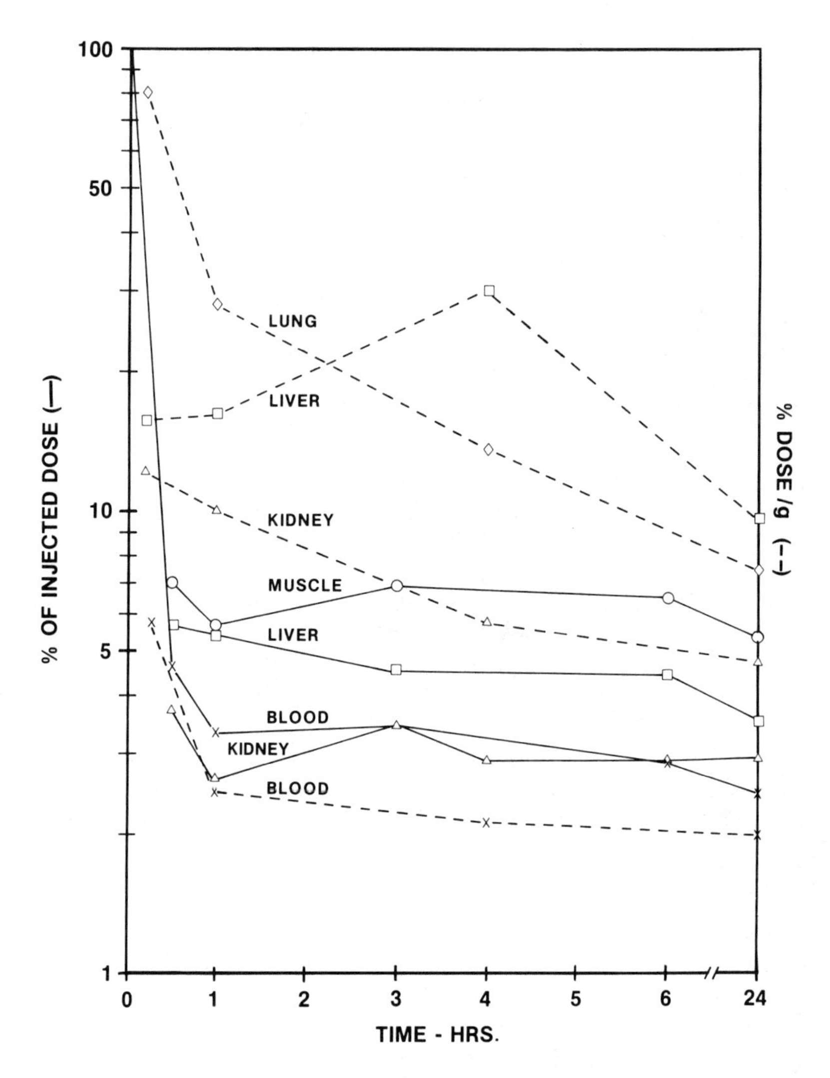

FIGURE 7.12 Kinetics of distribution of cis-platinum among tissues in the rat. (From Ref. 120.) Comparative distribution of CuKTS (-----) from Ref. 125.

cytosolic platinum remains in kidney but unbound to macromolecules. Since it seems inert to reaction, this may comprise cis-platinum bound to small molecule metabolites. When these amounts of platinum are normalized per milligram of protein in each cell fraction, cytosol, microsomes, and nuclei

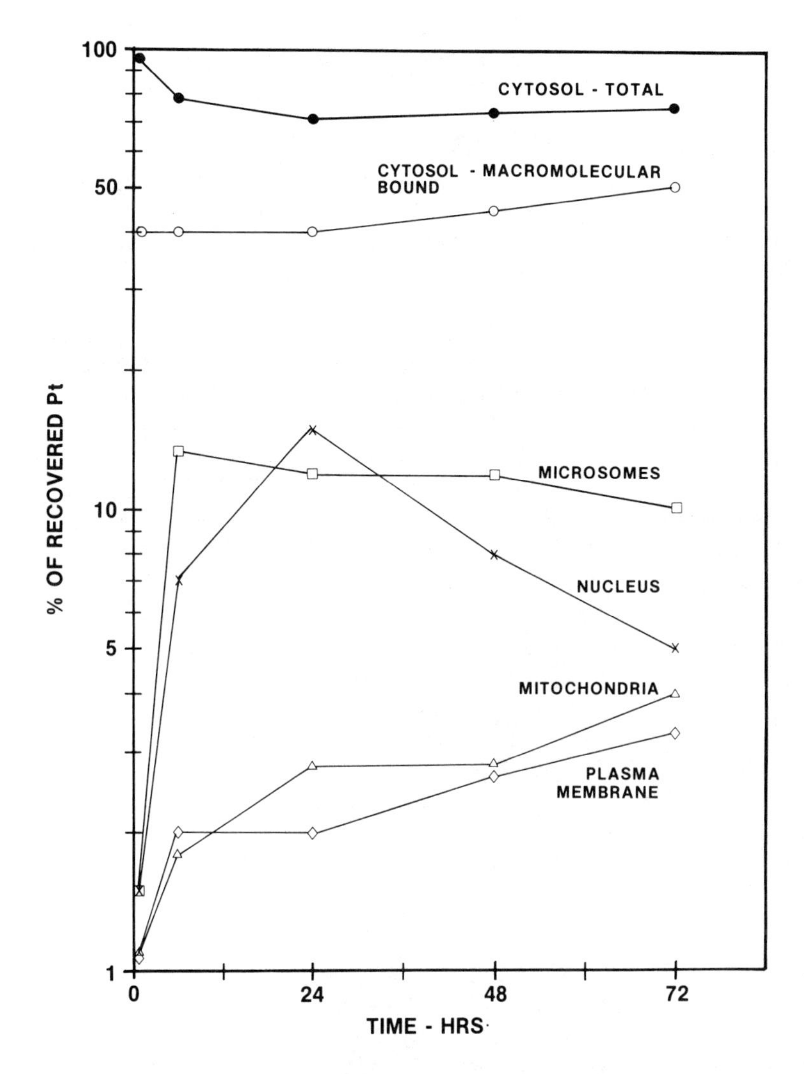

FIGURE 7.13 Kinetics of distribution of cis-platinum among components of rat kidney. (From Ref. 122.)

all contain similar concentrations of platinum. Past studies have focused almost exclusively on nuclear or nucleic acid binding of platinum complexes. However, it is clear from Figs. 7.11 and 7.13 that these compounds also interact irreversibly over short times with proteins. This may be expected because proteins contain an abundance of potential nitrogen (amine and imidazole) and sulfur (thiol, disulfide, and thioether) ligands, which can form kinetically stable bonds with Pt(II) (Table 7.5 and Fig. 7.10) [112].

C. Reactions of cis-Platinum with Nucleic Acids

The reactions of platinum complexes with nucleic acids have been intensively studied, for as discussed below the mechanism of antitumor activity of cis-platinum is thought to involve its binding to DNA. Although a number of investigations have centered on the structure of platinum-nucleic acid

TABLE 7.5 Rate Constants for the Reaction of Platinum Complexes with Nucleic Acids and Nucleosides

	$k(M^{-1}/sec \times 10^3)$	
Complex	37°C	24°C
$PtenCl_2$ [a]		
Guanine	10	
7-Methylguanosine	24	
Guanosine	106	
Poly G	150	
Adenine	8	
Adenosine	6	
AMP	330	160
Poly A	410	162
DNA (two rate constants)	100, 6	
cis-$Pt(NH_3)_2(Cl_2$ [b]		
DNA		
In 5 mM $NaClO_4$		320 [c]
In 0.15 M NaCl	~8 [d]	

[a]Refs. 127 and 128.
[b]Ref. 119.
[c]Rate constant for reaction of $Pt(NH_3)_2Cl(H_2O)$ with DNA in 5 mM $NaClO_4$, pH 5-6.
[d]Calculated, assuming pseudo-first-order reaction for 7% reaction of cis-platinum with 0.1 mM DNA over 24 hr.

adducts [126], relatively few have quantitatively described the kinetics of the reactions [119, 127, 128]. Some of the results are given in Table 7.5. The presence of the sugar and perhaps phosphate groups enhance the reactivity of the bases. Single- or double-stranded polynucleotides react as well or better than monomers. All of the reactions are slow and under pseudo-first-order conditions would have $t_{1/2}$ values of hours. A principal problem in relating the results of Robins to cellular conditions is that reactions were carried out in $NaClO_4$ solution in the absence of Cl^- [127, 128]. According to Johnson et al., the monoaquo form reacts with DNA directly or after loss of the second chloride, which yields the highly reactive diaquo species [119]. Using rate constants from Fig. 7.10 and from this study, one can calculate the pseudo-first-order k_{obs} for the reaction of cis-platinum with DNA as described in equation 21 as a function of chloride concentration in the medium. In 0.15 M NaCl it is 7×10^{-7} sec^{-1}, in good agreement with the observed value of 8×10^{-7} sec^{-1} (Table 7.5):

$$\mathrm{Pt(Cl)(Cl)} \underset{k_{-1}[Cl^-]}{\overset{k_1}{\rightleftharpoons}} \mathrm{Pt(Cl)(OH_2)} \underset{k_{-2}[Cl^-]}{\overset{k_2}{\rightleftharpoons}} \mathrm{Pt(OH_2)(OH_2)}$$

$$\mathrm{Pt(Cl)(OH_2)} \xrightarrow{k_3[DNA]} \text{products} \xleftarrow{k_4[DNA]} \mathrm{Pt(OH_2)(OH_2)} \qquad (21)$$

At 0.004 M NaCl, the rate constant is an order larger. However, in either case the reactions have half-times of greater than 14 hr. Since the binding of cis-platinum to proteins and DNA seems to occur at a more rapid rate in vivo, further studies will be necessary to determine whether in vitro results can quantatively model the kinetics of binding in cells and biological fluids.

The sites of reaction of cis-platinum with DNA have been the subject of many investigations [113, 126]. Crystal structures of many adducts of cis-platinum with bases, nucleosides, and nucleotides have been obtained. Numerous studies of solution interactions between cis-platinum and nucleic acids constituents have also been carried out. However, the nature of the important bound adducts of cis-platinum to DNA remains a subject of intense examination.

Buoyant density measurements have shown that platinum is bound to DNA in proportion to its G-C base pair content [129, 130]. After incubation of equivalent amounts of cis-platinum and DNA, the buoyant density of poly dG-poly dC was found to be much greater than poly d(G-C). This suggests a requirement for adjacent guanosine or cytosine residues on the same DNA strand.

This conclusion has received support and been refined in two recent experiments. Kelman and Buchbinder used the restriction endonuclease

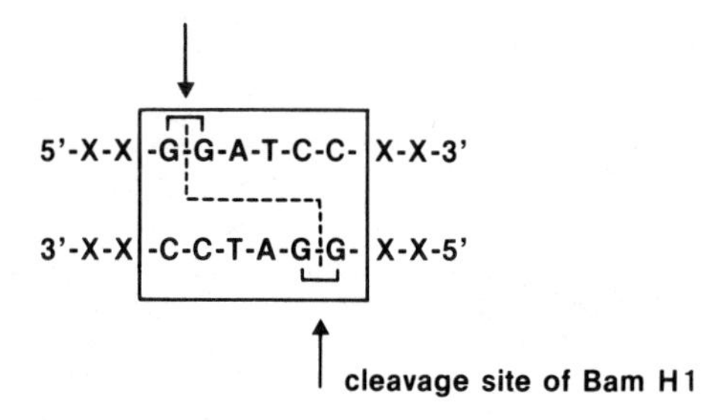

FIGURE 7.14 Action of Bam H1 endonuclease on λ DNA. (Ref. 131.) Proposed binding sites of cis-platinum (⌐¬). Recognitions sequence for endonuclease in box. Cleavage sites of endonuclease (→).

Bam H1 to cleave specifically bacteriophage λ DNA having the recognition sequence 5'-G-G-A-T-C-C-3' (Fig. 7.14). Separation of cleaved platinum-treated DNA into electrophoretically detectable fragments was prevented by the presence of bound platinum. Although such evidence is consistent with the formation of intrastrand cross-links between adjacent guanine residues, interstrand cross-links between nucleotide bases on the opposing strands straddling the recognition sequence could yield the same results. Other workers have used a specific restriction endonuclease to cleave plasmid pSM1 DNA containing bound platinum to support the binding of cis-platinum to a $(dG)_n \cdot (dC)_n$ sequence with $n \leq 4$ [132].

That the binding sites for cis-platinum may be guanine or adjacent guanine residues is consistent with the readily available sites of reaction of base pairs in double-stranded DNA. One can envision N^7-O^6 chelation to a single base or N^7-N^7 binding to adjacent residues (Fig. 7.15). However, chelation of cis-platinum by adenine or neighboring adenines at the N^6-N^7 binding of adjacent adenine and guanine groups also appears plausible. There is also no evidence from kinetic data (Table 7.5) to suggest a specificity of reactions of cis-platinum with guanine bases in polynucleotides.

The emphasis on adjacent cis reaction sites stems from the effort to find a molecular basis for the activity of cis- but not trans-$Pt(NH_3)_2Cl_3$ [133]. Whereas the cis complex can chelate two groups on the same base or consecutive bases trans-platinum can only do this in an interchain configuration. Recent studies confirm that the kinetics and total extent of binding of the cis and trans isomers to DNA are similar [119]. Thus, assuming that DNA is the critical site for antitumor activity, it appears that a particular type of adduct and not simply the random binding of platinum to bases in DNA is critical for cytotoxicity.

D. Cellular Effects of cis-Platinum

Soon after the determination of antitumor activity of cis-$Pt(NH_3)_2Cl_2$, several reports appeared on its inhibition of macromolecular synthetic

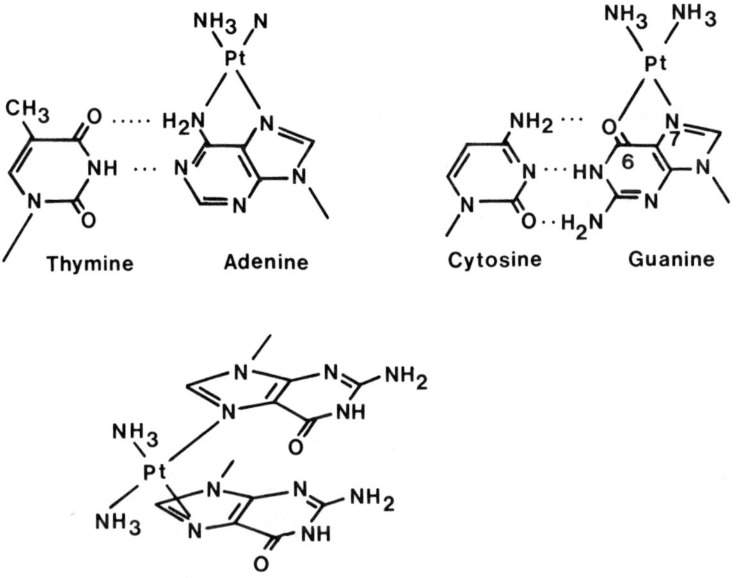

FIGURE 7.15 Plausible binding sites of *cis*-platinum to DNA bases.

processes. Harder and Rosenberg compared the effect of a variety of *cis*- and *trans*-platinum complexes on DNA, RNA, and protein synthesis in cultures of human annion AV_3 cells [134]. *cis*-Dichloroplatinum compounds previously found to be effective in inhibiting growth of sarcoma S180, or inducing filamentous growth in *Escherichia coli*, were the best inhibitors of long-term DNA synthesis. The trans isomers were always less effective than the cis complexes at comparable concentrations and were frequently without significant effect in the concentration range tested. DNA synthesis was more sensitive than RNA or protein synthesis; in all cases, the effects increased gradually over a period of hours. Placement of platinum-treated cells into fresh medium after a 4-hr exposure could not reverse DNA synthesis inhibition [134, 135]. The authors showed that these effects were not an artifact of reduced precursor uptake by cells, nor due to a direct inhibition of DNA polymerase [136]. Howle and Gale observed similar effects with Ehrlich ascites tumor [137]. Roberts and his co-workers also confirmed these results in HeLa cells in culture [138]. Cells treated with *cis*-platinum at a concentration of 8 μM show a 90% inhibition of colony formation, whereas about 160 μM of the trans complex is needed for the same effect . Most important, it was shown that the degree of inhibition of DNA synthesis correlated with the depression of colony formation and that under these conditions, RNA and protein synthesis were unaffected.

Thus the linkage of cytotoxicity with specific effects on DNA synthesis and the two of these with the reactivity of cis-platinum with DNA has led to the hypothesis that DNA is the critical molecular target for cis-platinum.

The missing piece in the puzzle is a convincing chemical basis to distinguish the functional effects of cis- and trans-platinum on DNA. As described above, both bind approximately as well to DNA [119, 139]. When bound, both inhibit to about the same extent in vitro deoxynucleotide polymerization using poly [d(A-T)·d(A-T)] and poly [d(G-C)·d(G-C)] [140]. Both depress RNA polymerase activity with calf thymus DNA with only a three- to fourfold difference in efficiency [141]. The key reaction is not simply to place blocking groups generally throughout the DNA structure. Instead, there may be very specific control sites with sequences of bases highly favorable to reaction such as poly [d(G)·d(C)] to which cis-platinum must bind in order to halt DNA synthesis and then cell division.

VIII. OTHER COMPLEXES

Other metallic species are being actively investigated. Of particular interest are gallium nitrate and tetra-μ-carboxylatodirhodium (II) complexes. Recent reviews of their chemistry and antitumor activity have appeared [7].

APPENDIX

1. Half-Time for Approach to Equilibrium, $t_{1/2}$ (142)

$$\mathrm{Pt}\langle^{\mathrm{Cl}}_{\mathrm{Cl}} + H_2O \rightleftharpoons \mathrm{>Pt}\langle^{\mathrm{Cl}}_{\mathrm{OH_2}} + \mathrm{Cl}^-$$

or

$$(\mathrm{Pt(NH_3)_2ClH_2O}) + H_2O \rightleftharpoons (\mathrm{Pt(NH_3)_2(OH_2)_2}) + \mathrm{Cl}^-$$

$$A + B \underset{k_{-1}}{\overset{k_1}{\rightleftharpoons}} C + D$$

Let $B = H_2O$, $D = \mathrm{Cl}^-$, $[C_0] = O$, $[D_0] \gg [A_0]$:

$$\frac{d[A]}{dt} = -k_1[A] + k_{-1}[C][D_0]$$

$$\frac{d[A]}{dt} = -k_1[A] + k_{-1}([A_0] - [A])[D_0]$$

$$\ln \frac{k_1[A]}{(k_1 + k_{-1}[D_0])[A] - k_{-1}[A_0][D_0]} = (k_1 + k_{-1}[D_0]t$$

at $t = t_{1/2}$ $\quad [A] = \dfrac{[A_0] + [A_{equilibrium}]}{2}$

$$t_{1/2} = \frac{1}{k_1 + k_{-1}[D_0]} \ln \frac{2\,k_1[A_0]}{(k_1 - k_1[D_0][A_0]) + (k_1 + k_{-1}[D_0][Aeq])}$$

or

$$t_{1/2} = \frac{1}{k_1 + k_{-1}[D_0]} \ln \frac{2}{1 - \frac{[D_0]}{K} + (1 + \frac{[D_0]}{K}) \frac{[Aeq]}{[A_0]}}$$

where $K = k_1/k_{-1}$.

2. Relaxation Time, τ (143)

$$\tau = \frac{1}{k_1 + k_{-1}[D_0]} \qquad \frac{1}{k_1 + k_{-1}[D_0]}$$

3. Kinetics of Reaction of cis-$Pt(NH_3)_2Cl_2$ and cis-$Pt(NH_3)_2(Cl)(OH)$ Complexes with Nucleophile (B)

$$>Pt(Cl)(Cl) \underset{k_{-1}[Cl_o^-]}{\overset{k_1}{\rightleftharpoons}} >Pt(Cl)(OH_2) + Cl^-$$

$$>Pt(Cl)(Cl) \xrightarrow{k_3[B]} >Pt(Cl)(B) \xleftarrow{k_2[B]} >Pt(Cl)(OH_2)$$

$$\frac{d[>PtCl_2]}{dt} = \left\{ \frac{k_1 k_2 \; [B]}{k_{-1}[Cl_o^-] + k_2[B]} + k_3[B] \right\} \left[>Pt\begin{matrix} Cl \\ Cl \end{matrix} \right]$$

Using the rate constants from Fig. 7.10,

$$k_{obs} = \frac{2.5 \times 10^{-5} k_2[B]}{7 \times 10^{-3}[Cl^-] + k_2[B]} + k_3[B]$$

If $k_2[B] \gg 7 \times 10^{-3}[Cl^-]$, the equation reduces to the form of k_{obs} frequently observed for reactions of square-planar complexes

$$k_{obs} = k_1 + k_3[B]$$

In this case $[Cl^-]$ would have no effect on k_{obs}. However, the substitution pathway involving k_3 may be significant, depending on the nature and concentration of B.

4. Kinetics of Reaction of cis-$Pt(NH_3)_2Cl_2$ with DNA Bases (119)

$$>Pt(Cl)(Cl) \underset{k_{-1}[Cl^-]}{\overset{k_1}{\rightleftharpoons}} >Pt(Cl)(OH_2) \underset{k_{-2}[Cl^-]}{\overset{k_2}{\rightleftharpoons}} >Pt(OH_2)(OH_2)$$

$$>Pt(Cl)(OH_2) \xrightarrow{k_3[DNA]} \text{Pt-bound DNA} \qquad >Pt(OH_2)(OH_2) \xrightarrow{k_4[DNA]} \text{Pt-bound DNA}$$

$$\frac{d[>PtCl_2]}{dt} = \frac{k_1[DNA][>PtCl_2]}{k_{-1}[Cl^-] + k_2 + k_3[DNA] - \dfrac{k_2 k_{-2}[Cl^-]}{k_{-2}[Cl^-] + k_4[DNA]}}$$

$$\left(\frac{k_2 k_4}{k_{-2}[Cl^-] + k_4[DNA]} + k_3\right)$$

Using the rate constants from Fig. 7.10, $k_3 = 0.3\ M^{-1}/sec$ and $k_4 = 0.015\ sec^{-1}$ from Ref. 119, and $[DNA] = 0.1\ mM$,

$k_{obs([Cl^-] = 0.15M)} = 7.1 \times 10^{-7}\ sec^{-1}$ Only the k_3 binding step is significant

$k_{obs([Cl^-] = 0.004)} = 1.3 \times 10^{-5}\ sec^{-1}$

$k_{obs}([Cl^-] \to 0) = k_1 = 2.5 \times 10^{-5}\ sec^{-1}$ The rate-limiting step is the initial solvolysis of cis-dichlorodiamine Pt(II)

In no case does k_4 contribute significantly to the magnitude of the observed rate constant.

ACKNOWLEDGMENTS

Support to write this review came from NIH Grant CA-22184, Biomedical Research Support Grant RR-07181, and the University of Wisconsin-Milwaukee. This is Publication 125 from the Laboratory for Molecular Biomedical Research.

REFERENCES

1. A. Furst, Chemistry of Chelation in Cancer, Charles C Thomas, Springfield, ILL., 1963.
2. F. A. French and B. L. Freedlander, Cancer Res., 18: 1298 (1958).
3. F. A. French and B. L. Freedlander, Cancer Res., 21: 505 (1960).
4. D. H. Petering and H. G. Petering, in Handbook of Experimental Pharmacology (A. C. Sartorelli and D. G. Johns, eds.), Vol. 38, Pt. II, Springer-Verlag, New York, 1975, p. 841.
5. B. Rosenberg, in Metal Ions in Biological Systems (H. Sigel, ed.), Vol. 11, Marcel Dekker, New York, 1980, p. 127.
6. D. H. Petering, in Metal Ions in Biological Systems (H. Sigel, ed.), Vol. 11, Marcel Dekker, New York, 1980, p. 197.
7. M.J. Cleare and P. C. Hydes, in Metal Ions in Biological Systems (H. Sigel, ed.), Vol. 11, Marcel Dekker, New York, 1980, p. 1.
8. S. B. Horwitz, E. A. Sausville, and J. Peisach, in Bleomycin: Chemical, Biochemical, and Biological Aspects (S. M. Hecht, ed.), Vol. 11, Marcel Dekker, New York, 1979, p. 170.
9. D. H. Petering and H. G. Petering, in Molecular Basis of Environmental Toxicity (R. S. Bhatnagar, ed.), Ann Arbor Science, Ann Arbor, 1980, p. 449.
10. H. G. Petering, H. H. Buskirk, and G. E. Underwood, Cancer Res., 24: 367 (1964).
11. J. A. Crim and H. G. Petering, Cancer Res., 27: 1278 (1967).
12. E. Mihich and C. A. Nichol, Cancer Res., 25: 1410 (1965).
13. H. G. Petering, H. H. Buskirk, and J. A. Crim, Cancer Res., 27: 1115 (1967).
14. G. J. Van Giessen, J. A. Crim, D. H. Petering, and H. G. Petering, J. Natl. Cancer Inst., 51: 139 (1973).
15. D. H. Petering, Biochem. Pharmacol., 23: 567 (1974).
16. D. H. Petering, Bioinorg. Chem., 1: 255 (1972).
17. D. T. Minkel, K. Poulsen, S. Wielgus, C. F. Shaw III, and D. H. Petering, Biochem. J., 191: 475 (1980).
18. E. Underwood, Trace Elements in Human and Animal Nutrition, Academic Press, New York, 1971, pp. 19, 67, 214.
19. P. S. Hallman, D. D. Perrin, and A. E. Watt, Biochem. J., 121: 549 (1971).

20. D. H. Petering, Bioinorg. Chem., 1: 273 (1972).
21. D. A. Winkelmann, Y. Bermke, and D. H. Petering, Bioinorg. Chem., 3: 261 (1974).
22. D. T. Minkel and D. H. Petering, Cancer Res., 38: 117 (1978).
23. D. T. Minkel, L. A. Saryan, and D. H. Petering, Cancer Res., 38: 124 (1978).
24. D. T. Minkel, C. Chan-Stier, and D. H. Petering, Mol. Pharmacol., 12: 1036 (1976).
25. D. Solaiman, L. A. Saryan, and D. H. Petering, J. Inorg. Biochem., 10: 135 (1979).
26. B. A. Booth and A. C. Sartorelli, Mol. Pharmacol., 3: 290 (1967).
27. C. Chan-Stier, D. T. Minkel, and D. H. Petering, Bioinorg. Chem., 6: 203 (1976).
28. J. Koch, S. Wielgus, B. Shankara, L. A. Saryan, C. F. Shaw, and D. H. Petering, Biochem. J., 189: 95 (1980).
29. H. Ohtake, K. Hasegawa, and M. Koga, Biochem. J., 174: 999 (1978).
30. D. H. Petering and L. A. Saryan, Biol. Trace Element Res., 1: 87 (1979).
31. R. W. Brockman, J. R. Thomas, M. J. Bell, and H. E. Skipper, Cancer Res., 16: 167 (1956).
32. F. A. French and E. J. Blanz, Jr., Cancer Res., 25: 1454 (1965).
33. E. J. Blanz, Jr. and F. A. French, Cancer Res., 28: 2419 (1965).
34. R. C. DeConti, B. R. Toftness, K. C. Agrawal, R. Tomchick, J. A. R. Mead, J. R. Bertino, A. C. Sartorelli, and W. A. Creasey, Cancer Res., 32: 1455 (1972).
35. F. A. French, E. J. Blanz, Jr., S. C. Shaddix, and R. W. Brockman, J. Med. Chem., 17: 172 (1974).
36. A. C. Sartorelli, K. C. Agrawal, A. S. Tseftsoglou, and E. C. Moore, Adv. Enzyme Regul., 15: 117 (1977).
37. F. A. French, A. E. Lewis, A. H. Sheena, and E. J. Blanz, Jr., Fed. Proc., 24: 402 (1965).
38. I. H. Krakoff, E. Etcubanas, C. Tan, K. Mayer, V. Bethune, and J. H. Burchenal, Cancer Chemother. Rep., Pt. 1, 58: 207 (1974).
39. A. C. Sartorelli, Biochem. Biophys. Res. Commun., 27: 26 (1967).
40. A. C. Sartorelli, K. C. Agrawal, and E. C. Moore, Biochem. Pharmacol., 20: 3119 (1971).
41. E. C. Moore, M. S. Zedeck, K. C. Agrawal, and A. C. Sartorelli, Biochemistry, 9: 4492 (1970).
42. (a) S. Hopper, Fed. Proc., 33: 1747 (1974); (b) S. Hopper, Fed. Proc., 34: 641 (1975).
43. L. A. Saryan, E. Ankel, C. Krishnamurti, D. H. Petering, and H. Elford, J. Med. Chem., 22: 1218 (1979).
44. W. E. Antholine, P. Gunn, and L. E. Hopwood, Int. J. Radiat. Oncol. Biol. Phys., 7: 491 (1981).

45. K. C. Agrawal, B. A. Booth, E. C. Moore, and A. C. Sartorelli, Proc. Am. Assoc. Cancer Res., 15: 73 (1974).
46. W. Antholine, J. Knight, H. Whelan, and D. H. Petering, Mol. Pharmacol., 13: 89 (1977).
47. W. E. Antholine, J. M. Knight, and D. H. Petering, Inorg. Chem., 16: 569 (1977).
48. E. Ankel and D. H. Petering, Biochem. Pharmacol., 29: 1833 (1980).
49. L. A. Saryan, K. Mailer, C. Krishnamurti, W. E. Antholine, and D. H. Petering, Biochem. Pharmacol., 30: 1595 (1981).
50. D. H. Petering, in Inorganic and Nutritional Aspects of Cancer (G. N. Schrauzer, ed.), Plenum Press, New York, 1978, p. 179.
51. J. M. Knight, H. Whelan, and D. H. Petering, Bioinorg. Chem., 11: 327 (1979).
52. M. Ishizuka, H. Takayama, T. Takeuchi, and H. Umezawa, J. Antibiot., A20: 15 (1967).
53. H. Umezawa, M. Ishzuka, K. Kimura, J. Iwanaga, and T. Takeuchi, J. Antibiot., A21: 592 (1968).
54. S. K. Carter and S. T. Crooke (eds.), Bleomycin: Current Status and New Developments, Academic Press, New York, 1978.
55. H. Suzuki, K. Nagai, E. Akutso, H. Uamaki, N. Tanaka, and H. Umezawa, J. Antibiot., 23: 473 (1970).
56. R. Ishida and T. Takahashi, Biochem. Biophys. Res., Commun., 66: 1432 (1975).
57. D. Solaiman, W. E. Antholine, L. A. Saryan, and D. H. Petering, Lloydia, 39: 470 (1976).
58. K. Takahashi, O. Yoshioka, A. Matsuda, and H. Umezawa, J. Antibiot., 30: 861 (1977).
59. E. A. Sausville, J. Peisach, and S. B. Horwitz, Biochemistry, 17: 2740 (1978).
60. E. A. Sausville, R. W. Stein, J. Peisach, and S. B. Horwitz, Biochemistry, 17: 2746 (1978).
61. S. M. Hecht (ed.), Bleomycin: Chemical, Biochemical, and Biological Aspects, Springer-Verlag, New York, 1979.
62. J. C. Dabrowiak, J. Inorg. Biochem., 13: 317 (1980).
63. E. A. Rao, L. A. Saryan, W. E. Antholine, and D. H. Petering, J. Med. Chem., 23: 1310 (1980).
64. Y. Sugiura, K. Ishizu, and K. Miyoshi, J. Antibiot., 32: 453 (1979).
65. D. Solaiman, E. A. Rao, W. E. Antholine, and D. H. Petering, J. Inorg. Biochem., 12: 201 (1980).
66. D. Solaiman, E. A. Rao, D. H. Petering, R. C. Sealy, and W. E. Antholine, Int. J. Radiat. Oncol. Biol. Phys., 5: 1519 (1979).
67. W. E. Antholine, D. Solaiman, L. A. Saryan, and D. H. Petering, J. Inorg. Biochem., 17: 75 (1982).
68. R. M. Burger, J. Peisach, W. E. Blumberg, and S. B. Horwitz, J. Biol. Chem., 254: 10906 (1979).

69. W. E. Antholine and D. H. Petering, Biochem. Biophys. Res. Commun., 91: 528 (1979).
70. R. K. Gupta, J. A. Ferretti, and W. J. Caspary, Biochem. Biophys. Res. Commun., 89: 534 (1979).
71. T. Takita, Y. Muraoka, T. Nakatani, A. Fujii, Y. Umezawa, H. Naganawa, and H. Umezawa, J. Antibiot., 31: 801 (1978).
72. J. C. Dabrowiak, F. T. Greenaway, and R. Grulich, Biochemistry, 17: 4090 (1978).
73. N. J. Oppenheimer, L. O. Rodriquez, and S. M. Hecht, Biochemistry, 18: 3439 (1979).
74. R. Lenkinski and J. Dallas, J. Am. Chem. Soc., 101: 5902 (1979).
75. N. J. Oppenheimer, L. O. Rodriquez, and S. M. Hecht, Proc. Natl. Acad. Sci. USA, 76: 5616 (1979).
76. E. S. Mooberry, J. L. Dallas, T. T. Sakai, and J. D. Glickson, Int. J. Peptide Protein Res., 15: 365 (1980).
77. Y. Sugiura, J. Am. Chem. Soc., 102: 5208 (1980).
78. R. P. Pillai, R. E. Lenkinski, T. J Sakai, J. M. Geckle, N. R. Krishna, and J. D. Glickson, Biochem. Biophys. Res. Commun., 96: 341 (1980).
79. W. E. Antholine and D. H. Petering, Biochem. Biophys. Res. Commun., 90: 384 (1979).
80. W. E. Antholine, D. H. Petering, L. A. Saryan, and C. H. Brown, Proc. Natl. Acad. Sci. USA, 78: 7517 (1981).
81. Y. Sugiura and T. Kikuchi, J. Antibiot., 31: 1310 (1978).
82. C. M. Vos, G. Westera, and D. Schipper, J. Inorg. Biochem., 13: 165 (1980).
83. R. P. Sheridan and R. K. Gupta, J. Biol. Chem., 256: 1242 (1981).
84. R. M. Burger, S. B. Horwitz, J. Peisach, and J. B. Wittenberg, J. Biol. Chem., 254: 12299 (1979).
85. R. M. Burger, J. Peisach, and S. B. Horwitz, J. Biol. Chem., 256: 11636 (1981).
86. L. F. Povirk, Biochemistry, 18: 3989 (1979).
87. W. J. Caspary, C. Niziak, D. A. Lanzo, R. Friedman, and N. R. Bachur, Mol. Pharmacol., 16: 256 (1979).
88. M. Chien, A. P. Grollman, and S. B. Horwitz, Biochemistry, 16: 3641 (1977).
89. L. F. Povirk, M. Hogan, and N. Dattagupta, Biochemistry, 18: 96 (1979).
90. A. P. Grollman and M. Takeshita, Adv. Enzyme Regul., 18: 67 (1980).
91. L. F. Povirk, M. Hogan, N. Dattagupta, and M. Buechner, Biochemistry, 20: 665 (1981).
92. Y. Sugiura and K. Ishizu, J. Inorg. Biochem., 11: 171 (1979).
93. R. P. Pillai, N. R. Krishna, T. J. Sakai, and J. D. Glickson, Biochem. Biophys. Res. Commun., 97: 270 (1980).

94. L. H. Oberley and G. R. Buettner, FEBS. Lett., 97: 47 (1979).
95. R. M. Burger, A. R. Berkowitz, J. Peisach, and S. B. Horwitz, J. Biol. Chem., 255: 11832 (1980).
96. J. A. Fee, in Metal Ion Activation of Dioxygen (T. G. Spiro, ed.), Wiley-Interscience, New York, 1980, p. 209.
97. A. D. Nunn and J. Lunec, Eur. J. Cancer, 14: 857 (1978).
98. A. Banergee and W. F. Benedict, Cancer Res., 39: 797 (1979).
99. B. Barlogie, B. Drewinko, J. Schumann, and E. J. Freireich, Cancer Res., 36: 1182 (1976).
100. J. Fujimoto, Cancer Res., 34: 2969 (1974).
101. M. Miyaki, T. Ono, S. Hori, and H. Umezawa, Cancer Res., 35: 2015 (1975).
102. I. V. Chapman and F. Alalawi, Int. J. Radiat. Oncol. Biol. Phys., 35: 2015 (1975).
103. J. J. Roberts and A. J. Thomson, Prog. Nucleic Acid Res. Mol. Biol., 22: 71 (1979).
104. A. W. Prestayko, J. C. D'Aoust, B. F. Issell, and S. T. Crooke, Cancer Treat. Rev., 6: 17 (1979).
105. B. Rosenberg, L. Van Camp, and T. Krigas, Nature, 205: 698 (1965).
106. B. Rosenberg, L. Van Camp, J. Trosko, and V. H. Mansour, Nature, 222: 385 (1969).
107. B. Rosenberg and L. Van Camp, Cancer Res., 30: 1799 (1970).
108. T. A. Connors and J. J. Roberts (eds.), Platinum Coordination Complexes in Cancer Chemotherapy, Springer-Verlag, Berlin, 1974.
109. Proceedings of the Third International Symposium on Platinum Coordination Complexes in Cancer Chemotherapy, J. Clin. Hematol. Oncol., 7: 1-827,
110. Symposium on Coordination Chemistry and Cancer Chemotherapy, Biochimie, 60: 829-935, 1978.
111. Proceedings of the National Cancer Insitute Conference on cis-Platinum and Testicular Cancer, Cancer Treat. Rep., 63: 1431-1699, 1979.
112. M. E. Howe-Grant and S. J. Lippard, in Metal Ions in Biological Systems (H. Sigel, ed.), Marcel Dekker, New York, 1980, p. 63.
113. B. de Castro, T. J. Kistenmacher, and L. G. Marzilli, in Trace Elements in the Pathogenesis and Treatment of Inflammation (K. D. Rainsford, K. Brune, and M. W. Whitehouse, eds.), Birkhäuser Verlag, Basel, 1981, p. 436.
114. G. R. Gale, in Handbook of Experimental Pharmacology (A. C. Sartorelli and D. G. Johns, eds.), Vol. 38, Pt. II, Springer-Verlag, New York, 1975, p. 829.
115. F. R. Hartley, The Chemistry of Platinum and Palladium, Applied Science Publishers, Barking, Essex, England, 1973, Chap. 11.

116. R. G. Wilkins, The Study of Kinetics and Mechanism of Reactions of Transition Metal Complexes, Allyn and Bacon, Boston, 1974, pp. 223-235.
117. G. Siebert, Subcell Biochem., 1: 277 (1972).
118. B. Rosenberg, Biochimie, 60: 859 (1978).
119. N. P. Johnson, J. D. Hoeschele, and R. O. Rahn, Chem.-Biol. Interact., 30: 151 (1980).
120. W. Wolf and R. C. Manaka, J. Clin. Hematol. Oncol., 7: 79 (1977).
121. R. C. Manaka and W. Wolf, Chem.-Biol. Interact., 22: 353 (1978).
122. D. D. Choie, A. A. del Campo, and A. M. Guarino, Toxicol. Appl. Pharmacol., 55: 245 (1980).
123. G. R. Gale, C. R. Morris, L. M. Atkins, and A. B. Smith, Cancer Res., 33: 813 (1973).
124. R. G. Pearson, H. Sobel, and J. Songstad, J. Am. Chem. Soc., 90: 319 (1968).
125. B. Pastakia, L. M. Lieberman, S. J. Gatley, D. Young, D. H. Petering, and D. Minkel, J. Nucl. Med., 21: 67 (1980).
126. L. G. Marzilli, Prog. Inorg. Chem., 23: 255 (1977).
127. A. B. Robins, Chem.-Biol. Interact., 6: 35 (1973).
128. A. B. Robins, Chem.-Biol. Interact., 7: 11 (1973).
129. P. J. Stone, A. D. Kelman, and F. M. Sinex, Nature, 251: 736 (1974).
130. P. J. Stone, A. D. Kelman, F. M. Sinex, M. M. Bhargava, and H. O. Halvorson, J. Mol. Biol., 104: 793 (1976).
131. A. D. Kelman and M. Buchbinder, Biochimie, 60: 893 (1978).
132. G. L. Cohen, J. A. Ledner, W. R. Bauer, H. M. Ushay, C. Caravana, and S. J. Lippard, J. Am. Chem. Soc., 102: 2487 (1980).
133. M. J. Cleare, J. Clin. Hematol. Oncol., 7: 1 (1977).
134. H. C. Harder and B. Rosenberg, Int. J. Cancer, 6: 207 (1970).
135. J. J. Roberts, in Platinum Coordination Complexes in Cancer Chemotherapy (T. A. Connors and J. J. Roberts, eds.), Springer-Verlag, Berlin, 1974, p. 79.
136. H. C. Harder, R. G. Smith, and A. F. Leroy, Cancer Res., 36: 3821 (1976).
137. J. A. Howle and G. H. Gale, Biochem. Pharmacol., 19: 2757 (1970).
138. J. M. Pascoe and J. J. Roberts, Biochem. Pharmacol., 23: 1347 (1974).
139. H. C. Harder, in Platinum Coordination Complexes in Cancer Chemotherapy (T. A. Connors and J. J. Roberts, eds.), Springer-Verlag, Berlin, 1974, p. 98.
140. H. C. Harder and R. G. Smith, J. Clin. Hematol. Oncol., 7: 401 (1977).
141. R. C. Srivastava, J. Froehlich, and G. L. Eichhorn, Biochimie, 60: 879 (1978).
142. S. Benson, The Foundation of Chemical Kinetics, McGraw-Hill, New York, 1960, pp. 29-30.
143. R. G. Wilkins, The Study of Kinetics and Mechanism of Reactions of Transition Metal Complexes, Allyn and Bacon, Boston, 1974, p. 35.

8

SYNTHETIC POLYANIONIC POLYMERS WITH INTERFERON-INDUCING AND ANTITUMOR ACTIVITY

RAPHAEL M. OTTENBRITE

Virginia Commonwealth University
Richmond, Virginia

GEORGE B. BUTLER

University of Florida
Gainesville, Florida

I. INTRODUCTION

Both natural and synthetic water-soluble polymers are known to manifest broad and varied biological activity [1-6]. In most instances, these polymers are anionic or cationic in nature and thus exhibit polyelectrolytic behavior. The polyanionic polymers in particular have been found to demonstrate a broad range of physiological properties, many of which have been studied extensively by oncolognists and virologists [7, 8]. When given to test animals prior to viral or tumoral challenge, the anionic polymers have significant inhibitory effects on bacteria, fungi, viruses, tumors, and enzymes. Their prolonged prophylactic activity has identified these agents for potential clinical applications and established an impetus for scientists to determine the fundamental role of anionic polymers in effecting host resistance to a variety of pathophysiology.

These polymeric drugs are water soluble, which is important for transport within the host and systemic administration, as insoluble suspensions injected into blood vessels can cause colloidoclasmic shock, resulting in major hypersensitive toxicity [9]. These macromolecules can be distributed in the host system through blood or lymphatic circulation, adsorption on cell surfaces, and cellular transport effected by mobile phagocytic cells. In order to be compatible with blood circulation, these agents cannot cause thrombosis, destroy cellular elements, alter plasma proteins, deplete electrolytes, or cause acute or delayed toxic or immune allergic responses.

It appears that those anionic polymers that exhibit the best biological activity behave similarly to certain proteins, glycoproteins, and polynucleotides which are known to modulate a variety of biological responses related to bacteria and fungi, such as enhanced immune response, inhibition of adjuvant arthritis, and anticoagulation [10].

The most important property of anionic polymers presently under investigation is the antineoplastic potential, which appears to be related to mitotic inhibitory effects. The major mechanism that many synthetic polyanions exhibit against tumor growth and certain antiviral effects appears to be by macrophage activation [11]. Macrophages activated by these anionic agents seem to play an important role in antineoplastic host defenses [12], which is related to their ability to act as adjuvants for enhancing antitumor resistance.

Several basic similarities seem to be prevalent in those synthetic anionic polymers that exhibit biological activity. These properties include defined molecular weight, a large charge density, chain rigidity, and lipophilicity. For optimum results polymers should have a large enough molecular weight to delay body clearance (>1000), yet stay below the kidney threshold (<50, 000). Large nonbiodegradable materials in the host present serious long-term physiological problems. Consequently, an ideal approach might involve the fabrication of biodegradable polymers that would retain their biological active structure long enough to elicit specific activity and then be converted to harmless, easily eliminated metabolites.

II. INTERFERON-INDUCING EFFECTS OF IONIC POLYMERS

Naturally occurring polyanions and synthetic anionic polymers have been reported to induce interferon as well as effect resistance to tumors and microorganisms [13]. The natural polymers include polysulfates, polyphosphates, polynucleotides, and some polysaccharides. The synthetic polyanions investigated are mostly polycarboxylates, such as homocarboxylic acids, maleic anhydride copolymers, other copolymers with carboxylic acid functionality, and oxidized oxyamylose.

Some of the activities elicited by these agents are:

1. Increased host resistance to bacteria, fungi, parasites, and viruses
2. Increased host resistance to tumors and enhancement of antibody production
3. Immunoregulation of cell-mediated immunity
4. Alteration of macrophage cells to cytotoxic activity
5. Induction of interferon
6. Alteration of coagulation process

Although the induction of interferon has been cited as a possible component leading to these biological activities [14,15], the mechanism or mechanisms involved is not understood. However, a number of the polyionic polymer features have been noted as necessary for significant interferon induction and antitumor and antiviral activity [1]. These include:

1. A relatively high number of polar groups with some carboxyl groups
2. Many lipophilic groups as part of or attached to the polymer chain
3. Specific molecular weights for antitumor and antiviral activity
4. A rigid and relatively stable polymer which is nonbiodegradable

The polar groups that have shown activity in conjunction with carboxylic acid groups are amides, imides, hydroxyls, ethers, and esters [1]. The molecular weight requirements are unusual and strongly indicate different mechanisms for antitumor and antiviral activity. For example, very little antiviral activity is observed below 30,000 MW and then only with high doses. Polymers with a MW of 50,000 or greater usually exhibit good antiviral activity as well as sustained activity (8-12 days) at low doses. However, as the molecular weight increases, so does the toxicity, particularly hepatomegalia, splenomegalia, and mixed microsomal enzyme activity [1]. On the other hand, antitumor activity appears to be more effective at the lower molecular weights which are less toxic. Recent studies have also indicated that a polymer with a rigid structure and lipophilic groups is more effective than those with more polar-type groups.

Interferon induction in vivo has been observed with a variety of polyanions. However, except for the polynucleotides, the synthetic polyanions are not major interferon inducers. Since only low levels of interferon are produced by synthetic polyanions, studies of the type of interferon produced have been limited (Tables 8.1 and 8.2).

The production of only small amounts of interferon have raised doubts as to whether interferon is actually responsible for the biological activities observed with these synthetic polyanions. The following data have been reported:

1. Polyanions with low or no induction of interferon can show equal activity to those with high interferon induction [16].
2. Polyanions have antiviral activity in animal species in which they do not induce detectable interferon [17].
3. Polyanionic treatment of animals with doses that do not induce interferon can provide antiviral activity [14].
4. Polyanionic treatment of animals with anti-interferon serum does not abort the antitumor or antiviral activity [18].
5. Polyanionic interferon induction kinetics do not correlate with duration of antiviral protection [15, 19].

Consequently, the biological effects observed for the synthetic polyanions seem much greater than what can be attributed to the interferon produced.

Although synthetic polyanionic polymers have been demonstrated to induce modest amounts of interferon in vivo, there is no clear evidence that this is the method that these agents use to invoke their biological activity. Further understanding of the complex relationship of synthetic polyanions must occur before these agents could be utilized in immunotherapy.

TABLE 8.1 Anionic Polymer and Copolymer Inducers of Interferon

Polymer	Approx. MW	Optimal dose (mg/kg)	Interferon titer (units/4 ml)
Maleic anhydride-co-ethylene	70,000	50	402
Maleic anhydride-co-propylene	30,000	500	250
Maleic anhydride-co-divinyl ether	17,000	125	500
Maleic anhydride-co-vinyl methyl ether	25,000	1000	80
Poly(acrylic acid)	70,000	100	91
Poly(methacrylic acid)	70,000	500	128

TABLE 8.2 Amidated Polymer and Copolymer Inducers of Interferon

Polymer[a]	Approx. MW	Optimum dose (mg/kg)	Interferon titer (units/4 ml)
MA/ethylene half-amide	100,000	100	<30
MA/propylene half-amide	30,000	100	145
MA/vinyl methyl ether half-amide	250,000	1000	55
MA/vinyl methyl ether half-amide	1,250,000	500	<10
MA/ethylene half-amide, half-ester	30,000	100	<30
Polyacrylamide	70,000	100	<30

[a]MA, maleic anhydride.

III. NATURAL AND MODIFIED NATURAL ANIONIC POLYMERS

Many natural polyanions inhibit fungi, bacteria, viruses, and tumors; consequently, any information about the mode of inhibition is important to our understanding the control mechanisms of normal and malignant growth. These polyelectrolytes are critical to cell function, blood partition, and cell secretion. Research indicates that these substances also serve an important role as antigenic markers at cell surfaces as orientors for cellular differentiation and cell recognition.

A. Heparin and Heparinoids

Heparin and heparinoids are among the most effective water-soluble polymeric anticoagulants. The antimitotic effect of heparin, heparinoids, and sulfomucopolysaccharides indicated that these polyanions also have a physiological growth-controlling function [20,21]. Subsequently, derivatives of natural polymers as well as synthetic polymers similar to heparin were found to possess antimitotic activity [22-24].

Heparinoids are sulfated polysaccharides that are related to heparin and prepared by partial degradation of natural polysaccharides followed by sulfonation or phosphorylation. Their physical properties are similar to heparin in high sulfate or phosphate anion content and water solubility. Heparin and heparinoids, although primarily developed clinically for their anticoagulant and lipolytic activity, have several other biological activities which have been reported by Regelson in reviews of the biological activity of polyanions [21,25,26]. The mucopolysaccharides are also naturally occurring carbohydrates, like heparin, but with fewer sulfate groups and weaker anticoagulant activity.

Several synthetic sulfonate polymers and copolymers have been prepared for biological activity studies. The sulfonate group is unique in that it apparently does not bind calcium or magnesium ions, as do carboxylates and phosphates. For example, a typical sulfonate polymer, such as poly (styrenesulfonic acid), is not precipitable by calcium or barium ions. The ability of these polyanions to maintain a high negative charge in the presence of calcium and/or magnesium ions is the apparent basis for the effectiveness of heparin and other polysulfonates as physiological agents. Ethylenesulfonic acid polymers and copolymers have especially marked advantages over other types of synthetic materials in this regard and are being clinically utilized [21,28]. However, poly(ethylenesulfonic acid) and poly(styrenesulfonic acid) have also been shown to displace histones bound to nucleic acid, resulting in stimulation of protein synthesis and ribonucleic acid polymerase activity.

Studies have shown that dextrans are generally ineffective as activators of macrophage and show neither significant antitumor effects against M109 lung carcinoma or any ability to activate the immune system like the carboxyl anionic polymers. In general, these sulfonated polysaccharides have not demonstrated the anticipated impediment to tumor or viral infestations. For example, Schultz et al. [29] studied the effect of dextran sulfate and diethylaminoethyl dextran (DEAE-dextran) sodium salts for their potential to produce growth-inhibitory macrophages and for their ability to enhance host resistance against a transplantable, spontaneous murine lung carcinoma M109. Dextran sulfate treatment inhibited M109 DNA synthesis and required 25 mg/kg to produce optimal macrophage stimulation. DEAE-dextran was totally ineffective in prolonging the life of animals with M109 tumors and did not activate macrophages [29]. It has been shown that dextran sulfate, poly(vinyl sulfate) [30] and poly(phloroglucinol phosphate) sodium salts [31] exert a potent inhibitory effect on herpes simplex. In a more recent study [32], dextran sulfate was reported to be active against vesicular stomatitis virus (VSR) as well as herpes simplex while poly(styrene sulfonate) was totally inactive. Poly(vinyl sulfate) had good activity against VSR and herpes and fair activity against Sindbis and vaccinia viruses [32]. Although some interferon activity has been observed for these polyions, it has not been significant. They also cause many clinical side effects such as hair loss, ulcerations of the gastrointestinal tract, and osteoporosis.

Since many polysaccharides are compatible with most biological systems, several derivatives have been made and tested for possible biological application. For example, Claes et al. [33] modified several polysaccharides to study their effectiveness as interferon inducers and potential antiviral agents. The modification involved oxidation of the anhydropyranose units to yield pendent carboxyl groups along a polyacetal backbone. This two-step oxidation involved the cleavage of the anhydropyranose units in the 2-position by iodate to produce aldehyde groups which were then further oxidized with sodium chlorite to the corresponding carboxylic acid groups. This modification was carried out in an attempt to produce agents that would exhibit antiviral activity similar to those observed for some synthetic polycarboxylic acids such as polyacrylic acid and polymethacrylic acid, which suffer from toxic effects and nonbiodegradability. These modified polysaccharides were designed to give a high carboxyl group density and a biodegradable backbone. The polysaccharides that were modified are listed in Table 8.3 together with some of their physicochemical properties and their physiological activity as interferon inducers and antiviral agents. It is apparent that chlorite-oxidized oxyamylose (COAM) exhibited the greatest activity. Further, COAM inhibited the cytopathic effect of vesicular stomatitis virus in mouse embryo [33]. Antiviral activity was only observed in those polymers with a molecular weight of 2×10^6 and at least 64% of the glucopyranose units oxidized. Billeau et al. [34] reported that intraperitoneal injection of COAM protected mice against mengo, vaccinia, Semliki forest, and influenza APR 8 viruses. COAM also inhibited spontaneous mammary carcinoma. Effective inhibition of tumor growth in mice by COAM with the Moloney strain of murine sarcoma virus has been reported by DeClerq and DeSomer [35]. Furthermore, when COAM was administered with an interferon inducer, a synergistic effect in inhibition of Friend leukemia virus was observed [36].

Another natural polyanion that has received considerable interest is bacterial endotoxin, a lipopolysaccharide (LPS). Endotoxin induces interferon in mice [37], rats [38], and rabbits [39] when administered intraperitoneally. In contrast to synthetic polyanions, which achieve a peak response in 24-48 hr, endotoxin yields maximum interferon production within a few hours [39]. Although endotoxin is a poor interferon inducer, it has the capacity to induce hyperactivity to a variety of strong interferon inducers. Usually, an interferon inducer makes the animal hyperactive to interferon production to a subsequent administration of the same inducer. Endotoxin, however, produces hyperactivity not only to itself but to other interferon inducers as well, such as viruses and polynucleotides, for a period of a week or more after administration [33,40,41].

Weinberg et al. [42] demonstrated that endotoxin has a potent effect on the induction of macrophage-mediated tumor cell cytotoxicity. Endotoxin also acts synergistically with macrophage-activating factors. Consequently, there exists the possibility that endotoxin contaminants in many agents tested may be responsible for the tumorcidal activity observed, thus leading to false implications [42].

TABLE 8.3 Interferon and Antineoplastic Activity of Some Oxypolysaccharides

Starting polysaccharide	Corresponding Co-oxypolysaccharide	Circulating interferon in mice[a] (units/ml)	Protection against vaccinia virus (% reduction in pox counts)	Protection against Mengo virus[a] (% surviving more than 2 weeks)
Amylose	Co-oxyamylose	1250	-63	75
Amylopectin	Co-oxyamylpectin	400	-85	67
Whatman cellulose powder	Co-oxycellulose	200	-53	58
Dextran 150	Co-oxydextran 150	30	-46	42
Dextran 500	Co-oxydextran 500	30	-76	42
Dextran 2000	Co-oxydextran 2000	30	-73	42
Xylan	Co-oxyxylan	30	-12	33
Alginic acid	Co-oxyalginic acid	30	-42	58
Polygalacturonic acid	Co-oxypolygalacturonic acid	30	-28	28

[a]Compared to polyacrylic acid having values of; 100-500 in column 3, -55 in column 4, and 17% in column 5.

Source: Data from Ref. 33.

IV. NUCLEIC ACIDS

Since nucleic acids and enzymes play such a large role in the replication of cell materials for mitosis, a considerable amount of research has been conducted in this area to control virus replication. On the molecular level, analogs of nucleic acids are capable of forming complexes with adenine, cytosine, uracil, thymine, and guanine. Through complexation, these nucleic acid analogs are potential inhibitors of biosynthesis and require nucleic acids as templates [43]. The polyvinyl analogs of nucleic acids are the few polymers that have been tested in living systems to investigate their bioeffects [44]. The most thoroughly investigated is polyvinyladenine, which has been reported as being effective against viral leukemia, chemically induced leukemia, and infection by other viruses [45]. The inhibition of viruses by complexation of nucleic acids with their polymer analogs is apparently virus specific [44]. For example, poly(9-vinyladenine) seems to inhibit viral replication through the reverse transcriptase step [46], while poly(9-vinylpurine) is ineffective. The synthesis and evaluation of several nucleic acids are thoroughly covered in Chap. 9.

V. SYNTHETIC POLY(CARBOXYLIC ACID) POLYMERS

Synthetic polymers with carboxylic acid functionality have been found to exhibit an inhibitory effect on viruses, bacteria, tumors, and enzymes [1-3, 6]. These polyions have a broad range of biological activity and have received considerable interest by researchers in the areas of oncology and virology. The prolonged protective action of these synthetic polyanions when given prior to virus inoculation has tremendous clinical potential. Consequently, a great deal of interest in the fundamental role of polyanions in controlling host resistance to a variety of pathophysiology has been established.

Several synthetic polyanions are known to produce a wide spectrum of effects on immune reactivity [47]. They have been shown to induce the production of interferon [48, 49], modify reticuloendothelial function [50], and to invoke immunoadjuvant [51], antiviral [52], and antitumor activity [53]. The antineoplastic properties of these polyanionic polymers have been attributed largely to their ability to activate macrophages [54].

These synthetic anionic polymers have been evaluated and found viable for numerous biological responses [6]. Further studies indicated that the more important features of the carboxylic polymers for interferon induction, antiviral activity, and growth inhibition are a high density of carboxylate groups attached to a long-chain polymeric backbone [55]. The molecular weight should be greater than 1000 and the carboxyl groups can be in alternate or adjacent positions. Polyanionic polymers, in general, have been found to be fairly stable and not readily biodegradable, which may account for their prolonged activity as well as some observed adverse toxicities [56].

A. Poly(carboxylic acid) Homopolymers

Only a few homopolymers with poly(carboxylic acid) groups have been studied for biological activity. These include poly(acrylic acid) (PAA) [57] poly(methacrylic acid) (PMAA), poly(ethacrylic acid) (PEA), poly(maleic acid) (PMA), and poly(itaconic acid) (PIA). Poly(acrylic acid) was demonstrated to give 100% protection against Semliki forest virus [58], to produce T/C (ratio of the mean survival time of the treated group to that of the control group) survival times of 132% for sarcoma 180 [59], to protect against vaccinia virus with a 55% reduction in pox count [64], and to be effective against herpes simplex virus type 2 and APR influenza virus [60]. Both PAA and PMAA are poor interferon inducers but were instrumental in effecting 25-35% survivors against lethal doses of Mengo virus [61] as well as significant inhibition of sarcoma 180 (Table 8.4). PMAA was also reported to form strong interactions between molecules similar to natural biopolymers at moderate molecular weights [62].

Poly(methacrylic acid) (PMAA) was found to be more effective than PAA against vaccinia and Sindbis virus [60]. PMAA effected significant inhibition of Sindbis virus multiplication with more pronounced effects 24 hr prior to infection. An inhibition of 80-90% of vesicular stomatitis virus adsorption was also observed when 24-hr pretreatment with PMAA was used. The finding that PMAA exerts inhibition of Sindbis-RNA with no effect on

TABLE 8.4 Inhibition of Ascites Sarcoma 180 by Poly(acrylic acid) and Poly(methacrylic acid)

$$\left[\begin{array}{c} R \\ | \\ -C- \\ | \\ C=O \\ | \\ X \end{array} -CH_2- \begin{array}{c} R \\ | \\ C \\ | \\ C=O \\ | \\ X \end{array} -CH_2- \right]_n$$

Average MW		Polyacrylic acid	Polymethacrylic acid	Acrylamide
	R	H	CH_3	H
	X	OH	OH	NH_2
2,000	Inhibition	50/50	50/54	-
25,000		37/25	26/19	-
65,000		50/19	58/25	800/1
80,000		72/10	61/40	400/19

polio virus suggests that the mode of interaction is with specific RNA metabolisms [63].

We have found that poly(ethacrylic acid), recently synthesized by Tirrell [64], was more active against Lewis lung carcinoma than PAA or PMAA and almost as active as pyran [65]. Poly(ethacrylic acid)-induced macrophages have higher 5'-nucleotidase levels than pyran or thioglycollate [65].

Hydrolyzed poly(maleic anhydrine) (PMA) homopolymer exhibited activity similar in most respects to the activity of pyran copolymer with some notable differences [66]. PMA-induced phagocytic activity did not cause significant depression in RES, nor was the activity molecular weight dependent. None of the PMA fractions induced thymic changes; however, PMA was slightly less effective against Friend leukemia virus [67]. Interestingly, supernatant fluids of peritoneal exudate cells from mice pretreated with PMA transferred protection against Friend leukemia. Poly (itaconic acid), not very extensively studied, exhibited activity against ascitic sarcoma 180 with 145% T/C [67].

B. Poly(amino acids)

Several poly(amino acid) homopolymers and copolymers have also been evaluated for interferon activity. Poly L-aspartic acid, polylysine, poly L- and poly D-glutamic acid, poly(lysine-co-DL-alanine), poly(lysine-co-DL-tyrosine), and poly(lysine-co-DL-glutamic acid) all showed no significant interferon activity [68].

C. Polyanions with Maleic Anhydride and Other Carboxylic Acid Copolymers

Maleic anhydride has been commonly used as a comonomer in the preparation of many carboxylic polyanions [69]. Because of the polarity of this monomer it is an excellent electron acceptor and therefore can complex readily with other π-systems. Consequently, there have been several reports of 1:1 copolymer compositions of maleic anhydride with such monomers as styrene, acrylic acid, furan, vinyl acetate, bicyclo[2.2.1]hept-2-enes, and methacryl ester. It was further found that the polymer composition was generally independent of initial monomer ratios. These findings have led to investigations of the possible formation of charge-transfer complexes prior to polymerization as a method of controlling copolymer compositions.

El-Saied et al. [70] in their study of the dependence of copolymer composition on the mole ratio of the monomer mixture of maleic anhydride (MA) and acrylic acid (AA) found that in an excess of MA a consistent 1:1 copolymer was obtained. However, an excess of AA resulted in two polymers being formed; one was a 1:1 copolymer and the other was a polyacrylic acid homopolymer. The authors proposed that the formation of a charge-transfer complex between MA-AA occurred. This complex appears to make the copolymerization of these two entities occur more readily than in the free state. El-Saied et al. [71], in further investigations, modified the polarity of the MA double bond by adding an inert electron donor naphthalene (NPH). It was reasoned that a reduction of the polarity of MA would increase its tendency to undergo homopolymerization (it is generally known that MA does not homopolymerize readily). It was found that when NPH was introduced that more MA was incorporated into the copolymer with no incorporation of NPH. It was concluded that in the presence of NPH, two complexes, MA-AA and MA-NPH, are formed and both complexes activated MA to polymerize. With the loss of the π bond of MA, on polymerization of the MA-NPH complex breaks down and only MA is incorporated into the polymer chain.

In another study by Potter and Zutty [72], MA reportedly formed an alternating 1:1 copolymer with a number of bicyclo[2.2.1]hept-2-enes. The monomer ratios were varied and only alternating 1:1 copolymers were observed. Nyjtray and Hardy [73], who also reported the copolymerization of MA with norbornene derivatives, did not report this phenomenon.

Carboxylic acid monomers other than maleic anhydride have also been established as forming 1:1 copolymers. For example, fumaric acid with acrylic acid [73] and itaconic acid with aconitic acid [74] were disclosed as yielding alternating 1:1 copolymers. Two primary effects have been postulated to account for the 1:1 composition: hydrogen-bonded complexes and a combination of frontier orbital and secondary orbital interactions [74].

One of the most widely investigated polyanions, from the biological standpoint, is the hydrolyzed form of the 1:2 regularly alternating cyclocopolymer of divinyl ether (DVE) and maleic anhydride (MA), commonly known in literature as "pyran copolymer," "pyran," DIVEMA, or, more recently, MVE [1,6]. The synthesis and structure of this molecule has been thoroughly discussed by Butler [6,75].

The phenomenal breadth of the physiological properties of this material has been well established and emphasizes not only its antitumor, antiviral, and interferon-generating action, but its antibacterial and antifungal properties as well [6]. Pyran has been under investigation in cancer chemotherapy for several years and is designated as NSC 46015 by the National Cancer Institute. It performs a variety of biological activities and has elicited the interest of several researchers in a number of different areas. Pyran copolymer is an inducer of interferon [76-79]; it has activity against a number of viruses [76-83], including Friend leukemia [81], Rauscher leukemia [82], Moloney sarcoma [83], polyoma [84], vesicular stomatitis [85], Mengo [86], encephalomyocarditis [88], MM, and foot-and-mouth disease [89]. It has antibacterial [90-92] and antifungal activity [90], it stimulates immune response [87-93], it inhibits adjuvant disease [94], it is an interesting anticoagulant [95], and it shows promise in removing plutonium from the liver [96]. However, the toxicity of the copolymer, although much lower than that of other anionic polymers which have been investigated, was apparently still too high for it to be used extensively in clinical investigations [97, 98]. More recently, studies have shown that low-molecular-weight fractions and the calcium salt of the polymer are much less toxic, stimulating further clinical investigation of this drug (Table 8.5) [99].

Poly(maleic anhydride-co-divinyl ether) is often referred to as "pyran" because during polymerization, a cyclic six-membered ether unit (pyran) is formed. This material was first prepared by Butler [100], who discovered that the linear monomers maleic anhydride and divinyl ether combined in a 2:1 ratio to form repeating cyclic units along the polymer backbone. The mechanism became known as a cyclopolymerization process and a six-membered ring was initially postulated [100-104]. Analysis confirmed the 2:1 copolymer ratio and the pyran structure was widely accepted.

TABLE 8.5 Biological Activity of Various Samples of Pyran

				Antitumor	
Sample	MW	SGPT[a]	Phagocytic index[b]	Ehrlich[c] (% inhibition)	Lewis lung[d] (T/C)
Control		30	0.044		
A	2,500	34	0.105	60	>130
B	3,000	48	0.073		>171
C	3,900	30			>133
D	5,200	54			125
E	6,900	46	0.055	43	
F	14,700	52	0.075	61	
G	19,600	93	0.014	45	
H	25,000	132			
I	44,800	96	0.010		
NSC 46015	22,500	>200	0.021	67	>117
XA 124-177	32,200	>200	0.015	53	

[a]Serum glutamic pyruvate transaminase, Sigma Frankel units.
[b]From first-order rate of carbon clearance, 24 hr after injection.
[c]Decrease in weight of tumor compared with control.
[d]Mean survival time, percent of control.
Source: Data from Ref. 99.

Recently, extensive studies of free-radical cyclization of monomers and polymers indicate that five-membered rings instead of six-membered rings are formed preferentially. Samuels [106] has reported that quantitative structural analysis supported the formation of a five-membered structure. ^{13}C nuclear magnetic resonance (NMR) spectroscopic analyses by Chu and Butler [107], Kunitake and Tsukino [108] and later by Freeman and Breslow [109] indicated that the structure is very complex, with both five- and six-membered rings being present as well as some branching. The ratio of five- to six-membered rings formed during cyclopolymerization has been found to be related to the reaction conditions; for example, higher temperatures and more polar solvents seem to favor the six-membered ring formation. Breslow [110], also one of the pioneers of the synthesis of pyran, has developed a method of preparing pyran with a narrow molecular weight distribution. The procedure involves photoinitiation of the monomers in the presence of acetone-THF solution. Using the right solvent ratios, these researchers reported being able to obtain nine different molecular weights, ranging from 2500 to 45,000 and having $\overline{M}_W/\overline{M}_\eta$ ranging from 1.6 to 2.6. This is compared to NSC 46015 prepared by the slurry method with a MW of 22,500 and $\overline{M}_W/\overline{M}_\eta$ of 3.7 [80].

In Table 8.6 are listed a number of carboxylic acid copolymers and their anticancer activity. More recently, we have evaluated several polyanionic copolymers of maleic anhydride [111]. A number of these polymers were as effective or more effective than pyran against Lewis lung carcinoma (Fig. 8.1) and Ehrlich ascites tumor cells (Table 8.7). The polymers were prepared as low molecular-weight materials and fractionated by ultrafiltration methods. They were characterized by ^{1}H and ^{13}C NMR as 1:1 alternating copolymers. The more effective polymers appear to be those with a higher degree of lipophilicity.

The copolymerization of monomers not involving maleic anhydride produces copolymers in which the monomers are added randomly or in block sequences. For example, Hodnett et al. [212] prepared a number of polymeric carboxylic acids with different solubilities in water. These polymers were evaluated against sarcoma 180 ascites tumor of mice. Maximum antiviral effectiveness was obtained by the polymers with the least number of carboxylic acid groups ionized at pH 7. Animal toxicity of these polymers, however, decreased with increased carboxylic acid group content of the polymer.

Hodnett prepared five copolymers of acrylic acid and isobutyl vinyl ether. Homopolymerization attempts with free-radical initiators of isobutyl vinyl ether yielded only oligomers; macromolecules were obtained only with a cationic initiator. Since acrylic acid polymerizes readily by free-radical initiation, the concentration of isobutyl vinyl ether had to be kept high in order to get appreciable amounts of this monomer into polymerization process. Acrylic acid was also copolymerized with β-(N, N-dimethylamino)ethylmethacrylate and isooctyl vinyl ether. The former copolymer

TABLE 8.6 Antitumor Activity of Some Carboxyl-Containing Polymers and Copolymers[a]

NSC no.	Polymer or copolymer	Tumor	Dose (mg/kg)	T/C (%)
D59196	DVE-MA	LE	45.0	122
D59199	1,4-Pentadiene-MA	SA	30.0	49
D59200	p-(2-Vinyloxy-2-ethoxy-O-benzaldehyde-MA)	CA	100	55
84645	$DVSO_2$-methacrylic acid	LE	400	101
84649	1,4-Pentadiene-MA $[\eta] = 0.18$	LE	50.0	95
84650	1,4-Pentadiene-MA $[\eta] = 0.26$	LL	10.0	43
99425	1,4-Pentadiene-MA-$BrCCl_3$ (telomer)	LE	100	146
99426	1,4-Pentadiene-MA-$BrCCl_3$ (telomer)	LE	200	97
99427	DVE-MA-$BrCCl_3$ (telomer)	LE	200	107
104,304	4-Vinylcyclohexane-MA	WM	100	92
119165	Furan-itaconic anhydride	LE	200	97
119166	Furan-MA	LE	270	105
119167	Furan-MA-(half-amide)	LE	177	105
119168	Furan-itaconic anhydride (half-amide)	LE	177	137
133,788	DVE-citraconic anhydride	LE	132	103
133789	β-Chloroethyl vinyl ether-citraconic anhydride	LE	37.5	117
133790	β-Chloroethyl vinyl ether-MA	LE	75.0	119
133791	2,5-Dihydrofuran-MA	LE	400	110
133792	2-Methyl-4,5-dihydrofuran-MA	LE	200	107
148129	Isoprene-MA	PS	0.29	118
148130	2-Methylenenorbornene-MA	LE	200	93
148131	2-Ethylidenenorbornene-MA	LE	80.5	98

TABLE 8.6 (Continued)

NSC no.	Polymer or Copolymer	Tumor	Dose (mg/kg)	T/C (%)
148132	2-Vinylnorbornene-MA	LE	80.5	106
184133	Butadiene-MA	LE	1.56	109

[a]$DVSO_2$, divinyl sulfone; DVE, divinyl ether; MA, maleic anhydride; LL, Lewis lung carcinoma; LE, L1210 lymphoid leukemia; CA, adenocarcinoma 755; SA, sarcoma 180; WM, Walker carcinosarcoma 256; PS, P388 lymphocytic leukemia.

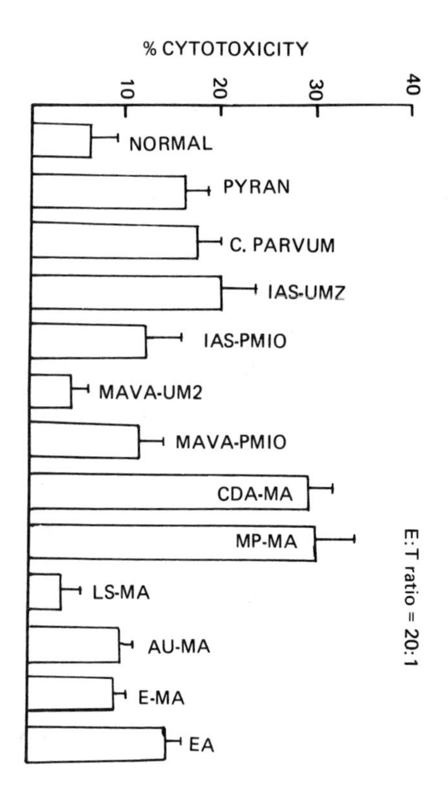

FIGURE 8.1 Induction of cytotoxic macrophages with polyanionic compounds determined by morphological assay.

TABLE 8.7 Effect of Copolymers Against Ehrlich Ascites Tumor Cells[a]

a. Effect of Maleic Anhydride Copolymers

Polymer	10,000-30,000 Molecular weight		1000-10,000 Molecular weight	
	Cells/pc x 10^8	Percent control	Cells/pc x 10^8	Percent control
Saline	1.52	100	2.17	100
Pyran	0.74	49	0.63	30
MA-co-acrylic Acid	1.8	118	1.25	58
MA-co-styrene	0.76	45	0.15	7
MA-co-methacry-lic acid	1.42	93	1.31	60
MA-co-allyl phenol	1.31	86	0.35	16
MA-co-allyl suc-cinic anhydride	1.32	87	0.91	42
MA-co-1,3-dioxepin	1.43	94	0.63	30
MA-co-isobutenyl succinic anhydride	1.21	80	1.33	61

b. Effect of 2,3-Dicarboxynorborn-5-ene Copolymers

Copolymer	10,000-30,000 Molecular weight		1000-10,000 Molecular weight	
	Cells/pc x 10^8	Percent control	Cells/pc x 10^8	Percent control
Control	1.52	100	2.17	100
Pyran	0.74	49	0.64	30
Maleic anhydride	1.64	1.08	0.16	7

TABLE 8.7 (Continued)

	10,000-30,000 Molecular weight		1000-10,000 Molecular weight	
Copolymer	Cells/pc x 10^8	Percent control	Cells/pc x 10^8	Percent control
Acrylic acid	1.06	1.06	0.48	22
Vinyl acetate	0.89	41	0.76	34
Vinyl alcohol	0.85	56	0.71	32

[a] 10^6 Ehrlich ascites cells were inoculated intraperitoneally into mice. Five days after inoculation, animals were sacrificed and total peritoneal exudate cells were counted with a hemocytometer.

was very nontoxic (LD_{50}) of 600 mg/kg for mice) and produced a 45% increased survival time against sarcoma 180 ascites, while the latter was more toxic and less effective (Table 8.8).

Many other copolymers with carboxylic acid groups have been reported, but only a few of these have been evaluated for biological activity. Examples of some that have been prepared and evaluated are listed in Table 8.6. A novel type of polyanion has been developed with N-substituted triazolinediones and styrene or isoprene in a two-step reaction [113]. The resulting disubstituted urazoles have been shown to have pKa 6, in comparison to corresponding carboxylic acids that have pKa 5. Extension of the reaction to bistriazolinedione led to polymeric structures and to the corresponding polyanions. Other polyurazole anions have also been prepared via the reaction of N-substituted triazolinediones with preformed polymers containing allylic halogen [114]. This reaction is quite versatile in that it occurs rapidly at room temperature and can be used to effect any degree of substitution desired. The antineoplastic activity is listed in Table 8.9.

VI. HALF-AMIDES AND IMIDE COPOLYMERS

It was hypothesized that inhibition of tumor growth may be a function of the density and distribution of ionic charges within the polyelectrolyte molecule [1-6]. Consequently, the structure of the divinyl ether-maleic anhydride and similar copolymers were modified by postreaction of the preformed copolymers. For example, conversion of the divinyl ether-maleic anhydride copolymer to a variety of imides [6] was readily accomplished with certain amines. Thus the polymer structure was modified either via partial or total conversion of the anhydride units to select imide units which may also

TABLE 8.8 Effect of Some Acrylic Acid Copolymers on Sarcoma 180

Polymer	Polymer name	Formula	LD_{50} (mg/kg)	T/C (%)
I	Acrylic acid	(AA)	39	132
II	Poly(acrylic acid-isobutyl vinyl ether)	$(AA)_x \cdot (IBVE)_{0.035x}$	25	165
IIII		$(AA)_x \cdot (IBVE)_{0.046x}$	82	171
IV		$(AA)_x \cdot (IBVE)_{0.29x}$	13	150
V		$(AA)_x \cdot (IBVE)_{0.43x}$	3.5	111
VI		$(AA)_x \cdot (IBVE)_{0.73x}$	3.5	122
VII	Poly(isobutyl) ether	$(IBVE)_x$	—	—
VIII	Poly(itaconic acid)	$(TACA)_x \cdot (H_2O)_{0.7x}$	425	145
IX	Poly(acrylic acid-itaconic acid)	$(AA)_x \cdot (ITCA)_x \cdot (H_2O)_{0.4x}$	300	192
X	Poly(acrylic acid-β-(N, N-dimethyl-amino) ethyl methacrylate	$(AA)_x \cdot (DMAEM)_x$	600	145
XI	Poly(acrylic acid-isoocytl vinyl ether)	$(AA)_x \cdot (IOVE)_{0.15x}$	10.5	125

Source: Data from Ref. 112.

possess other functional groups capable of enhancing the effectiveness of the material as an antitumor agent. Other physiological characteristics of the material may be modified in a similar manner by careful selection of co-reactants.

The first study [115] involved two classes of synthetic polymers: the homopolymer, polyacrylic acid, and the copolymer, poly(ethylene-co-maleic

TABLE 8.9 Effects of Polyurazoles on P388 Lymphoma and Lewis Lung Carcinoma-Infected Mice

	Mice bearing P338 lymphoma			Mice bearing Lewis lung carcinoma	
	Dose (mg/kg)	N	MST (days)	Dose (ng/kg)	MST
Saline	—	16	9.8	—	28.1
Polyisoprene modified with N-phenyltriazolinedione	25	8	11.0	25	29.1
	50	8	Toxic	50	Toxic
	75	8	Toxic	75	Toxic
Polyisoprene modified with N-methyltriazolinedione	25	8	10.0	25	30.2
	50	8	9.5	50	33.3
	75	8	8.9	75	36.9
Poly(styrene-co-isoprene) with N-phenyltriazolinedine	25	8	10.9	25	34.1
	50	6	11.3	50	33.3
	75	7	11.4	75	36.4
	25	8	11.3	25	29.9
Poly(styrene-co-butadiene) with N-phenyltriazolinedine	50	8	11.3	50	Toxic
				75	Toxic

anhydride). The charge density and solution configuration of these compounds were varied over a wide range by proper choice of substituents on the backbone of the molecule and by substitutions on the carboxyl groups. The hydrolyzed poly(ethylene-co-maleic anhydride) (HEMA) had the dicarboxylic structure and the ammoniated poly(ethylene-co-maleic anhydride) (AEMA) had the half amide-half acid form. The principal tumor in this study was sarcoma 180. When activity was observed with sarcoma 180, a wider range of tumor systems, including Krebs 2 carcinoma, leukemia L-1210, and carcinoma 755, were evaluated.

The following derivatives of poly(ethylene-co-maleic anhydride) EMA were prepared: the dicarboxylic acid-HEMA, the ammonium salt of AEMA, the amide acid form of AEMA, the EMA diamide, and hydrolyzed and amidated propylene and isobutylene-maleic anhydride copolymers. Molecular weights ranged from approximately 2000 to 120,000. The evaluation against sarcoma 180 showed that the diamide of EMA had a much lower tumor inhibitory activity and toxicity than HEMA or AEMA. As the molecular weight increased up to 80,000-100,000, toxicity of the dicarboxylic acid HEMA increased. The dicarboxylic acid propylene and isobutylene copolymers tested were more toxic and less tumor-inhibitory than the corresponding half-acid amide compounds.

Another series of polymers, consisting of polyacrylic acid, polymethacrylic acid, and polyacrylamide, showed analogous biological activity (Table 8.10). Here, too, the completely amidated product had negligible antitumor activity but had lower toxicity than carboxyl-containing compounds of similar molecular weight. Hence it appears that some carboxylic groups are necessary for significant tumor inhibition. The difference between the two series in position of carboxyl groups on the polymer backbone (which still has the same charge density per repeating unit) did not greatly alter the antitumor activity of the compound.

The activity of low molecular weight (2000-3000) HEMA and AEMA against several tumors were compared (Table 8.11). The half-amide, half-acid AEMA form was clearly more effective as an antitumor agent and showed a broader spectrum of activity. Polymers of MW 20,000-30,000 displayed the same pattern of tumor inhibition.

The monomers of HEMA and AEMA, such as succinic acid, succinamic acid, succinimide, and succinamide, were also evaluated for activity; no significant activity against sarcoma 180 was observed, indicating the necessity for the polymeric structure for tumor inhibition. These studies indicate that tumor inhibition by polyanions may be dependent on functional group density and distribution and that a certain carboxamide-carboxyl balance may broaden the scope of activity against a variety of tumors.

Sharabash et al. [116] investigated the copolymerization of furan and maleic anhydride. The resultant 1:1 FMA copolymer was evaluated as NCS 119166 and its half-amide half-ammonium salt as NCS 118167. At doses of 400 mg/kg FMA exhibited a 40% increase in survival time and the half-amide a 30% increase against L1210. In another study [117], it was shown that low-molecular-weight FMA had much less hepatomeglia, spleenomeglia, LD_{50}, and hexobarbital sleeping times than the polydisperse pyran XA-124-177 sample. It was found that this sample of FMA was not very effective against Lewis lung carcinoma and was totally ineffective against encephalomyocarditis.

The copolymer of furan and itaconic anhydride and its half-amide, half-ammonium salt were also synthesized. Evaluation against L1210 indicated a 50% increase in survival time at doses of 600 mg/kg for the diacid. Divinyl ether and citraconic anhydride also exhibited about a 30% increase in survival time against L1210 lymphoral leukemia. A number of divinyl ether maleimide copolymers and their anticancer activities are listed in Table 8.12.

Recently, Fields et al. [118, 119] have prepared a low-molecular-weight ethylene-maleic anhydride copolymer derivatized to contain both a half-amide, half-carboxylate salt function and an imide function. The synthesis was carried out by first preparing a low-molecular-weight alternating copolymer of ethylene and maleic anhydride. The anhydride groups of

TABLE 8.10 Inhibition of Ascites Sarcoma 180 by Modified Poly(ethylene-co-maleic anhydride)

$$\left[-\underset{R_1}{\overset{R_2}{\underset{|}{\overset{|}{C}}}} - CH_2 - \underset{\underset{X}{|}}{\underset{C=0}{\underset{|}{\overset{H}{C}}}} - \underset{\underset{Y}{|}}{\underset{C=0}{\underset{|}{\overset{H}{C}}}} - \right]_n$$

Molecular weight		Hydrolyzed ethylene	Ammoniated ethylene	Ethylene amide-acid	Diamide ethylene	Hydrolyzed propylene	Ammoniated propylene	Hydrolyzed isobutylene	Ammoniated isobutylene
	R_1	H	H	H	H	H	H	CH_3	CH_3
	R_2	H	H	H	H	CH_3	CH_3	CH_3	CH_3
	X	OH	NH_2	NH_2	NH_2	O(Na)	NH_2	O(Na)	NH_2
	Y	OH	ONH_4	OH	NH_2	O(Na)	ONH_4	O(Na)	ONH_4
	Inhibition dose (mg/kg)								
2000-3000		54/200	80/300	70/400	—	-	59/400	13/19	79/50
20,000-30,000		72/100	81/50	78/100	38/800	15/9	67/50	-	77/40
60,000-70,000		55/10	65/50	69/100	-	39/19	59/50	23/9	65/25
80,000-100,000		46/4	83/75	58/25	-	-	-	-	-
120,000 and up		61/4	72/75	51/25	-	-	-	-	46/5

Source: Data obtained from Ref. 115.

TABLE 8.11 Antitumor Activity of Hydrolyzed Poly(ethylene-co-maleic anhydride) (HEMA) and Ammoniated Poly(ethylene-co-maleic anhydride) (AEMA)[a]

Tumor	Dose[a] (mg/kg)	Percent inhibition	
		HEMA	AEMA
Sarcoma 180	200	56	77
Krebs 2 carcinoma	200	34	55
L1210	200	12	65
Carcinoma 755	150	-17	58

[a]MW 2000-3000.

the copolymer were converted to half-amide, half-ammonium salt functions by reacting a solution of the polymer in acetone with a liquid ammonia-acetone mixture. This ammoniated copolymer was then converted to the partial imide. The product, coded NED 137, was shown to have 14-25 wt % of the succinimide rings. The NED 137 copolymer was evaluated for biological activity against several transplantable tumors. It was found to have relatively low acute toxicity in mice and rats with an LD_{50} of approximately 2500 mg/kg body weight. It inhibited Lewis lung carcinoma and several other murine solid tumors. It was indicative from this study that the antitumor activity of ammoniated ethylene-maleic anhydride copolymers could be increased by ring closure of a portion of the acid-amidated succinate groups along the polymer backbone. It is to be noted that the formation of the imide ring causes the polymer to be more rigid. This feature has been shown to increase antitumor activity in other polyanionic systems [1-6].

NED 137 has been potent as a tumor inhibitor and in preventing metastases of a methylcholanthrene-induced carcinoma of the bladder (FBCa) in F344 rats [120]. This tumor is known to metastasize to the lung within 1 week of tumor implantation. The survival of animals with in situ FBCa treated with NED 137 at 30 mg/kg showed prolonged survival as compared to control animals. All the treated animals were found to be free of pulmonary metastases when autopsied, while all the control animals had extensive pulmonary metastases.

The effect of NED 137 as an adjuvant to surgical excision of the tumor was examined. The treated animals were observed for tumor recurrence and survival time after excision versus untreated control animals. Tumor recurrence was 100% in the control animals, with subsequent death by 35

TABLE 8.12 Antitumor Activity of Some Poly(Divinylether-co-N-Substituted Malemides)[a]

NSC no.	Monomer or comonomers	Tumor	Dose (mg/kg)	T/C (%)
77033	DVE-N-phenylmaleimide	SA	500	71
84551	DVE-maleimide	LE	400	88
84652	DVE-N-methylmaleimide	SA	500	114
84653	DVE-N-ethylmaleimide	SA	500	113
84654	DVE-N-n-propylmaleimide	SA	500	106
84655	DVE-N-n-butylmaleimide	LE	100	100
84656	DVE-N-n-butylmeleimide	SA	500	112
84657	DVE-N-i-butylmaleimide	SA	500	82
84658	DVE-N-benzylmaleimide	LE	400	105
84659	DVE-N-α-naphthylmaleimide	SA	350	109
148134	DVE-p-carboxyphenylmaleimide	PS	3.12	110
217996	DVE-N-morpholinomethylmaleimide (10:1)	LE	100	100
266062	DVE-maleimide of d,l-alanine	PS	20.0	117
266063	DVE-maleimide of d,l-phenylalanine	PS	40.0	101
266064	DVE-maleimide of d,l-methionine	PS	10.0	112
266066	DVE maleimide of d,l-leucine	PS	7.5	125
266067	DVE-maleimide of glycine	PS	50.0	109
266226	DVE-maleimide of 1-phenylalanine	PS	45.0	105

[a]DVE, divinyl ether; LE, L12o0 lymphoid leukemia; SA, sarcoma 180; PS, P388 lymphocytic leukemia.

days after surgical excision. Autopsy of the control animals indicated massive lung metastases. The rats treated with NED 137, however, showed no local recurrences of tumor 60 days after tumor excision. Autopsy after 60 days indicated that NED 137-treated animals were free of pulmonary metastases [120]. Indefinite survival in these animals could be obtained with repeated administration of the drug. The investigators showed that the active antitumor effect was due to a component of the serum and was coprecipitable with the serum immunoglobins [121]. This response was transferred to normal animals by the serum of animals treated with NED 137. It was also noted that the experimental animals showed no acute or chronic toxicity from NED 137.

Subsequently, using the same bladder carcinoma, FBCa, the antitumor activity of NED 137 was compared with a series of known immunoadjuvants. These were Bacille Calmette-Guérin (BCG), Corynebacterium parvum, pyran, levamisole, and Freund's complete adjuvant (FCA) [121]. These adjuvants were administered after excision of tumor implants. A single intraperitoneal injection of NED 137 at 30 mg/kg body weight prolonged survival beyond 60 days with no evidence of recurrent or metastatic disease, whereas with the other adjuvants, animals survived a mean of 30-40 days with 100% local recurrence and a 60-90% incidence of pulmonary metastases.

In 1979, a modified phase I study of NED 137 in patients with gastrointestinal cancer was initiated at the University of Toronto and the Health Protection Branch, Federal Ministry of Health of Canada. Patients receiving NED 137 therapy were compared to a group of patients with metastatic gastrointestinal cancer who were studied over the period 1974-1978. This control group had received BCG and 5-fluorouracil (5-FU) or 5-FU alone as therapy. In terms of overall survival, these two groups have been compared by using corrected life survival curves [120, 121].

VII. MACROPHAGE ACTIVIATION BY CARBOXYLIC ACID POLYMERS

Initially, macrophages were considered as the "antigenic garbage disposal unit," concerned only with the phagocytosis and the degradation of antigen. In recent years, however, macrophages have undergone considerable reevaluation with regard to their role in the immune system. The function that macrophages play in the generation of the immune response has been extensively studied, and postulated mechanisms of macrophage activity in antibody production include antigen processing for "presentation" to the lymphocytes and antigen processing by elaboration of soluble factors. It has been reported that cell-mediate immunity is dependent primarily on the interaction between T lymphocytes and macrophages [122].

Macrophages are produced by rapidly dividing precursor cells in the bone marrow, and daughter cells are released into the bloodstream. This mononuclear system consists of several types of cells and are found distributed throughout the body. Once they leave the blood, the macrophage locate in the tissues of the liver, spleen, lymph nodes, lungs, and peritoneum. In these sites, they differentiate into the various types of fixed macrophages and function [123, 124]. Synthetic polyanionic immunopotentiators such as pyran and polyacrylic acid are known to enhance macrophage function as well as to induce resistance to tumor growth [125]. Under suitable conditions, macrophages can be transformed into "activated" macrophages, characterized by enlarged cells with undulating plasma membranes. Macrophage treated with these polyanionic polymer stimulants have shown cytotoxicity for cancer cells [126]. The immunopotentiator pyran causes an increase in the number of histocytes present in the connective tissue surrounding the Lewis lung tumor of mice [127]. In addition, increased numbers of tumor-associated macrophages are correlated with a decrease in metastasis in pyran-treated tumor-bearing mice [128]. The involvement of "factors" produced by activated macrophages in the tumoricidal event are receiving considerable attention [129-131].

Recent data indicate that macrophages activated by pyran are cytotoxic for tumor cells and have a new macrophage cell surface antigen. This new macrophage cell surface antigen was not detected on normal macrophages or macrophages elicited by glycogen or thioglycollate, which are also known to increase biochemical activity but are not cytotoxic for tumor cells [132]. The correlation of activated macrophage with cytotoxicity and in vivo antitumor activity provides a simple, rapid technique for analyzing macrophage activation. Moreover, this provides a model system for analyzing the chemical moiety associated with these agents which is responsible for antitumor activity and a powerful tool for quickly screening potentially active compounds.

The cytotoxicity of activated macrophages has been clearly demonstrated to be confined only to tumor cells [132-136] and has an insignificant or no effect on normal or natural cells such as mouse embryo cells [137] or murine kidney cells [134, 136]. The mechanism of activation of macrophages or the tumoricidal activity of activated macrophages is not understood. It has been observed that a population of aneuploid Lewis lung carcinoma cells, in the presence of activated macrophages, show reductive mitotic cell division resulting from tumor cells with 50% less DNA per cell [137]. This depletion of DNA leads to cell destruction since these cells no longer have the appropriate DNA to synthesize necessary molecules for cell division.

Cell cycle analysis has shown that drastic changes in DNA distribution occurs in Lewis lung cells cultivated with ionic polymer-activated macrophages [138]. Consequently, the use of anionic polymer activated macrophages resulted in (1) a high overall level of tumoricidal activity in vivo and in vitro, (2) the appearance of a tumor cell population with 50% of their normal DNA content, and (3) a shift of tumor cells from phase G_2M to G_1. These results indicate that a possible mechanism of activated macrophage tumoricidal activity involves the induction of tumor cells with a reduced DNA content.

In a more recent study, we prepared several polyanionic polymers of defined molecular weight, chain rigidity, lipophilicity, and surface charge to probe the mechanism of macrophage activation [139]. To assess the state of activation demonstrated by these polymer-elicited macrophages, their activities were compared to resident and thioglycollate, pyran, and

C. parvum elicited macrophages. For study, macrophages were lavaged from the peritoneal cavities of C57B1/6 mice who had received injections of polymers (50 mg/kg) or C. parvum (17.25 mg/kg) 7 days prior to harvests.

Macrophages elicited with itaconic acid-styrene copolymer (IAS), vinyl acetate-maleic anhydride (MAVA), cyclohexyl-1, 3-dioxepin-maleic anhydride copolymer (CDA-MA), 4-methyl-2-pentenoyl-maleic anhydride copolymer (MP-MA), and α-ethyl-acrylic acid homopolymer (EA) were cytotoxic to Lewis lung carcinoma in vitro. Macrophages elicited with styrene-maleic anhydride copolymer (S-MA), allylurea-maleic anhydride copolymer (AU-MA), and ethylene-maleic anhydride copolymer (E-MA) did not demonstrate significant antitumor activity (Fig. 8.1).

The enzyme profiles of macrophages elicited by the test polymers did not necessarily concur with previously reported profiles of activated macrophages [139]. All polymer-elicited macrophages demonostrated 5' activity which had previously been associated only with nontumoricidal, resident macrophages. Interestingly, the 5' activity of macrophages elicited with CDA-MA, MP-MA, and MAVA, which have significant antitumor activity, also possess the highest 5' activity of the polymers. In contrast, tumoricidal macrophages elicited with pyran and C. parvum have negligible 5' activity. Thus 5' activity may be used to discriminate between macrophages elicited by the test polymers and those of conventional activating agents.

Leucine aminopeptidase levels of macrophages may be used to identify maleic anhydride polymers that induce macrophage antitumor activity. To date, maleic anhydride copolymers that induce enhanced tumoricidal activity also induce a concomitant increase in LAP activity. In contrast, E-MA-, S-MA-, and AU-MA-elicited macrophages, which are not tumoricidal, demonstrate LAP levels similar to that of resident macrophage.

Thus far, it has been determined that whereas molecular weight generally plays a small role in activation, lipophilicity, chain rigidity, and enhanced surface charge all play a significant role associated with increased activation of macrophages.

VIII. CHANGES IN TUMOR CELL DNA EFFECTED BY ACTIVATED MACROPHAGES

The cytotoxicity of activated macrophage has been demonstrated to be confined to tumor cells and has an insignificant or no effect on normal or natural cells such as mouse embryo cells or murine kidney cells [140-144]. The mechanism of activation of macrophage or the tumoricidal activity of activated macrophage is not understood. It has been observed that a population of aneuploid Lewis lung carcinoma cells, in the presence of activated macrophages, show reduced cell division resulting from tumor cells with 50% less DNA per cell [144]. This depletion of DNA leads to cell destruction since these cells no longer have the appropriate DNA to synthesize necessary molecules for cell division.

As indicated in Table 8.13, a cell cycle analysis [145] has shown that in vitro Lewis lung cells are distributed such that 15% are in the resting phase (G_1), 52% in the DNA synthesis phase (S), and 33% are in cell division phases (G_2M). After treatment with pyran-"activated" macrophages, the tumor cells in the resting phase (G_1) rose to 74%, while synthesis (S) and cell division (G_2M) phases fell to 22% and 4%, respectively. The shift to G_1 phase was not seen with Lewis lung cells cultivated with normal macrophage or mouse embryo fibroblasts incubated with activated macrophages. Animals treated interaperitoneally with pyran produced a 30-fold inhibition of Ehrlich ascites tumor growth, with maximum inhibition of tumor growth occurring with pyran treatment 2 days prior to tumor cell inoculation.

Similar to the in vitro study using Lewis lung cells, it was observed that animals pretreated with pyran had no detectable Ehrlich ascites cells in phase G_2M and only a few in the S phase after 2 or 6 days, compared to pyran-untreated mice, which had 58% in the S phase and 22 in the G_2M phase [145]. Consequently, the use of pyran-activated macrophage resulted in a high overall level of tumoricidal activity both in vivo and in vitro, the appearance of a tumor cell population with 50% of their normal DNA content, and a shift of tumor cells from phase G_2M to G_1. These results indicate that a possible mechanism of activated macrophage tumoricidal activity involves the induction of tumor cells with a reduced DNA content.

TABLE 8.13 Change in DNA Distribution of Lewis Lung Cells Cultivated with Anionic Polymer Activated Macrophages

Lewis lung cultured[a] with activated macrophages for:	Percent DNA in phase		
	G_1	S	G_2M
0 hr	15	52	33
4 hr	16	52	32
8 hr	32	47	20
16 hr	62	34	4
24 hr	74	22	4

[a] Activated macrophages were obtained from mice injected intraperitoneally with 25 mg/kg of pyran 7 days before peritoneal lavage.

TABLE 8.14 Cell Cycle Analysis of Ehrlich Ascites Tumor Cells Before and After in Vivo Exposure to Anionic Polymer

Days following tumor inoculation[a]	Pyran treatment[b]	Percent DNA in phase		
		G_1	S	G_2M
2	-	20	58	22
2	+	98	2	0
6	-	36	47	17
6	+	98	2	0

[a]Mice were inoculated intraperitoneally with 1 x 10^6 Ehrlich ascites cells and killed on various days thereafter.

[b]Pyran was injected intraperitoneally (23 mg/kg) 2 days prior to tumor inoculation.

IX. IMMUNE ADJUVANT EFFECTS OF POLY(CARBOXYLIC ACID) POLYMERS

It has been reported that several agents are capable of modifying the immune response. More recently, it has been found that some of these immunoactivators also enhance the activity of certain anticancer agents. For example, Chirigos et al. [146] reported that pyran copolymer serves as an effective adjuvant to L1210 tumor cell vaccine, while pyran alone is ineffective against L1210. The best immunity to tumor challenge was produced by concomitant administration of L1210 vaccine with pyran.

The L1210 vaccine alone provided some degree of protection against the L1210 challenge with a 30% increase in median survival time. However, none of the animals survived beyond the test period. In contrast, an adjuvant effect was observed with various molecular weight pyrans [147]. All molecular weight fractions were effective; these ranged from 12,500 to 52,600. In each case, more than 50% of the animals survived more than 45 days. A major observation was that a marked protection was obtained when surviving animals were rechallenged 45 days after the first L1210 challenge. The mean survival time of these animals was greater than 70 days. Furthermore, when animals were first challenged 45 days after vaccination with L1210 vaccine-pyran regimen, the survival time was increased by 40% over control. These experiments indicate that an appreciable residence of protection can be obtained with this regimen.

Mohr et al. [148] observed that pyran (NSC 46015), a polydisperse material, actively induced host resistance and increased the survival time of LSTRA-bearing mice following BCNU chemotherapy. The survival time was extended to 70% of control. In a later study by Dean et al. [149], two pyran fractions were evaluated: a 15,500-MW sample and a 52,600-MW sample. Both samples demonstrated adjuvant activity and enhanced host resistance to LSTRA leukemia BCNU chemotherapy. These pyrans extended survival from 20-30% in the BCNU controls to 60-90% in the BCNU plus pyran-treated groups. Adjuvant activity was obtained with a simple dose of 5 or 25 mg/kg administered 6 or 13 days following BCNU treatment. A good correlation was obtained between adjuvant activity and remission in the LSTRA model to macrophage activation as measured in vitro with a microculture.

Przybyski et al. [150] covalently linked methotrexate to pyran copolymer to obtain a product with 25% methotrexate content. Antitumor evaluation of pyran-methotrexate in mice has shown a potentiated activity over either component individually or in a combination of pyran plus methotrexate against the highly resistant L1210 carcinoma at optimal equivalent doses and schedules. In addition to a sustained plasma pharmacokinetic effects of methotrexate, the pyran copolymer demonstrated an adjuvant effect of enhanced antitumor activity. In a further study, the relative immune activity of the pyran-methotrexate polymer in combination with an L1210 vaccine was evaluated [151]. The drug carrying copolymer was a potent immunoadjuvant with 60% survivors, which, however, was less than pyran alone with L1210 vaccine, which had 90% survivors.

X. DRUG CARRYING POLYANIONIC POLYMERS

Since polymers in biological systems diffuse slowly and are often absorbed at interfaces, the attachment of active pharmaceutical moieties to the structure of a macromolecular chain has been found to produce polymers with distinct pharmacological activity. It has become recognized that the binding of drugs to a polymer backbone can effect some desirable properties, such as synergistic effects, adjuvant effects, sustained therapy, slow drug release, prolonged activity, and drug latentation, as well as decreased drug metabolism and excretion.

Two very active antineoplastic drugs that have been incorporated into polymers are 5-fluorouracil and 6-methylthiopurine. The parent compounds of these active materials are the nucleic acids uracil and adenine, which have been converted to various monomer derivatives and polymerized [152]. These polymers exhibit inhibition of leukemia virus [153] and RNA polymerase [154] as well as other biological activity. While the acryolyl and carbamoyl derivatives of 6-methylthiopurine have been prepared, they have not been as extensively evaluated for biological activity as the uracil derivatives [155].

Umrigar et al. [156] copolymerized 1-(2-carbomethoxyacryloyl)-5-fluorouracil (CMAFU) with divinyl ether, styrene, and β-chloroethyl vinyl ether to yield the three corresponding copolymers with molecular weights in the range 5000-7500. The styrene copolymer (St/CMAFU) and chloroethyl vinyl ether copolymer (CEVE-DMAFU) were shown by analysis to be 1:1 alternating copolymers, while the DVE-CMAFU copolymer was 2:1 molar in DMAFU:DVE content. The biological evaluation of these copolymers by the National Cancer Institute are shown in Table 8.15. 5-Fluorouracil was released from these copolymers hydrolytically, respective rates of release being determined from dispersion in 0.5 M NaCl. Under these conditions, the monomer (CMAFU) released 5-FU almost instantly and completely. On the other hand, the St:CMAFU and DEVE:CMAFU copolymers were more resistant to hydrolysis and only gradually released 5-FU. DVE:CMAFU was hydrolyzed faster than the other two copolymers, but much slower than the monomer. The hydrophobic character of the St:CMAFU copolymer appears to be important for slow release of 5-FU.

More recently, a vinylcarbamyl of 5-fluorouracil was polymerized and found to be active against P388 leukemia [155]. Other derivatives, such as the allylcarbamyl acryloyl, although attempted, have not been successfully polymerized [152]. The inclusion of 5-fluorouracil in polymer matrices has been recently reported by Hoshida et al. [157] to provide controlled release of the drug.

Another active agent, methotrexate, N-[4-(N-methyl-2,4-diamino-6-pteridinyl-methylamino)-benzoyl] glutamic acid, is a widely used antitumor agent and a folic acid antagonist. Pryzbylski et al. [159] covalently bonded

TABLE 8.15 Evaluation of Polymers Containing 5-Fluorouracil

	Test/control survival time (%)		
Dose (mg/kg)	St/CMAFU (NSC 255081)	CEVE/CMAFU (NSC 255082)	DVE/CMAFU (NSC 255083)
400	94	129	112
200	192	165	189
	144	141	172
100	171	165	137
	127	127	140
50	133	123	125
25	115	117	105

this agent to various molecular weight samples of pyran. This copolymer was selected as a potential carrier for this agent because of its own established antitumor and immunostimulating activity. Bonding to pyran was accomplished by nucleophilic addition reactions of the pteridinyl-amino groups under mild conditions. The polymeric derivatives were purified by membrane filtration, solvent extraction, and reprecipitation, and were characterized by thin-layer chromatography, infrared, nuclear magnetic resonance, ultraviolet and mass spectrometry, and elemental analysis. The molar ratios of the DVE-MA repeating unit of the copolymer to methotrexate ranged from 2 to 3.5; by varying the reaction time from 24 to 96 hr, methotrexate residues introduced into the copolymer ranged from 3.0 to 42.6 mol %. The methotrexate was bonded at either the 2- or 4-amino group position of the pteridine ring. A methotrexate-substituted derivative of DVE-MA was evaluated by the National Cancer Institute (NSC 282447) for dihydrofolate reductase inhibitory activity in vitro. These preliminary studies showed inhibition of dihydrofolate reductase and cytotoxicity to L1210 lympohoid leukemia cells in vitro similar to free methotrexate.

In a more recent study of drug attachment to a polyelectrolytic polymer, Pryzbylski et al. o[159] made several methotrexate polymer derivatives. Poly(L-lysine), polyimmunoethylene, poly(vinyl alcohol), and carboxylmethylcellulose were synthesized and characterized with 3-15 mol % drug incorporated into the polymer chain. The pteridinyl amino groups of methotrexate were bound to pyran by nucleophilic addition reactions under mild conditions. All the polymers containing methotrexate were water soluble except poly(vinyl alcohol).

Butler and Zampini [158] prepared copolymers of DVE with maleimides of glycine (NSC 266067), d, l-phenylalanine (NSC 266063), d, l-alanine (NSC 266062), d, l-leucine (NSC 266066), d, l-methionine (NSC 266064) and 1-phenylalanine (NSC 266226). The methyl ester of the copolymer of DVE with the maleimide of d, l-alanine having inherent viscosity of 0.27 dl/g was found to have a number average molecular weight of 26,000, by size exclusion chromatography. These copolymers were evaluated against P388 lymphocytic leukemia by the National Cancer Institute. The results are recorded in Table 8.12.

The pyran copolymer substituted with methotrexate showed inhibition of dihydrofolate reductase and cytotoxicity to L1210 lymphoid leukemia cells in vitro, similar to the free drug [159]. The drug-attached polymer was significantly more effective against L1210 leukemia than were the free drug or the polymer alone. The polymer-drug showed activity against Lewis lung carcinoma, which is resistant to methotrexate.

In vitro studies were made on four polymer systems to which methotrexate was linked. These were evaluated for their ability to inhibit tetrahydrofolate dehydrogenase as well as inhibition of L5278Y leukemia cells [160]. Pyran copolymer-methotrexate and polyethyleneimine were only marginally effective, whereas carboxymethyl cellulose-methotrexate and poly(L-lysine)-methotrexate produced significant effects.

XI. CLINICAL STUDIES OF POLY(CARBOXYLIC ACID) POLYMERS

Most polyanions are water soluble at physiological pH and are easily administered either intravenously or intraperitoneally as a buffer saline solution. Pyran was clinically tested in phase I and phase II by intraperitoneal administration to advanced cancer patients who were no longer responding to other treatments [161]. Patients were taken off chemotherapy and radiation for 2 weeks prior to treatment with pyran NSC 46015, a polydisperse material [99]. The limiting toxicity was hypertension, temporary blindness, and sclerosis of blood vessels. Pyrexia, thrombocytopenia, leukopenia, and anticoagulant effects were observed but were not considered as seriously limiting toxicities. More recently a new clinical study has been carried out with a lower-molecular-weight and narrower-polydisperse pyran [110]. This is being administered as a less toxic calcium salt intraperitoneally rather than intravenously. Less drastic toxic effects were observed in phase I trials and the material is now being evaluated in phase II.

Another polycarboxylate that has been studied clinically is NED 137, a half-acid half-amide polymer with imide groups. A clinical study [40] consisted of 212 patients with a variety of tumor types, tumor burdens, and prior therapeutic treatments. The efficacy of NED 137 appears to depend on the tumor type and extent of the disease. It appears that patients with minimal disease residue were more responsive to NED 137.

In 1979, a modified phase I study of NED 137 in patients with gastrointestinal cancer was initiated at the University of Toronto and the Health Protection Branch, Federal Ministry of Health of Canada [40]. Patients receiving NED 137 therapy were compared to a group of patients with metastatic gastrointestinal cancer who were studied from 1974-1978. The control group had received BCG and 5-fluorouracil (5-FU) or 5-FU alone as therapy. Longer life spans were reported for patients receiving NED 137 with colorectal and pancreatic tumors than with 5-FU and BCG regimens.

XII. SUMMARY

As indicated in the literature cited, polyanions have a broad spectrum of biological activities. The most important of these are their antiviral and antitumor effects. Both of these effects seem to occur by different mechanisms since low-molecular-weight polyanions are effective as antitumor agent and only the high-molecular-weight polyanions are effective as antiviral agents. Although polyanions induce low levels of interferon, there does not seem to be any correlation to the biological effects observed.

The mode of activity of the polyanions appears to be through the activation of macrophages. These activated macrophages are able to differentiate between normal and neoplastic cells, as illustrated by their destruction of the latter. It has been further observed that the activated macrophages alter the amount of DNA in a tumor cell as well as change the relative distribution of the remaining DNA in the various cell phases.

It has been found that these polyanions are effective immune adjuvant agents. A much greater degree of effectiveness was observed when pyran was used in conjunction with other chemotherapeutic modalities.

The potential of using polyanions as drug carriers has been explored only in a preliminary manner. At present, the advantage of these materials is not only in providing a water-soluble vehicle for drug administration but also in increasing the time the drug is in the body. Most polyanions show a prolonged effect which lasts from 1 to 10 days.

Current studies show that toxicity and activity are related to molecular weight and structure. A number of polyanions have been developed that are more efficacious than pyran in that they are less toxic and more active on a similar dose basis. Structure is also related to the population of macrophages elicited. Pyran activates a new population of macrophages, whereas other polyanions appear to activate a resident population.

Other areas of interest for polyanion application are anti-inflammatory agents, enzyme-inhibition, anticoagulants, vaccines, and chemotherapeutic adjuvants. At the present time, it seems important that the biological scientists involved in evaluating these poly(carboxylic acid) polymers become more aware of the structural relationship to the activity observed and to go beyond testing only pyran, the structure of which is not completely established or necessarily repeated from batch to batch. This could be achieved by eliciting the expertise of available polymer chemists.

ACKNOWLEDGMENTS

The authors wish to acknowledge financial support of NIH under Grant No. 5-21370, and the contributions of Sissy Williams, James Creegan, Jeff Jones, and Tom Ma in helping prepare this manuscript.

REFERENCES

1. R. M. Ottenbrite, W. Regelson, A. M. Kaplan, R. Carchman, P. Morahan, and A. Munson, in Polymer Drugs (L. G. Donaruma and O. Vogl, eds.), Wiley, New York, 1978, p. 263.
2. A. M. Kaplan, R. M. Ottenbrite, W. Regelson, R. Carchman, P. Morahan, and A. Munson, in Handbook of Cancer and Immunology, Vol. 5 (H. Walters, ed.), Garland, New York, 1978, p. 135.
3. R. M. Ottenbrite and W. Regelson, in Encyclopedia of Polymer Science and Technology, Suppl. Vol. 2, Wiley, New York, 1977, p. 118.
4. L. G. Donaruma, Prog. Polym. Sci., 4: 1 (1974).
5. E. F. Razvodovskii, Adv. Polym. Sci., 281 (1972).
6. L. G. Donaruma, R. M. Ottenbrite, and O. Vogl (eds.), Anionic Polymeric Drugs, Wiley, New York, 1980.
7. W. Regelson, Interferon, 6: 353 (1970).

8. M. A. Chirigos (ed.), Control of Neoplasia by Modulation of the Immune System, Vol. 3, Raven Press, New York, 1977.
9. W. Regelson, Pharmacol. Ther., 15: 1 (1981).
10. W. Regelson, J. Polym. Sci., Polym. Symp., 66: 483 (1979).
11. A. M. Kaplan, in Anionic Polymeric Drugs (L. G. Donaruma. R. M. Ottenbrite, and O. Vogl, eds.), Wiley, New York, 1980, p. 227.
12. R. M. Schultz, J. D. Papamatheakis, W. A. Stylos, and M. A. Chirigos, Cell. Immunol., 25: 309 (1976).
13. P. S. Morahan, in Augmenting Agents in Cancer Therapy (E. M. Hersch, ed.), Raven Press, New York, 1981, p. 185.
14. M. C. Breining and P. S. Morahan, in Interferon and Interferon Inducers: Clinical Applications (D. A. Stringfellow, ed.), Wiley, New York,
15. M. C. Breining, A. E. Munson, and P. S. Morahan, in Anionic Polymeric Drugs (L. G. Donaruma, R. M. Ottenbrite, and O. Vogl, eds.), Wiley, New York, 1980.
16. P. S. Morahan, W. Regelson, and A. E. Munson, Antimicrob. Agents Chemother., 3: 16 (1972).
17. P. S. Morahan, D. W. Barnes, and A. E. Munson, Cancer Treat. Rep., 62: 1797 (1978).
18. D. S. Giron, R. Y. Liu, F. E. Hemphill, F. F. Pindak, and J. P. Schmidt, Proc. Soc. Exp. Biol. Med., 163: 146 (1980).
19. E. DeClerq and P. DeSomer, Proc. Soc. Exp. Biol. Med., 132: 699 (1969).
20. J. Runnstrom, Exp. Cell Res., 12: 374 (1956).
21. W. Regelson, in Water Soluble Polymers (N. M. Bakalas, ed.), Plenum Press, New York, 1973, p. 161.
22. B. Jacques, in Polyelectrolytes and Their Applications, Vol. 2 (A. Rembaum and E. Selegny, eds.), D. Reidel, Boston, 1975.
23. L. B. Jacques, in Progress in Medicinal Chemistry (G. Ellis and G. West, eds.), Butterworth, London, 1967.
24. H. P. Gregor, in Polyelectrolytes (E. Selegny, ed.), D. Reidel, Boston, 1965.
25. W. Regelson, Adv. Chemother., 3: 303 (1968).
26. W. Regelson, J. Polyan. Sci., C, 66: 483 (1979).
27. D. S. Breslow and G. E. Huke, J. Am. Chem. Soc., 76: 6399 (1954).
28. W. Regelson and J. F. Holland, Clin. Pharmacol. Ther., 3: 730 (1962).
29. R. M. Schultz, J. D. Papamatheakis, and M. A. Chirigos, in Immune Modulation and Control of Neoplasia by Adjuvant Therapy (M. A. Chirigos, ed.), Raven Press, New York, 1978, p. 459.
30. K. K. Takemoto and S. S. Spicer, Ann. N.Y. Acad. Sci., 130: 365 (1965).
31. A. Vaheri and J. S. Pagano, Virology, 27: 434 (1965).

32. P. DeSomer, E. De Clerq, A. Billiau, S. Schonne, and M. Claesen, J. Virol., 2: 878 (1968).
33. P. Claes, A. Billeau, E. DeClercq, J. Desmyter, E. Schonne, H. Vanderhaege, and P. DeSomer, J. Virol., 5: 313 (1970).
34. A. Billeau, J. Muyembe, and P. DeSomer, Appl. Microbiol., 21: 580 (1971).
35. E. DeClercq and P. DeSomer, Eur. J. Cancer, 8: 536 (1972).
36. M. H. Levy and E. F. Wheelock, J. Immunol., 114: 962 (1975).
37. W. R. Stinebring and J. S. Younger, Nature, 204: 712 (1964).
38. P. DeSomer and A. Billeau, Arch. Ges. Virusforsch, 19: 143 (1966).
39. M. Ho, Science, 146: 1472 (1964).
40. M. Ho, Y. Kono, and M. K. Breinig, Proc. Soc. Exp. Biol. Med., 119: 1227 (1965).
41. M. Ho, M. K. Breinig, B. Postic, and J. A. Armstrong, Ann. N.Y. Acad. Sci., 173: 680 (1970).
42. J. B. Weinberg, H. A. Chapman, and J. B. Hibbs, J. Immunol., 121: 72 (1978).
43. J. Pitha, Polym. Sci. Technol., 14: 203 (1981).
44. J. Pitha, M. Akashi, and M. Draminski, in Biomedical Polymers (E. Goldberg, ed.), Academic Press, New York, 1981.
45. J. Pitha, in Polymers in Biology and Medicine, Vol. I (L. G. Donaruma, R. M. Ottenbrite, and O. Vogl, eds.), Wiley, New York, 1981.
46. J. Pitha, K. Kociolek, and C. A. Apffel, Cancer Res., 39: 170 (1979).
47. A. K. Field, A. A. Tytell, G. P. Lampson, and M. R. Hilleman, Proc. Natl. Acad. Sci. USA, 58: 1004 (1967).
48. T. C. Merigan and W. Regelson, N. Engl. J. Med., 277: 1283-1287 (1967).
49. A. E. Munson, W. Regelson, W. Lawrence, and W. R. Wooles, J. Reticuloendothel. Soc., 7: 375-385 (1970).
50. L. G. Baird and A. M. Kaplan, Cell. Immunol., 20: 167-176 (1975).
51. P. S. Morahan, W. Regelson, and A. E. Munson, Antimicrob. Agents Chemother., 2: 16-22 (1972).
52. P. S. Morahan and A. M. Kaplan, Int. J. Cancer, 17: 82-89 (1976).
53. S. J. Mohr, M. A. Chirigos, F. S. Fuhrman, and J. W. Pryor, Cancer Res., 35: 3750-3654 (1975).
54. P. S. Morahan and A. M. Kaplan, Int. J. Cancer, 17: 82-89 (1976).
55. T. C. Merigan and M. S. Fenkelstein, Virology, 35: 363 (1968).
56. T. C. Merigan and W. Regelson, N. Engl. J. Med., 277: 1283 (1967).
57. T. C. Merigan, Nature, 214: 416 (1967).
58. A. Billeau, J. Desmyter, and P. DeSomer, J. Virol., 5: 321 (1970).
59. E. M. Hodnett, J. Amirmoazzami, and J. Tien Hai Tai, J. Med. Chem., 21: 652 (1978).
60. P. DeSomer, E. DeClercq, A. Billeau, E. Schonne, and M. Claesen, J. Virol., 2: 878 (1968).

61. T. C. Merigan and M. S. Finkelstein, Virology, 35: 363 (1968).
62. Z. Priel and A. Silverberg, J. Polym. Sci., A-2, 8: 713 (1970).
63. A. Billiau, J. Muyembe, and P. DeSomer, Nature, 232: 183 (1971).
64. D. A. Tirrell, IUPAC 28th Macromol. Symp. Proc., 1982, p. 372.
65. R. M. Ottenbrite, K. Kuus, and A. Kaplan, Polym. Prepr., 24(1): 25 (1983).
66. R. M. Ottenbrite, E. Goodell, and A. E. Munson, Polymer, 18: (1977).
67. A. E. Munson, J. M. Veager, S. E. Loveless, and R. M. Ottenbrite, J. Reticuloendothel. Soc., 18: 406 (1975).
68. S. St. Pierre, R. T. Ingall, M. S. Verlander, and M. Goodman, Biopolymers, 17: 1837 (1978).
69. B. M. Culbertson and B. C. Trivedo, Maleic Anhydride, Plenum Press, New York, 1982.
70. A. A. El'Saied, et al., Dokl. Akad. Nauk, USSR, 177: 380 (1967).
71. A. A. El'Saied, et al., Polym. Sci., USSR, 11: 314 (1969).
72. G. H. Potter and N. L. Zutty, U.S. Patent 3,280,080 (1967).
73. K. Nyitray and G. Y. Hardy, Acta Chem. Sci. Hung. Tonius, 52: 99 (1967).
74. G. B. Butler and A. F. Campus, J. Polymer Sci., A19: 545 (1970).
75. G. B. Butler, Acc. Chem. Res., 15: 370 (1982).
76. T. C. Merigan, Nature, 214: 416 (1967).
77. T. C. Merigan and W. Regelson, N. Engl. J. Med., 277: (1967).
78. T. C. Merigan, Ciba Foundation Symposium on Interferon (G. E. W. Wolstenholme and M. O'Connor, eds.), J. & A. Churchill, London, 1967, pp. 50-60.
79. E. DeClercq and T. C. Merigan, Arch. Intern. Med., 126: (1970).
80. W. Regelson, Adv. Exp. Med. Biol., 1: 315 (1967).
81. T. C. Merigan and M. S. Finkelstein, Virology, 35: 363 (1968).
82. E. DeClercq and T. C. Merigan, J. Gen. Virol., 5: 359 (1969).
83. P. S. Morahan and A. M. Kaplan, Int. J. Cancer, 17: 82-89 (1976).
84. M. A. Chirigos, W. Turner, J. Pearson, and W. Griffin, Int. J. Cancer, 4: 267 (1969).
85. M. A. Chirigos, Comparative Leukemia Research 1969, Bibl. Haemat. 36 (R. M. Dutcher, ed.), S. Karger, Basel, 1970, pp. 278-292.
86. J. P. Schmidt, F. F. Pindak, D. J. Giron, and R. R. Ibarra, Texas Rep. Biol. Med., 29: 133 (1971).
87. J. Y. Richmond, Infec. Immun., 3: 249 (1971). Arch. Gesamte Virusforsch., 36: 232 (1972).
88. G. B. Schuller, P. S. Morahan, and M. J. Snodgrass, 10th Nat. Meet. Reticuloendothel. Soc., 1973, Abstr., Vol. 28.
89. C. H. Campbell and J. Y. Richmond, Infect. Immun., 7: 199 (1973).

90. W. Regelson, A. Monson, and W. Wooles, Int. Symp. Stand. Interferon Interferon Inducers, London, 1969; Symp. Series Immunobiol. Stand., Vol. 14, S. Kager, Basel, 1970, pp. 227-236.
91. F. F. Pindal, Infect. Immun., 1: 271 (1970).
92. D. J. Giron, J. P. Schmidt, R. J. Ball, and F. F. Pindak, Antimicrob. Agents Chemother., 1: 80 (1972).
93. W. Regelson and A. E. Munson, Ann. N.Y. Acad. Sci., 173: 831 (1970).
94. M. A. Kapusta and J. Mendelson, Arthritis Rheum., 12: 463 (1969).
95. Y. Shamash and B. Alexander, Biochim. Biophys. Acta, 194: 449 (1969).
96. M. W. Rosenthal, Argonne National Laboratory, personal communication, 1978.
97. T. J. Leavitt, T. C. Merigan, and J. M. Freeman, Am. J. Dis. Child., 121: 43 (1971).
98. W. Regelson, Personal communication, 1979.
99. D. S. Breslow, Pure Appl. Chem., 46: 103-113 (1976); and Polym. Prepr., 22: 24 (1981).
100. G. B. Butler, Abstr., 133rd Nat. Am. Chem. Soc., Meet., San Francisco, April 1958, p. 6R.
101. G. B. Butler, Abstr. 134th Am. Chem. Soc. Meet., Chicago, September 7-12, 1958, p. 32T. This paper deals with some additional examples of the cyclopolymerization.
102. G. B. Butler, J. Polym. Sci., 48: 279 (1960).
103. G. B. Butler, U.S. Patent, 3,320,216 (May 16, 1967).
104. U. S. Patent Reissue 26,407 (June 11, 1968).
105. G. B. Butler, J. Macromol. Sci.-Chem., A5(1): 219 (1971).
106. R. J. Samuels, Polymer, 18: 452 (1976).
107. Y. C. Chu and B. G. Butler, J. Polym. Sci., Chem. Ed., 17: 859 (1979).
108. T. Kunitake and Tsukino, J. Polym. Sci., Chem. Ed., 17: 877 (1979).
109. W. J. Freeman and D. S. Breslow, in Biological Activities of Polymers (C. E. Carraher and C. G. Gebelein, eds.), ACS Symp. Ser. 186, American Chemical Society, Washington, D.C., 1982, p. 243.
110. D. S. Breslow, Polym. Prepr., 22: 24 (1981).
111. R. M. Ottenbrite, IUPAC, Macromol. Symp. Proc., Amherst, Mass., 1982, p. 366.
112. E. M. Hodnett, J. Amirmoazzami, and J. Tien Hai Tai, J. Med. Chem., 21: 652 (1978).
113. A. G. Williams and G. B. Butler, J. Polym. Sci., Chem. Ed., 17: 1117 (1979).
114. Compounds supplied by G. B. Butler and tested by A. E. Munson, Department of Pharmacology, Virginia Commonwealth University, Richmond, Va.

115. W. Regelson, S. Kuhar, M. Tumis, J. Fields, J. Johnson, and E. Gluesenkamp, Nature, 186: 778 (1960).
116. M. Sharabash, G. B. Butler, and J. T. Badgett, J. Macromol. Sci. Chem., A4: 51 (1970).
117. Program Analysis Branch, Drug Research and Development, National Institutes of Health, Bethesda, Md.
118. J. E. Fields, S. S. Asculai, and J. H. Johnson, Monsanto Company, St. Louis, Mo., U.S. Patent 4,255,537, March 10, 1981.
119. J. E. Fields, S. S. Asculai, J. H. Johnson, R. K. Johnson, unpublished observation, 1979.
120. R. E. Falk, L. Makowka, N. Nossal, J. A. Falk, J. E. Fields, and S. S. Asculae, Br. J. Surg., 66: 861-863 (1979).
121. R. E. Falk, L. Makowka, N. A. Nossal, L. E. Rotstein, and J. A. Falk, Surgery, 88: 126 (1980).
122. H. Wagnes, M. Feldmann, W. Boyle, and J. Schrader, J. Exp. Med., 136: 331 (1971).
123. N. I. Safout and M. Richter, Adv. Immunol., 12: 202 (1970).
124. E. R. Unanue, Adv. Immunol., 15: 95 (1972).
125. O. A. Holterman, E. Klein, and G. P. Casale, Cell. Immunol., 9: 339 (1973).
126. A. M. Kaplan, P. S. Morahan, and W. Regelson, J. Natl. Cancer Inst., 52: 1919 (1974).
127. M J. Snodgrass, A. M. Kaplan, and P. S. Morahan, Cancer Res., 55: 455 (1975).
128. S. A. Eccles and A. Alexander, Nature, 250: 667 (1974).
129. G. A. Currie and C. Basham, J. Exp. Med., 142: 1600 (1975).
130. H. Melson, J. Exp. Med., 140, 1085 (1974).
131. M. S. Meltzger and G. L. Bartlett, J. Natl. Cancer Inst., 49: 1439 (1972).
132. A. M. Kaplan and T. Mohanakumar, J. Exp. Med., 146: 1461 (1977).
133. G. Poste, R. Kirsh, W. E. Fogler, and I. J. Tidler, Cancer Res., 39: 881 (1979).
134. O. A. Holteman, E. Klien, and G. P. Casal, Cell. Immunol., 9: 339 (1973).
135. S. W. Russell, W. F. Doe, and C. G. Cochrane, J. Immunol., 116: 164 (1976).
136. G. A. Currie and C. Basham, Br. J. Cancer, 38: 653 (1978).
137. M. S. Melter, R. W. Tucker, and A. C. Breuer, Cell. Immunol., 17: 30 (1975).
138. A. M. Kaplan, K. M. Connolly, and W. Regelson, in The Host Invader Intraplay (H. Van Vendbosshe, ed.), Elsevier/North-Holland, Amsterdam, 1980, p. 479.
139. R. M. Ottenbrite, K. Kuus, and A. M. Kaplan, Polym. Prepr., 24(1): 25 (1983).

140. G. Poste, R. Kirsh, W. E. Fogler, and I. J Tidler, Cancer Res., 39: 881 (1979).
141. O. A. Holteman, E. Klien, and G. P. Casal, Cell. Immunol., 9: 339 (1973).
142. S. W. Russell, W. F. Doe, and C. G. Cochrane, J. Immunol., 116: 164 (1976).
143. G. A. Currie and C. Basham, Br. J. Cancer, 38: 653 (1978).
144. M. S. Melter, R. W. Tucker, and A. C. Breuer, Cell. Immunol., 17: 30 (1975).
145. A. M. Kaplan, K. M. Connoly, and W. Regelson, in The Host Invader Interplay (H. Van Vendbosshe, ed.), Elsevier/North-Holland, Amsterdam, 1980, p. 479.
146. M. A. Chirigos, W. A. Stylos, R. M. Schultz, and J. R. Fullen, Cancer Res., 38: 1085 (1978).
147. M. A. Chirigos and W. A. Stylos, Cancer Res., 40: 1976 (1980).
148. S. J. Mohr, M. A. Chirigos, and F. S. Fuhrman, Cancer Res., 35: 3750 (1975).
149. J. H. Dean, M. L. Padarathsingh, and L. Keys, Cancer Treat. Rep., 62: 1807 (1978).
150. M. Przbylski, W. P. Fung, H. Ringsdorf, and D. S. Zaharko, Proc. Am. Assoc. Cancer Res., 19: 2 (1978).
151. M. Przbylski, D. S. Zaharko, M. A. Chirigos, R. H. Adamson, R. M. Schultz, and H. Ringsdorf, Cancer Treat Rep., 62: 1837 (1978).
152. C. G. Gebelein, R. Morgan, R. Glowacky, and W. Baig, Polym. Sci. Technol., 14: 191 (1980).
153. V. E. Vengris, P. M. Pitha, L. L. Sensenbrenner, and J. Pitha, Mol. Pharmacol., 14: 271 (1978).
154. H. J. Chou, J. P. Froehlich, and J. Pitha, Nucleic Acids Res., 5: 691 (1978).
155. C. G. Gebelein, Org. Coatings Plastic Chem., 42: 422 (1980).
156. P. Umigar, S. Ohashi, and G. B. Butler, J. Polym. Sci. Chem. Ed., 17: 351 (1979).
157. M. Yoshida, M. Kamakura, and I. Kaetsu, Polymer J., 11: 775 (1979).
158. G. B. Butler and A. Zampini, J. Macromol. Sci. Chem., A11: 491 (1977).
159. M. Pryzyblski, E. Fell, and H. Ringsdorf, Macromol. Chem., 179: 1719 (1978).
160. W. P. Fung, M. Przbylski, H. Ringsdorf, and D. Zaharko, J. Natl. Cancer Inst., 62: 1261 (1979).
161. W. Regelson, B. I. Schnider, J. Colsky, K. B. Olson, J. F. Holland, C. L. Johnston, Jr., and L. H. Dennis, in Immune Modulation and Control of Neoplasia (M. A. Chirigos, ed.), Raven Press, New York, 1978, p. 469.

9

POLYNUCLEOTIDES WITH INTERFERON-INDUCING AND ANTITUMOR ACTIVITY

JOSEF PITHA and JOHN W. KUSIAK

National Institute on Aging
Baltimore City Hospitals
Baltimore, Maryland

I. INTRODUCTION

Nucleic acids and polynucleotides have been the focus of attention of both biologists and chemists since the late 1940s when they were identified as carriers of genetic information. Nevertheless, there have been only few practical applications of these compounds.

At the present time we are probably on the verge of a new era of nucleic acid use, an era of recombinant deoxyribonucleic acid (DNA) technology. This technology is based on methods that enable the design and assembly of genes in vitro and their entry into living systems. Technical advances have made it possible to synthesize extensive regions of either deoxyribonucleic or ribonucleic acid of any sequence desired through the use of a combination of chemical and enzymatic methods. These synthetic nucleic acids can then be duplicated in mass using bacterial or eukaryotic replication systems which may lead to the synthesis of corresponding proteins. Recombinant DNA technology will eventually lead to the use of bacterial systems for industrial biosynthesis of human peptide hormones and enzymes for therapeutic use.

In spite of these great advances there is only very limited direct therapeutic use for either DNA or polynucleotides; these compounds have not been included in any major pharmacopeia and their only use is an experimental one. There are fundamental biological reasons for this lack of direct application. In a multicellular organism there is continuously occurring death of a small fraction of cells and this leads to partial spillage of cellular nucleic acids into the circulation. For example, normal human serum contains 13 ng/ml of DNA. This amount may be increased in the presence of tumors up to a value of 150 ng/ml, and any pathological process, like viral infections, also leads to an increase in this value. This means that a majority of the cells are continuously exposed to both isologous and heterologous nucleic acids. If any of these nucleic acids penetrated into cell regions where they could be replicated or translated into proteins along with the inherent cellular nucleic acids, this would lead to a breakdown in cell regulation and possibly dedifferentiation of specialized cells.

Even though it is possible to prepare practically any sequence of nucleic acids, there are few reasons for doing so for direct therapeutic applications. Eukaryotic cells are well protected from entry of any nucleic acids from extracellular space and this protection can be broken only after cells are considerably damaged. This is one factor that makes a direct therapeutic application of nucleic acids limited. Another factor is the lack of ability to target a nucleic acid to the proper group of cells; thus any direct application of nucleic acids to an organism could result in indiscriminate effects.

These views are based on a realistic appraisal of the present accomplishments and hopefully proper solutions to these problems will be found in the future. To some extent it is possible to envisage such approaches. For example, a certain species of cells from a diseased individual may be explanted, grown, and multiplied in culture. This process could give enough of the cells for extracorporeal treatment with a suitable nucleic acid. Genetic or acquired metabolic errors of the cells in question could be corrected by such treatment and the toxicity of the treatment would not matter, since the treatment is outside the body. The cells that survived the treatment and contained the new genetic information could then be further grown in culture and then implanted back into the patient. One can envision such treatment for cells that are supposed to produce a hormone but do not do so; the treatment would lead to cells with an orderly hormone production. Nevertheless, considerable technical advances are required before such a process can be attempted since any endocrine gland contains various cells producing different hormones, and also very little is known about the regulation of hormone synthesis. Furthermore, the implanted cells could multiply in an uncontrolled manner and lead to an overproduction of a hormone which potentially is an even more damaging phenomenon than its underproduction.

Presently, there are two direct therapeutic applications of polynucleotides that are at least in experimental use. One such application is based on induction of interferon. The exposure of cells either in vitro or in vivo to polynucleotides causes an inducted synthesis of new glycoproteins, called collectively interferons. A recent report [1] indicates that the human genome probably contains information for the synthesis of a series of as many as 8-10 homologous interferon molecules which seem to differ in sequence both in their signal peptides and in their mature forms (approximately 80% homology). Interferons were discovered due to their ability to protect cells against a variety of viruses, but they also have important effects on the immune system as well as direct antitumor effects. The synthesis of interferon is only a temporary event, since it is terminated in normal cells within a few hours, unless the regulation of protein synthesis is interefered with in a process called superinduction. In addition to interferon induction, polynucleotides also induce cells to synthesize other new protein and these proteins may be associated with the establishment of the antiviral state [2]. The two effects of these proteins, their ability to combat viral infections and their antitumor effects, are most promising therapeutically. The second potential application of polynucleotides is their immunoadjuvant capacity. This has been experimentally used in antitumor treatments. Since these two applications have direct relevance to polymer chemists they are reviewed in the latter part of this chapter, accomplishments of gene synthesis are mentioned only in a narrative manner. A few of the aspects of structure and nomenclature which are essential for understanding this chapter are recapitulated in Figure 9.1.

II. SYNTHESIS OF NUCLEIC ACIDS

Both interferon induction and adjuvant effects can be achieved with simple homopolymeric polynucleotides. These can easily be prepared by enzyme-catalyzed polycondensation, and the enzymes and many monomers and polymers are commercially available. Detailed studies of structure-activity relationships have been done both for interferon induction and adjuvant effects of polynucleotides. The results have been, from a chemical point of view, rather disappointing. None of the rare or chemically modified polynucleotides proved to be significantly better than the easily accessible parent compounds. These findings eliminate the necessity to review in this chapter the fine accomplishments in polynucleotide chemistry. These accomplishments have been mainly achieved in the preparation of synthetic

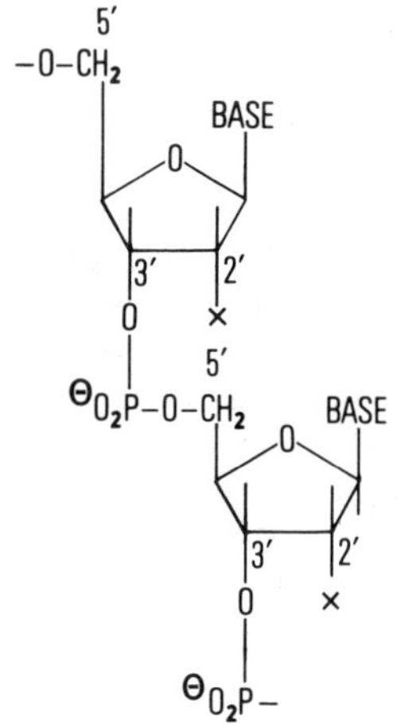

FIGURE 9.1 Segment of single-stranded nucleic acid structure. In polyribonucleosides or RNA, x = OH, in poly deoxyribonucleotides or DNA, x = H. Unit consisting of base and sugar residue is called nucleoside, unit consisting of base, sugar, and phosphate residue is called nucleotide. Two nucleotides joined by phosphodiester bond is called dinucleotide. Bases are heterocyclic residues and were named in that way due to their nitrogen content; the common bases are uracil, thymine, cytosine, adenine, guanine, and hypoxanthine. Uracil or thymine can form a hydrogen-bonded complex (called a Watson-Crick type base pair) with adenine. Cytosine can form a Watson-Crick base pair with guanine or hypoxanthine. The base pairing between the bases in two different strands is capable of holding these strands together, thus leading to the formation of a double-stranded structure.

and semisynthetic nucleic acids of defined sequences. However, a brief overview will be given as a perspective of the present technology.

The stepwise chemical synthesis of oligonucleotides of both the ribo- and deoxyribo- series has recently been completely redesigned. The methods formerly used were based on the so-called phosphodiester principle. Nucleoside phosphate with suitably protected groups was condensed with another nucleoside or oligonucleotide which was fully protected but possessed one free hydroxy group. The condensation was achieved by dehydrating agents such as various carbodiimides and 2,4,6-triisopropylbenzenesulfonyl chloride. Such a condensation resulted in the formation of a new phosphodiester bond and the product, a protected oligonucleotide, carried an electronegative charge. This compound, after deprotection, was purified in aqueous media by chromatography on ion exchange resin. This purification step was quite lengthy and takes one or two laborious days.

Considerable improvement has been obtained by redesigning the synthesis; one method does not deprotect the substrate to give a polar product and the other methods produce electroneutral derivatives of oligonucleotides. Such nonpolar and electroneutral compounds can be purified by a fast and effective process used in ordinary organic synthesis. There are two approaches producing electroneutral derivatives of oligonucleotides. The first one is termed the phosphotriester method. In this approach an additional protecting substituent is introduced onto the phosphate group of nucleoside phosphate. This substituent must have the property of being easily eliminated; for example, 2-cyanoethyl group may be used, which is easily removed by hydrolysis or 2,2,2-trichloroethyl group, which is unstable in reducing conditions. Such a protected phosphodiester is then condensed with a free hydroxy group on a protected nucleoside or nucleotide derivative. This condensation leads to a phosphotriester derivative that does not have an ionic charge. After purification, the triester is deprotected into the desired oligonucleotide fragment. The second approach involves protected 3'-chlorophosphinylnucleosides which are prepared by using dichlorophosphites. These phosphite derivatives are condensed with a free hydroxy group located suitably on protected nucleoside or nucleotide derivatives; the reaction is usually very fast. The product is nonionic and can be effectively purified by chromatographic methods and later deprotected and oxidized into a phosphodiester derivative. The above principles, when combined with the use of other newly developed protecting groups, enable speedy and effective synthesis. Furthermore, the synthesis can be automated using solid-phase methods originally designed for synthesis of peptides.

Direct chemical condensation of nucleotides into oligomers and polymers not employing the stepwise approach has been used only rarely. All of these methods result in low yields of oligomer mixtures that are difficult to separate and consequently are of little preparative interest. In the deoxy series short linear or cyclic oligonucleotides having 3'→5' phosphodiester groups can be generated. In the ribo series, unless the 2'-hydroxyl is protected all known condensations resulted in a 2'→5' phosphodiester bond. The only exception is oligomerization of nulceoside 2',3'-cyclic phosphates catalyzed by zinc ions which produce the natural 3'→5' bonds.

Synthesis of oligonucleotides and polynucleotides that involves enzymes has also advanced considerably. In the past, four groups of enzymes were routinely used. Polynucleotide phosphorylase catalyzes an equilibrium reaction between riboside diphosphate and polynucleotide. This has been the enzyme of choice both for laboratory and industrial production of polyribonucleotides. For the preparation of polydeoxyribonucleotides another enzyme, deoxyribonucleotidyl transferase, has been used. This enzyme catalyzes an equilibrium between the deoxyribonucleoside triphosphate and polydeoxyribonucleoside. Ribonucleases, which are usually used to hydrolyze polynucleotides, under suitable conditions catalyze the reverse condensation reaction, but their use for this purpose was and continues to be limited. All of the above enzymes effect direct condensation, a condensation process that does not require a template. The fourth group of enzymes that were and continue to be of importance in the mass synthesis of nucleic acids are template-dependent polymerases. In the past mainly DNA-dependent DNA or RNA polymerases were known and used; however, presently all the possible directions are covered by various enzymes available from viral, bacterial, or eukaryotic materials. These enzymes can copy DNA into new DNA, DNA into RNA, and RNA into DNA.

This armament of enzymes has been considerably enlarged mainly in the direction enabling the synthesis of polynucleotides of known sequences. The basis for such development was an advance in sequencing extensive regions of nucleic acids. This advance was accomplished by the discovery of a new group of bacterial nucleases, site-specific restriction endonucleases. These enzymes have very high specificity, requiring the presence of a certain symmetry in base sequence in double-stranded DNA, which they then split in a manner leaving short single-stranded fragments (so-called cohesive ends) at the ends. As a result of such treatment, genetic material can be split into segments containing a moderate number of base pairs on the order of hundreds. Effective methods of separation and sequencing have been developed for such segments. Thus it is possible to isolate extensive fragments of DNA from natural sources and elucidate their sequence.

Fragments of natural nucleic acids and oligonucleotides prepared by the synthetic methods mentioned above can then be used as building blocks to obtain larger segments. To effect this, all of the fragments must be joined together by phosphodiester bonds; consequently, the proper cohesive ends must be created on all the building blocks. Cohesive ends are short single-stranded segments on one building block that can form base pairs with the complementary sequences on another building block. When suitable cohesive ends are not available from the cleavage by restriction endonucleases, they must be added in some other way. This may be done by adding a homopolymer end by the enzyme mentioned above, terminal deoxynucleotidyl transferase. By this process a larger segment of DNA is assembled in which the individual fragments are joined together only by base pairs, not phosphodiester bonds. The conversion of these segments into double-stranded DNA, where the strands are properly joined by phosphodiester bonds, is accomplished using enzymes called ligases.

In some cases the desired biological message can be more easily isolated in RNA than in DNA form, for example, as a single-stranded messenger RNA of a specific protein. Use of an ezyme called reverse transcriptase enables the eventual conversion of information in such single-stranded RNA into double-stranded DNA form.

With the use of such in vitro procedures, minute quantities of DNA can be obtained that carry distinct and meaningful biological messages, for example, all the necessary information for biosyntheses of a desired hormone. As a next step it is necessary to enter this information into living cells and make them use it. This can be achieved by joining the prepared DNA (also termed passenger) to a DNA vehicle (also termed vector or replicon) that can carry the passenger along the replicative process. This vehicle DNA can replicate in living cells even with foreign DNA inserted into it. Plasmids and bacteriophages, which have the ability to replicate in bacterial cells, are usually used as vehicles. For eukaryotic cells SV40 virus and polyoma virus were used as vehicles.

The fully assembled DNA, with both the passenger and vehicle parts, is then introduced into a host, which may either be bacteria or eukaryotic cells. The entry process has a very low efficiency and only a small fraction of the cells treated are transformed so as to receive and actively use the entered information. These cells fortunately can replicate and eventually can be separated from nontransformed cells and grown (cloned) in quantity. Thus cell division can be used for replication of the synthetic or semisynthetic fragment of DNA that was prepared in vitro. Furthermore, the replication can be used to make the transformed cells synthesize the RNA and proteins encoded by this DNA fragment. Methods used in recombinant DNA research have been recently summarized [3].

III. CHARACTERISTICS OF SYNTHETIC POLYNUCLEOTIDE INDUCERS OF INTERFERON

Synthetic polyribonucleic acids are a class of potent inducers of interferon activity both in vitro and in vivo. The understanding of the requirements for interferon induction has been based on a systematic investigation of these synthetic polynucleotides. Potent synthetic polynucleotide inducers examined up to the present time have a rather wide range of chemical and structural features, but nearly all of them are polyribonucleotides with double-stranded structure. Furthermore, certain physicochemical properties of these synthetic polynucleic acids correlate well with the ability of these derivatives to induce interferon activity including (1) molecular weight; (2) melting temperature, the characteristic temperature at which double strands dissociate into single strands; and (3) resistance to nuclease attack. There are several recent reviews on interferon induction [4]. This review will concentrate on some of the chemical properties and structural requirements of synthetic polynucleotides that may be of interest to polymer chemists.

In the late 1960s it was shown that double-stranded RNAs from either viruses [5] or mycophages [6] were inducers of interferon activity which caused viral resistance in vitro and in vivo and inhibited tumor growth in vivo. However, it was found that double-stranded RNAs from procaryotic [7] and eukaryotic [8] cells were also capable of inducing interferon activity. A most important observation was that a synthetic double-stranded polynucleotide , polyriboinosinic acid, and polycytidylic acid (poly I·poly C) induced resistance against certain viruses in a number of cell cultures and that this resistance was due to the induction of interferon activity [9]. Subsequently, it was shown that poly I·poly C produced resistance to viral infections [10] and inhibited tumor growth in mice [11], although this same complex was apparently much less effective in humans. Much work since the late 1960s has focused on synthesizing highly potent and nontoxic inducers of human interferon. This approach has lost importance since recent advances in recombinant gene technology have potentially made possible the manufacture of large amounts of interferon. However, the advantages and disadvantages of exogenously supplied or endogenously produced interferons are not completely known at the present time.

A. Molecular Weight

Studies of the interferon induction by poly I·poly C duplexes have shown that as the molecular size of the complex decreases below a critical value, interferon induction also decreases rapidly [12]. This same phenomenon seems to hold true for different naturally occurring double-stranded RNAs [13]. In another approach to establish the effect of molecular weight, the size of each individual homopolymer was varied while the size of the other polymer was constant. The length of the poly I homopolymer was found to be more important than the length of the poly C homopolymer in inducing interferon activity [13, 14]. However, in the case of poly A·poly C, although there is a direct relationship between increasing molecular weight of the complex and increasing interferon inducing activity, the importance of the length of one homopolymer over the other seems secondary. In general, between the molecular weight range from approximately 10,000 to about 120,000, an increase in the molecular weight of the complex leads to an increase in antiviral activity. Beyond this range, no consistent interpretation of the data is possible.

B. Structural Stability

It seems that the double-stranded structure of polynucleotides is a necessary requirement for interferon induction. Those polynucleotides that are capable of forming classical Watson-Crick base pairing seem to be most potent [15]. Not only polynucleotides made up of homopolymers, such as poly I·poly C or poly A·poly U, but also heterocopolymers, such as those containing alternating inosine and cytidine residues in both strands of double-stranded structures, are also inducers of interferon activity [16]. It was shown [14, 17, 18] that polynucleotides with a melting temperature greater than 60°C were required for maximal antiviral activity, that those with melting temperatures below 40°C were inactive, and those with melting temperatures between 40 and 60°C were intermediate in inducing interferon activity.

C. Resistance to Ribonuclease Treatment

Closely related to and reflecting structural stability as measured by melting temperatures is the resistance of polynucleotide duplexes to degradation by ribonuclease treatment. Usually, the more resistant a duplex is to ribonuclease, the better an inducer of interferon it becomes. Nevertheless, some highly ribonuclease resistant synthetic polynucleotide duplexes are no better interferon inducers than poly I·poly C. Replacement of the oxygen atom in the phosphodiester group of polynucleotides by a sulfur atom increases their resistance to ribonuclease treatment and also increases somewhat the interferon-inducing capability of the polynucleotides; unfortunately, the toxicity is also increased [19,20]. Furthermore, preincubation of some polynucleotides at 37°C seems to increase, in parallel, their resistance to degradation by ribonucleases and their ability to induce interferon activity [19-21]. Not only is ribonuclease resistance a reflection of double-helical structural stability, it is a most important consideration in in vivo induction of interferon activity. Because of the ubiquitous nature of ribonuclease activities in the extra- and intracellular space, a stable inducer of interferon would seem to be required for optimization of induction. It has been shown [22] that while poly I·poly C is relatively inactive in producing interferon in primates, ribonuclease-resistant complexes of poly-L-lysine and carboxymethylcellulose with poly I·poly C were capable of producing high levels of interferon in these species.

D. Requirement for 2'-Hydroxyl Group

The necessity of a 2'-hydroxyl group on the ribose moiety is one of the most important requirements for interferon induction activity by polynucleotides. Substitution of the 2'-OH group in double-stranded polyribonucleotides with hydrogen leads to the corresponding DNA-RNA or DNA complexes rendering these polyncuelotides inactive as interferon inducers [23]. Substitution of the 2'-OH with other substituents (such as -F, -Cl, $-N_3$, $-OCH_3$, -O-CO-CH_3), often increase the melting temperature of the complex and substantially increases the resistance to ribonuclease attack, both of these effects are associated with increased interferon inducing activity; however, these modifications were found to reduce interferon activity from 10- to 10,000-fold [13].

E. Other Alterations of the Backbone of Polynucleotides

As was previously mentioned, altering the backbone structure of polynucleotides causes a reduction in their interferon, inducing activity. Nevertheless poly(1-vinylcytosine), when complexed with poly(inosinic acid), was found to be a potent inducer of interferon activity [24]. Thus, in contrast to most other examples, the presence of an extremely modified backbone in one member of a polynucleotide duplex still allowed for the induction of interferon activity. This surprising activity was explained by the ability of poly(1-vinylcytosine) to enhance the low induction capacity of poly I by increasing the uptake of this polynucleotide by cells in the same manner that certain poly-basic molecules such as DEAE-dextrans are able to do [24-26]. Also tested were poly D- and poly L-lysines that were substituted with cytosine residues. It was shown that these polybases potentiate the otherwise very weak inducing activity of poly I. Since these polybases also potentiated the inducing activity of poly C, the potentiation is not due to base-pair formation [27].

F. Substitutions in Heterocyclic Bases

A recent review article lists a large series of synthetic polynucleotides that have at least some capacity for inducing antiviral activity both in vivo and in vitro [28]. Many substitutions enhance the interferon-inducing capacity of the complexes, for example, substitution by bromine in position 5 of cytidine in the poly I·poly C or the substitution of a methyl group in position 5 of uridine in poly A·poly U. Nevertheless, there are some modifications of the bases which abolish activity, such as the replacement of nitrogen by carbon atoms in poly I or poly A strands of their corresponding duplexes. Another interesting point about these different modified heterocyclic base substitutions is that most of these duplexes incorporating modified bases have an increased melting temperature, an increased resistance to ribonuclease degradation, possess a 2'-hydroxyl group on ribose, and have appropriate molecular size. Each of these characteristics alone is sufficient for increasing induction activity, yet they still fail to induce interferon activity. Thus it appears that an empirical approach to discovering effective inducers of interferon activity is still necessary, and no failure-proof generalization of structure-activity relationship seems to hold for the various modifications tested.

G. Base Mismatching

The base mismatching, such as replacement of cytidine by uridine, in double-stranded complexes potentially affects their structure; at low ionic strength the mismatched bases simply loop out from the regular structure. This process leads to a considerable distortion of structure. At high ionic strength or when there are only very few mismatchings, these loops are eliminated by the formation of anomalous base pairs. A high proportion of loops decrease the inducing activity of double-stranded polynucleotides when tested in cells in vitro [24]. Also, the results from the in vivo studies show that with an increasing proportion of mismatched base there is a decrease in the interferon-inducing activity [29].

A very small percentage of mismatching in double-stranded complexes of polynucleotides nevertheless does not lead to cancellation of the interferon-inducing activity [30]. This phenomenon has been used for separating the interferon induction activity of polynucleotides from their numerous and serious toxic side effects [31]. According to this line of reasoning, a polynucleotide with some mismatching may have considerable antiviral activity which occurs rapidly, but its low resistance to ribonucleases brought about by the mismatching could reduce chronic toxicity, which is much slower to develop [30, 31]. The results seem to support this hypothesis in that certain toxic aspects of polynucleotides including mitogenicity, pyrogenicity, thymic atrophy, anemia, and reduced antibody production, while antiviral activity remained similar to that of poly I·poly C. Most of the mismatched polynucleotides tested were derivatives of poly I·poly C altered in the poly C chains with uridine or guanosine substituted to provide the mismatching.

IV. OTHER EFFECTS OF SYNTHETIC POLYNUCLEOTIDES

In addition to the ability to induce interferon activity, polynucleotides may have direct effects on tumors, and other multiple effects on the cellular and humoral immune system. The direct mechanism is difficult to prove due to a multiplicity of polynucleotide effects. Nevertheless, that was the explanation for effects of poly I·poly C on carcinogen-induced skin tumors [32]. Further evidence for a direct effect of polynucleotides on tumor growth comes from studies performed in mice in which their immune system was suppressed either by sublethal radiation or by use of antilymphocyte antiserum [33, 34]. Since in these cases tumor growth was inhibited by polynucleotides even in the absence of a functional immune system, there is probably a direct nonimmune component of inhibition of tumor growth. In a more recent study poly I·poly C was shown to inhibit the growth of tumors developing at the site of injection of L929 cells [35]. In this study nude mice were utilized which were athymic and thus had a defective component in their immune system. Furthermore, mouse interferon injected into these mice at concentrations comparable to those elicited by poly I·poly C failed to inhibit tumor growth, indicating that the antitumor effect of poly I·poly C was not elicited by the induction of interferon. As an explanation it was suggested that a direct cytotoxic effect of poly I·poly C is responsible since it had been shown much earlier that this polynucleotide duplex was directly toxic in a number of cell lines [36].

Polynucleotides also have the potency to influence the immune system and thus cause a variety of biological effects. The immunoresponse of an organism depends on the proper and timely interaction of cells of more than six different types. Polynucleotides usually affect any cell type with a bell-shaped concentration dependence—that is, the effects are maximal at some polynucleotide concentration and decrease towards the higher concentration, at which polynucleotides start to be toxic. Since each type of cell involved in immunoresponse has a different response curve to a polynucleotide, the concentration and timing of effects is also different, and the phenomenon is of considerable complexity. Bearing this in mind it is easy to understand that changes in the amount and timing of a dose of polynucleotide can lead either to an inhibition or acceleration of tumor growth. The importance of the regulation of the immunoresponse has led to many studies of the effects polynucleotides exercise on this system; these studies were summarized elsewhere [37]. In short, polynucleotides and their complexes enhance the capacity to form antibodies in animals; the stimulation of macrophages and lymphocytes of immunosystem has been considered as a mechanism of this enhancement. Double-stranded complexes of polyribonucleotides seem to be more effective than single strands, the difference probably being due to the very fast degradation of the latter. A complex of poly A·poly C has been found more effective than poly I·poly C in the majority of studies. In contrast, triple-stranded polyribonucleotide complexes were found ineffective for interferon induction but do affect the immunosystem. More recent mechanistic studies are focusing on the responses of individual cell types to polynucleotides. On this level, polynucleotides show distinct similarities to polycarboxylates [38,39], which are reviewed in Chap. 8.

REFERENCES

1. D. V. Goedell, D. W. Leung, T. J. Dull, M. Gross, R. M. Lawn, R. McCandliss, P. H. Seeburg, A. Ullrich, E. Yelverton, and P. W. Gray, Nature, 290: 20 (1981).
2. N. B. K. Raj and P. M. Pitha, Proc. Natl. Acad. Sci. USA, 77: 4918 (1980).
3. R. Wu (ed.), Methods in Enzymology: Recombinant DNA, Vol. 68, Academic Press, New York, 1979.
4. W. A. Stewart (ed.), Interferons and Their Action, CRC Press, Cleveland, Ohio, 1977.
5. A. A. Tytell, G. P. Lampson, A. K. Field, and M. R. Hilleman, Proc. Natl. Acad. Sci. USA, 58: 1719 (1967).
6. W. J. Kleinschmidt, L. F. Ellis, R. M. Van Frank, and E. B. Murphy, Nature, 220: 167 (1968).
7. R. B. Wickner, Bacteriol. Rev., 40: 757 (1976).
8. E. De Maeyer, J. De Maeyer-Grignarel, and L. Montagnier, Nature New Biol., 229: 109 (1971).
9. A. K. Field, A. A. Tytell, G. P. Lampson, and M. R. Hilleman, Proc. Natl. Acad. Sci. USA, 61: 340 (1968).
10. E. De Clercq, M. R. Nuwer, and T. C. Merigan, J. Clin. Invest., 49: 1565 (1970).
11. H. B. Levy, L. W. Law, and A. S. Rabson, Proc. Natl. Acad. Sci. USA, 62: 357 (1969).
12. G. P. Lampson, A. K. Field, A. A. Tytell, M. M. Nemes, and M. R. Hilleman, Proc. Soc. Exp. Biol. Med., 135: 917 (1970).
13. E. De Clercq, in Top. Curr. Chem., 52: 173 (1974).
14. P. M. Pitha and W. A. Carter, Nature New Biol., 234: 1105 (1971).
15. E. De Clercq, R. D. Wells, R. C. Grant, and T. C. Merigan, J. Mol. Biol., 50: 83 (1971).

16. C. Colby and M. J. Chamberlin, Proc. Natl. Acad. Sci. USA, 63: 160 (1969).
17. E. De Clercq and T. C. Merigan, Nature, 222: 1148 (1969).
18. J. F. Niblack and M. B. McCreary, Nature, 233: 52 (1971).
19. E. De Clercq, F. Eckstein, and T. Merigan, Science, 165: 1137 (1969).
20. E. De Clercq, F. Eckstein, H. Sternbach, and T. C. Merigan, Virology, 42: 421 (1970).
21. E. De Clercq, R. D. Wells, and T. C. Merigan, Nature, 226: 364 (1970).
22. H. B. Levy, G. Baer, S. Baron, C. E. Buckler, C. J. Gibbs, M. J. Iadarola, W. T. London, and J. Rice, J. Infect. Dis., 132: 434 (1975).
23. J. Vilcek, M. H. Ng, A. E. Friedman-Kien, and T. Kraweiw, J. Virol., 2: 648 (1968).
24. J. Pitha and P. M. Pitha, Science, 172: 1146 (1971).
25. A. Billian, C. E. Buckler, F. Dianzani, C. Uhlendorf, and S. Baron, Proc. Soc. Exp. Biol. Med., 132: 790 (1969).
26. L. Noronha-Blob and J. Pitha, Biochim. Biophys. Acta, 519: 285 (1978).
27. P. M. Pitha and J. Pitha, J. Gen. Virol., 24: 385 (1974).
28. P. F. Torrence and E. De Clercq, Pharmacol. Ther., 2A: 1 (1977).
29. S. Matsuda, M. Kida, H. Shirafuji, M. Yoneda, and H. Yaoi, Arch. Gesamte Virusforsch., 34: 105 (1971).
30. W. A. Carter, J. O'Malley, M. Beeson, P. Cunnington, A. Kelvin, A. Vere-Hodge, J. L. Alderfer, and P. O. P. Ts'o, Mol. Pharmacol., 12: 440 (1976).
31. W. A. Carter, P. M. Pitha, L. W. Marshall, I. Tazawa, S. Tazawa, and P. O. P. Ts'o, J. Mol. Biol., 70: 567 (1972).
32. K. Elgj and M. Degre, J. Natl. Cancer Inst., 54: 219 (1975).
33. J. C. Fisher, S. R. Cooperband, and J. A. Manniek, Cancer Res., 32: 889 (1972).
34. D. Webb, W. Braun, and O. J. Plescia, Cancer Res., 32: 1814 (1972).
35. E. De Clercq, Cancer Res., 37: 1502 (1977).
36. A. M. Badger, S. R. Cooperband, and J. A. Green, J. Natl. Cancer Inst., 49: 613 (1972).
37. O. Plescia and W. Braun (eds.), Nucleic Acids in Immunology, Springer-Verlag, New York, 1968.
38. R. M. Schultz, J. D. Papamatheakis, J. Luetzeler, P. Ruiz, and M. A. Chirigos, Cancer Res., 37: 358 (1977).
39. R. M. Schultz, J. D. Papamatheakis, J. Luetzeler, and M. A. Chirigos, Cancer Res., 37: 3338 (1977).

10

INTERFERON: ITS APPLICATION AND FUTURE AS AN ANTINEOPLASTIC AGENT

PAUL E. CAME*

HEM Research Incorporated
Rockville, Maryland

WILLIAM A. CARTER

Herbert L. Orlowitz Institute for Cancer and Blood Diseases
Hahnemann University of the Health Sciences
Philadelphia, Pennsylvania

I. INTRODUCTION

Only a few years ago most members of the scientific community knew, or thought they knew, exactly what interferon was. More recently, however, came a recognition that there were at least three major antigenic types--now termed α, β, and γ (alpha, beta, and gamma). The α type is the molecular species obtained predominantly from leukocytes induced with live or inactivated viruses, the β type is mainly obtained from cultured fibroblasts induced with synthetic double-stranded polynucleotides or viruses, and the γ type (immune or type 2 interferon) is the predominant antigenic type found when leukocytes are induced with mitogens, specific antigens, or antibody directed against the T-cell population of leukocyte preparations. Moreover, it is now recognized that there are at least a dozen subtypes of α interferon,

*Present affiliation: Heidrick and Struggles, Inc., Chicago, Illinois

possibly four or five subtypes of β and one—possibly more—subtypes of interferon.

In addition to the major types and subtypes of native interferons, which differ in their amino acid sequence, and the "cloned" interferons resulting from the genetic transfer procedures of molecular biologists who now can produce some, if not most, of the polypeptide variants of mammalian interferons by expressing these genes in bacterial hosts. In the molecular cloning approach, the particular interferon gene of interest has been first isolated, then covalently coupled to a bacterial expression vector (usually bacteriophage), and then finally inserted into the recipient bacterial cell with appropriate "promoters" to facilitate interferon production. These bacterial-derived interferons display amino acid sequences which are nearly identical to native interferons, that is, those obtained from fibroblasts in culture or fresh leukocytes. However, it is not yet known if the absence of carbohydrate moieties and attendant possible differences in the secondary or tertiary structure of the protein will make the cloned interferons biophysically as well as biologically significantly different from native (natural) interferon. Given fundamental differences in initiation mechanisms of protein synthesis and modes of secretion of the nascent (newly formed) polypeptide, it would seem surprising if prokaryotic cells were able to produce perfect copies of nature's own work. Recent advances in amino acid sequence analysis and disulfide bond location, coupled with studies to determine the sequence and location of the carbohydrate moiety, should facilitate the detailed comparison of at least some interferons.

The recent recognition that there are three major types of interferons and the subsequent revelation that there are often long common stretches of amino acid sequences now gives credence to the real possibility that the active sites of these molecules may be the sugar region of the carbohydrate-poor types from leukocytes or interferon beta—which is richly embellished with sugar moieties (core and peripheral complex oligosaccharides)—the polypeptide is 165-166 amino acids in length. The amino acid composition of the polypeptides are similar and certain sequences are shared; the shared sequences are also observed in certain nonhuman interferons, indicating the biological importance of these structural domains during evolutionally divergence processes [1]. Additionally, there are similarities in the noncoding regions of the genes that code for the synthesis of interferons and much is yet to be learned about their roles.

Cloned interferon gamma is composed of some 20 fewer amino acids and has a lower molecular weight than either alpha or beta. However, like beta, natural gamma interferon is greatly enriched in carbohydrate moieties. Thus, in the last few years we have come to understand that the term "interferon" is, in many respects, analogous to the term "antibiotic" —namely, there are many types and subtypes as well as a variety of sources in nature. Zoon and Wetzel [2] have recently reviewed the comparative structures of the known mammalian interferons. As additional information becomes available, it is possible that there will soon also be a variety of synthetic approaches to the production of interferon polypeptide, either the entire molecular structure or—more likely in the short term—synthesis of the active-site domain [1].

Even with amounts of interferon sufficient for chemical analysis, the current short supply of clinical grade drug of any of the three types and many subtypes of interferon makes it difficult for us to predict with precision what promise "interferon" may hold as an antineoplastic agent in specific neoplastic disorders. One observes that the analogous question was poised in 1936: What is the future of antibiotics in the treatment of infectious diseases? It was only with the realization that there were many families of antibiotics (penicillins, tetracyclines, macrolides, aminoglycosides, etc.) and that each family—indeed, each member of the family—exerted its own specific and distinct antimicrobial spectrum as well as characteristic pharmacokinetic profile, that meaningful answers as to their future values could be framed. Similarly today, we are confronted with a closely parallel situation where we recognize that numerous varieties of native interferons exist; even before these interferons can be clinically evaluated their number is being enlarged by still more interferon polypeptides derived by recombinant DNA processes. An important realization is the fact that cloned interferons do not obviously reflect the heterogeneous subtypes seen with interferons that are produced naturally (fibroblast and leukocyte cultures). Accordingly, setting aside the possible subtle differences in primary structures when the interferon genes are expressed in bacteria, it is likely that the biological (therapeutic?) spectrum of activity may be significantly more narrow for the cloned interferons.

The initial reports of antitumor activity of interferon in animals were conducted with impure or partially purified natural interferon preparations obtained from cell cultures or from animal serum or tissues while the majority of the human studies have been conducted with natural leukocyte interferon obtained from Kari Cantell, Helsinki, Finland, or by use of his production method. Fewer studies with natural fibroblast interferon have taken place to date and such studies have involved relatively few patients. More recently, clinical studies using interferon preparations obtained through recombinant DNA technology have been initiated with larger patient groups, but few published data describing their antitumor activity have appeared thus far. Type II interferon, also called immune (gamma) interferon, has only just become available in sufficient quantities for human pilot studies. In retrospect, it seems unfortunate that the initial clinical trials with natural leukocyte or fibroblast interferons were conducted with two major limitations: impure preparations were employed and therapy was started without clear knowledge of a maximum tolerated dose or the dose that activates maximally the relevant limbs of the immune defense processes against cancer. An understanding of the immunodulatory effect of interferons had not yet been fully developed and the efficacious regimens are not yet completely unraveled in appropriate animal models. Notwithstanding this paucity of pharmacological information and the impure preparations employed, some surprisingly encouraging results have already been seen in the clinic. We earnestly believe that the results will grow even more impressive as the clinical pharmacologist becomes progressively better armed with facts regarding the multiplicity of interferon's actions and the ability of different molecular species to target selectively to various diseased tissues in the human body.

II. ANIMAL STUDIES

The initial evidence suggesting that interferon possessed antitumor as well as antiviral activity stemmed from experiments conducted in mice and these results have been summarized by Gresser and Tovey [3] and Stewart [4]. At the time these studies were conducted, purified interferons were unavailable; however, the preparations were obtained from a variety of sources, including cell culture, serum from mice injected with various interferon inducers, and homogenates of mouse tissues. Furthermore, the chromatographic and other methods employed to remove large amounts of the impurities (i.e., to purify partially the interferon preparations) were varied and essentially guaranteed that the antitumor effects observed were not primarily due to the impurities but to the interferon molecule itself. This interpretation has been borne out subsequently by various studies, showing the similar spectrum of biological activity by a variety of homogeneous (completely pure) interferons.

One of the early and convincing reports of antitumor activity was conducted in mice suffering from lymphoid leukemia. Gresser et al. [5] injected interferon preparations into AKR mice which resulted in a diminished incidence of disease and an increased survival time. The interferon preparation employed in this first study which demonstrated an inhibitory effect against a spontaneous malignancy had been prepared from extracts of virus-infected mouse brains. Shortly thereafter, Kassel [6] reported that interferon prepared from suspensions of L cells, when administered intravenously, mediated an oncolytic effect in AKR mice suffering from leukemia. Not long after these studies of antitumor activity in "spontaneous" leukemias, another "spontaneous" tumor model was studied by Came and Moore [7]. They reported that a strain of mice, in which approximately 90% of the females develop mammary adenocarcinomas by 1 year of age, were protected from neoplasia development by treatment with a serum interferon preparation. In this study, the interferon was prepared by injecting Newcastle disease virus into mice and subsequently exsanguinating the animals at a time when they exhibited peak serum interferon levels. The serum from these animals contained interferon, which was used to treat the females at risk of developing mammary cancer. While these spontaneous tumors models were being studied, a variety of similar experiments were either under way or completed in animal models in which the tumors were induced by injection with oncogenic viruses or by exposure to irradiation. The latter results have been reviewed in detail by Krim and Sanders [8].

These investigations and others, including the 1960 study by Atanasui and Chany [9] showing that interferon delayed the appearance of tumors in hamsters injected with polyomer virus, certainly provided some of the impetus for the carefully designed clinical studies now being conducted with purified interferon preparations. Studies now under way will define rigorously optimal dose levels and therapeutic regimens.

III. HUMAN TRIALS

At the present time, numerous clinical trials with interferons, both natural and recombinant DNA derived, are under way. The results of only a few trials are published, but more information should appear soon.

A. Natural Interferons: Leukocyte or Alpha, Fibroblast or Beta, and Immune or Gamma Interferons

Leukocyte Interferon

1. Osteogenic Sarcoma: The first and most extensive trial with alpha interferon is an ongoing study conducted at the Karolinska Institute employing interferon obtained from leukocytes induced with Sendai virus. In this pioneering investigation, patients with osteogenic sarcoma are treated intramuscularly: some of these patients have been followed for as long as 10 years and still receive interferon therapy. There is an unmistakable trend in increased survival resulting from initial treatment consisting of 3.0 million units (MU) daily followed by chronic administration three times weekly. At present, approximately 50% of the patients in the interferon group are alive, whereas only about 25% of the control group are surviving after 5 years. Details of the design of this trial can be found in a report by Strander [10]. During the course of this important study, some of the results came under constructive scrutiny and questions were raised because the initial limb of the trials was not done under double-blind conditions [11]. However, as the trial continues, modifications of the patient selection and randomization scheme have apparently resolved the questions that arose in the early clinical trials.

More recently, Caparros and colleagues [12] treated 11 cases of metastatic osteogenic sarcoma and one patient with chondrosarcoma for a minimum of 30 days with a dose ranging from 3 to 10 MU daily by the intramuscular route. Although none of the 10 evaluable patients with osteogenic sarcoma showed an objective response by standard clinical and roentgenographic evaluation, the patient with chondrosarcoma had a marked response accompanied by an increased NK (natural killer) cell activity. This patient has continued to be stable for 1 year.

2. Non-Hodgkin's Lymphoma: In another study with alpha interferon, in which the primary objective was to determine how well natural leukocyte interferon was tolerated, patients with non-Hodgkin's lymphoma received doses of interferon ranging from 5 to 10 MU per day for 1 month [13].

There was no statistically significant evidence of antitumor activity in this trial, possibly due to the small number of patients. However, the overall trend suggested a beneficial effect: regression of tumors occurred in three of six patients, although in certain patients the disease progressed during therapy. In one instance in which no response was seen to treatment with 3-6 MU daily, the patient was subsequently treated with 30 MU daily intravenously and responded [14]. Gutterman and his colleagues [15] had also observed favorable responses to treatment with 3-9 MU daily in a proportion of lymphoma patients.

3. Juvenile Laryngeal Papilloma and Warts: A trial using natural alpha interferon was conducted at the Karolinska Hospital and included seven children with severe disease [16]. Prior to treatment, tumor progression occurred in all cases. During treatment with three intramuscular injections of 3 MU per injection, the tumors decreased in size. When treatment was halted, the tumors increased in size but upon reinitiation of therapy they once again shrank and in one case there was complete disappearance of tumor. No serious side effects were observed. More recently, in a study at the University of Iowa School of Medicine, 15-20 children with laryngeal papilloma were treated intramuscularly with 3 MU three times weekly and the results are encouraging (McCabe and Clark, personal communication, 1982). Another condition also thought to be caused by papilloma viruses, human warts, has been shown to respond to injections of alpha interferon [17]. In their report, two patients with extensive warts which were stable for 2 years or more were treated with natural leukocyte interferon by intramuscular injection and intralesional injection. The intramuscular administration produced a softening and decreased volume of each patient's warts. Progressive disappearance of bilateral plantar warts occurred in a cancer patient being treated with leukocyte interferon [18].

4. Multiple Myeloma: At least 36 patients suffering from this disease have been treated at Karolinska Hospital, Stockholm; M. D. Anderson Hospital, Houston; and the Rega Institute, Leuven; at dosages ranging from 3 to 9 MU daily administered intramuscularly. In some patients, the condition clearly improved as evidenced by complete or partial tumor regression [15, 19,20]. In more recent studies, there also have been instances where prompt worsening of disease parameters occurred with interferon therapy [20]. The mechanism by which the myeloma progressed is not yet understood, but it seems to have occurred in patients being treated concomitantly with established chemotherapeutic agents.

Recently, some updated data have become available and Osserman and others [20] reported results obtained with two protocols involving multiple myeloma patients. In protocol I, 18 cases were previously untreated and three were in relapse after responding to prior chemotherapy. Leukocyte interferon therapy was initiated with 3 MU daily and if significant granulocytopenia was not achieved after 1 month, the dose was increased to 6 MU daily. Treatment was continued for 6 months unless the disease was clearly progressive. Under this regimen, objective evidence of disease regression was seen in 4 of 21 cases. In these cases there was a 20-70% reduction in the monoclonal protein and a decrease in skeletal symptoms. In three cases there was an increase in hemoglobin. The effects were maximal at 4-6 weeks and, with one exception, there was no further improvement.

In protocol II, daily intramuscular injection of 3 MU was given for 3 months in addition to ongoing chemotherapy in patients in partial remission. One of the three patients entered into the study, one had been treated for 2 months according to protocol I. The three patients subsequently received continuous low-dose cyclophosphamide, and when 3 MU of interferon was resumed there was a prompt lessening of all disease parameters. In the second case, the addition of 3 MU of interferon to cyclophosphamide produced a transient decrease in monoclonal protein but exacerbated the anemia. In the third case, the addition of 3 MU daily also produced anemia as well as leukopenia and thrombopenia.

5. Mammary Carcinoma: Gutterman and colleagues [15] have treated 17 patients with breast cancer recurrence with 3-9 MU daily for several weeks to 4 months via the intramuscular route. Approximately 25 have been treated similarly in the trial being sponsored by the American Cancer Society. A statistically significant reduction in the volume of tumors was seen in about 20-30% of the patients. Habif (personal communication, 1983) treated five women with recurrent breast cancer lesions by intralesional administration. Tumor regression or carcinolytic effects were observed in each patient. These observations and others have prompted Habif to seek an in vivo laboratory test, such as human tumor engraftment into athymic mice, to identify mammary tumors on an individual basis that are sensitive to interferon.

6. Malignant Melanoma: Interferon alpha has been given to 35 patients at doses of 1, 3, or 9 MU daily for over 1 month. Using a reduction of tumor mass as evidence of activity, six of these patients showed partial tumor regression. However, some 20 patients did not respond to treatment and only minor shrinking of tumor size occurred in two patients. The details of this study can be found in a report by Krown and colleagues [21].

7. Renal Cell Carcinoma: In a preliminary study by Quesada and colleagues [22], it was shown that renal cell carcinoma may be sensitive to native alpha interferon. From 3 to 36 MU was given daily by the intramuscular route to 15 patients. In three responders to 3 MU the dose was escalated to 18 MU twice weekly, and one showed another minor response. Disease progressed in 5 of the 13, although four of six responders remained stable for a prolonged period. The findings described above and summarized in Table 10.1.

Natural Fibroblast or Beta Interferon

Most of the initial studies with leukocyte interferon were conducted with material from the facility in Finland. Unlike the situations with leukocyte material, quantities of beta interferon sufficient for clinical trials have only recently been produced and these lots came from numerous production units.

TABLE 10.1 Clinical Studies with Natural Alpha or Leukocyte Interferon

Disease	Number of patients	References	Results and comments
Osteogenic sarcoma	48	10, 18	Increased survival
Osteogenic sarcoma (metastatic)		12	No objective response
Non-Hodgkin's lymphoma	18	13-15	Favorable response in a proportion of patients
Juvenile laryngeal papilloma	22	16; McCabe and Clark, personal communication, 1982	Highly significant activity; early results are encouraging
Multiple myeloma	36	15, 19, 20, 23	Some patients responded
Mammary carcinoma (recurrences)	30	Habif, personal communication, 1983; 15	Significant reduction in tumor volume
Malignant melanoma	35	21	About 20% of patients showed partial tumor regression
Renal cell carcinoma (stage IV)	13	22	Suggestive of activity
Warts	2	17	Warts disappeared or diminished in size

Cultured diploid fibroblasts, the source of this type of natural interferon, have not been widely adopted as a substrate for interferon production primarily because until recently there was no technology available for growing the massive numbers of cells required to produce quantities of interferon sufficient for trials. Several organizations have, however, recently produced sufficient beta interferon using roller bottles and other culture methods. Most of the clinical grade beta interferon has been produced by Toray Industries, Inc., Japan; Rentschler Laboratories, Germany; Rega Institute for Medical Research, Belgium; HEM Research, Inc., and Roswell Park Memorial Institute, United States; and Searle Laboratories, England. The results of controlled clinical studies are not yet available since only a few patients with any single histologic type of cancer have been treated; however, limited phase I studies have been undertaken by Billiau et al. [23] and Horoszewicz et al. [24]. Furthermore, it is not clear whether the producers of this interferon employed the same or similar production and processing techniques. Although doses exceeding 20 MU daily were not given, the interferon appeared to be free of serious side effects. More recently, Hawkins and co-workers [25] found dose-limiting side effects with 10 MU of native beta interferon produced at Rosewell Park Memorial Institute when given intravenously. These side effects were partially controlled with antipyretics. A repetitive intravenous schedule appears safe.

In Japan, some 40 patients with diverse diseases such as viral warts; melanoma; brain, breast, ovarian, and gastric cancer; lymphoma; and other malignancies have been treated. The beta interferon was administered by various routes, including intravenous infusion, intralesionally, and intramuscularly. In one study involving 25 patients, 3 MU was administered daily for at least 30 consecutive days and some patients were treated with twice that dose by drip infusion. Most of these patients (13 of 15) developed mild transient fever and evidence of low-level hematologic and hepatic toxicity was reported. Ten of the patients showed an increase in NK (natural killer) cell activity 12-24 hr after initiation of treatment. In only three of the patients was their underlying malignancy stabilized, and in 11 there was progression [26].

In another study by Shimoyama and associates [27], 10 patients were given from 1.5 to 6.0 MU daily intravenously for 8-30 days; other drug schedules employed included intratumoral injection daily or weekly with 0.6-9.0 MU. The side effects included low- to high-grade fever after both intravenous or intratumoral injection. Two patients treated intratumorally, one suffering from lymphoma and other from rhabdomyosarcoma, showed evidence of tumor regression.

In a trial conducted by Ishihara and Hawasaka [28], eight patients with malignant melanoma were treated by intratumoral administration. The dosage started at 0.6 MU and escalated to 1.5 MU every 48 hr. There was a significant reduction of the tumor size in seven of the eight patients. Histopathological findings showed abundant lymphocyte infiltration into the tumor and surrounding tissue. In another study involving patients with medulloblastoma and four with glioblastoma, Nagai et al. [29] reported that intravenous therapy with 0.3-3.0 MU two or three times weekly to a total dosage of up to 20-200 MU over 2 months resulted in an improvement of both cases of medulloblastoma. Two of the glioblastoma patients showed improvement; patients experienced temporary elevation of temperature but not exceeding 38.5°C.

Studies with beta interferon in the United States have been limited. The earliest were reported by Carter and colleagues at Roswell Park Memorial Institute, Buffalo, New York. These clinical evaluations [30, 31] of beta interferon involved intralesional treatment of 17 patients: six with melanoma, six with breast cancer, and one each with prostatic carcinoma, renal cell carcinoma, transitional cell and squamous cell carcinoma, and cancer of the larnyx. All of these patients had easily measurable cutaneous or subcutaneous metastatic lesions. The lesions were injected daily and of 19 tumors treated, 14 regressed, generally within 10-14 days. Histological examination of biopsied tissue specimens from the injected nodules showed an infiltration of lymphocytes and macrophages suggestive of enhanced lymphocyte function. Most lesions were injected with approximately 0.5 MU daily. Importantly, no fever was associated with the treatment, indicating that beta interferon preparations obtained following hydrophobic affinity chromatography are largely free of side effects [32].

In addition to these 17 patients treated intralesionally, an additional 13 were treated by the subcutaneous, intramuscular, and intravenous routes with up to 25 MU daily. In two other patients with acute lymphocytic leukemia, treatment with approximately 0.6 MU via the intrathecal route was given. The number of patients treated by the various routes and the total amounts of interferon administered is shown in Table 10.2. All injections were well tolerated and there was no pyrogenicity associated with intramuscular or subcutaneous administration of 25 MU daily. A slight increase in temperature (38.5°C) of 3 hr duration was seen with intravenous administration of approximately 3 MU. Carter and colleagues [33] did not observe allergic skin responses, granulocytopenia, thrombocytopenia, coagulopathy, or untoward effects on kidney or liver function during these studies. Similarly, fibroblast interferon given intrathecally at a dose approximating 0.6 MU was also well tolerated.

On a disease-by-disease analysis, the following have also been reported:

1. Warts: Scott and Csonka [34] treated 11 male patients with genital warts by injecting fibroblast interferon and placebo into the bases of two similar warts. The diminution in the size of the treated warts compared with the changes seen in the controls suggested that the 300 units of interferon inhibited the growth. In one patient, with a wart on his penile shaft, injection with interferon caused the wart to disappear within 2 weeks, whereas an untreated meatal wart increased in size. It is of interest that Strander and Cantell [18] reported earlier that bilateral plantar warts disappeared in a patient who was treated with leukocyte interferon for cervical carcinoma.

2. Malignant Melanoma: In the United States, the initial evaluation of beta interferon in melanoma was reported by Carter's group [30] and involved intralesional treatment of six patients with melanoma. All of these patients had cutaneous or subcutaneous metastatic lesions which were readily measurable. The nodules were injected daily, usually receiving approximately 0.5 MU, and most regressed within 10-14 days. Histological examination of biopsied tissues consistently showed an infiltration of lymphocytes and macrophages, suggestive of enhanced lymphocyte function.

TABLE 10.2 Individual Patients in Clinical Trials with Natural Human Fibroblast Interferon at Roswell Park Memorial Institute: Phase I Study

Patient diagnosis	Length of treatment (days)	Total dosage (MU)
A. Intramuscular and subcutaneous administration		
1. Hepatitis B[a]	82	85
2. Hepatitis B	84	85
3. Breast cancer	88	120.5
4. Hepatitis B	32	247
5. Melanoma[b]	66	739
B. Intravenous administration		
1. Melanoma[b]	15	117
2. CML	12	89
3. Hepatoma	2	24
4. Neuroblastoma	14	71
5. Adrenal cortical cancer	3	12.1
6. Breast cancer	23	24.2
7. Bladder cancer	25	15.2
8. Renal cell cancer[b]	80	87.0
C. Intrathecal administration		
1. Acute lymphatic leukemia	23	13.9
2. Acute lymphatic leukemia	29	31.8

[a]Partial response.

[b]Same patient.

Source: Ref. 31.

In a study by Ishihara and Hayasaka [28] eight patients with malignant melanoma were treated by intratumoral administration of fibroblast interferon at dosages starting at 0.6 MU and escalating to 1.5 MU every 48 hr. There was a significant reduction of tumor size in seven of eight patients. Histopathological findings showed abundant lymphocyte infiltration into the tumor and surrounding tissue.

3. Mammary Carcinoma: In an unpublished study (Pouillart et al., personal communication, 1982), 11 patients with metastatic breast cancer were treated with eight intramuscular injections of 6 MU administered every 5 days. The treatment period was 40 days. In 10 of 11 patients, the skin nodules showed either a decrease in size or central necrosis accompanied by an inflammatory reaction suggestive of therapeutic activity. The NK

(natural killer) cell activity was significantly increased following the first injection, although the magnitude of the increase on subsequent administrations was not as pronounced. The injections did not cause irritation or inflammation and only one of the 11 patients developed a fever.

4. Brain Tumor: Six cases of malignant brain tumors (two medulloblastoma and four glioblastoma) were treated with natural fibroblast interferon [29]. The patients were treated intravenously with 0.3-3.0 MU twice or three times weekly for more than 2 months, resulting in a total dosage of 20-200 MU. In the two medulloblastoma cases, the treatment followed partial surgical removal of the tumor and was reported to result in significant tumor reduction. Computerized axial tomography (CAT) evaluation revealed reductions of volume of 85.2% and 79.6%, and beta interferon injections were continued for over a year in both cases. Furthermore, cultures of cells from one of the cases were shown to be sensitive to growth inhibition by the inclusion of interferon in the culture medium.

Two of the four cases of glioblastoma did not respond, but partial remission was seen with the other two. These authors suggested that other routes of administration, such as intrathecal or local, be developed to increase the drug concentration surrounding the tumor tissue.

The possibility of using the intrathecal route may offer an expanded usage for interferons and is noteworthy in that patients with acute lymphocytic leukemia have received natural beta interferon intrathecally. Murphy [31] and Jacobs and colleagues [35] also treated 10 patients suffering from multiple sclerosis once weekly by intrathecal administration. In both studies the patients tolerated the injections without serious side effects. More recently, Salazar (unpublished data) has evaluated several lots of interferon for tolerance by injecting the material into monkeys intracisternally. His study has shown that some beta interferon preparations are tolerated very well at multiples of the dose employed by the Jacobs team [35].

5. Multiple Myeloma: Few data on the effect of beta interferon on this disease have been published, but in one study by Billiau and colleagues [36], of two patients who did not respond, a subsequent course on leukocyte interferon brought about a reduction of Bence-Jones proteinuria approximating 25% in one of the two patients. These data, when viewed with the findings of Osserman et al. [20], suggest that a greater understanding of dose, regimen, and possible drug interactions may be required before either beta or alpha interferons can be used effectively in this disease. The clinical results with beta interferons are shown in Table 10.3.

Natural Immune or Gamma Interferons

There are no published reports of clinical trials with native immune interferon at this time but several groups have now produced and purified enough to initiate pilot clinical projects. Laboratory studies have been conducted which suggest that immune interferon might have certain advantages over alpha or beta interferons, but sufficient comparative data are not at hand to predict reliably whether immune interferon will be of special value. Such

TABLE 10.3 Clinical Studies with Natural Beta or Fibroblast Interferon

Disease	Number of patients	References	Results and comments
Malignant melanoma	14	28, 30	Significant reduction of nodule volume by intralesional treatment
Mammary carcinoma	11	Pouillart et al., personal communication, 1982	Skin nodules were decreased in size in 10 of 11 patients treated intramuscularly
Brain tumor	6	29	Both gliomas and two of four medulloblastomas responded
Warts	11	34	Size of warts diminished by injecting the base of the wart

studies suggest that gamma interferon might be used, especially in conjunction with beta interferons, to obtain a synergistic antitumor effect.

B. Recombinant DNA-Derived Interferons

At present, data are just beginning to appear concerning the clinical activity of interferon derived from bacteria. These "cloned" interferons are being examined in a variety of laboratories, moreover, to determine if they will display the same characteristics as the native of natural interferons. There are several major laboratories producing "cloned" interferons, of which the most visible are Cetus Corporation, Berkeley; Biogen, Geneva; Genentech, South San Francisco; and Schering-Plough Corporation, Bloomfield, New Jersey.

A recent review by Weck and Came [37] describes the comparative biological activities of the native and cloned interferons. Many of the biological activities seen with natural or native interferons, particularly the antiviral activity seen in cell culture and in certain animal models are also observed with the cloned interferons. Also many of the antigenic properties are qualitatively indistinguishable between the natural and the bacterial derived interferon proteins. The amino acid composition and sequence of the native and cloned interferons appear to be essentially identical. However, the cloned varieties of interferon lack carbohydrate moieties, which we believe may contribute important distinguishing characteristics to the natural interferons. The role of the carbohydrate embellishment is not yet completely understood but, by analogy to other glycoproteins, it may be expected to contribute stability to the tertiary structure of interferons, as well as influence its pharmacokinetics, such as by governing the avidity of binding to receptor sites on both virus infected or cancer cells. In short, carbohydrates may contribute a variety of subtle differences between human cells and bacterial-derived interferons. These differences obviously remain to be fully unraveled. Clearly, only further comparative studies with quantitiative models will reveal the extent to which the sugar moieties found attached to the polypeptides of natural interferons may modulate their role as members of the natural host defense systems. In the interim, clinical trials with cloned interferons will evaluate the various interferon polypeptides in their "pure" state (i.e., unembellished with sugar groups).

In a phase I study conducted by Sherwin et al. [38] approximately 70 patients with a variety of hematologic and nonhematologic malignancies were treated with either recombinant leukocyte A interferon or natural lymphoblastoid interferon. The bacterial derived product was a single molecular species (by polyacrylamide gel analysis) of alpha interferon with a specific activity of 2×10^8 units/mg. In contrast, the natural lymphoblastoid interferon preparation contains eight physicochemically distinct alpha interferon subtypes which differ in their physical, antigenic, and biological properties [39]; these forms display specific activity of 5×10^7 units/mg in the preparations used clinically. The recombinant interferon has been given intramuscularly and the native material has been administered intravenously: both were given in escalating doses. The cloned interferon was given at a maximum dose of 118 MU and the native material at doses of up to 50 MU per day. The side effects of each were similar and consisted of fever, chills, fatigue, anorexia, myalgias, and—less frequently—nausea, vomiting, and headache. Dose-dependent leukopenia was common but corrected upon drug discontinuation. Transient hepatic transaminase elevations were also seen but generally at the higher doses [40,41]. With the natural lymphoblastoid interferon preparations, occasional episodes of hypertension and hypotension have been noted. It is tempting to speculate that these side effects, apparently never observed with any other interferons, might derive from the fact that the producing cell has been transformed with a putatively oncogenic virus, Epstein-Barr (EB) virus. Integration of the virus into the interferon-producing cell may "reprogram" the expression of other genc products, possibly accounting thereby for novel low-level products (vasoreactive moieties?) which account for certain unexpected findings in the clinical preparations. Approximately 25% of the patients treated with bacteria-derived protein demonstrated tumor regressions, and one of eight patients treated with native lymphoblastoid interferon achieved a partial response. Thus both preparations have antitumor activity in vivo.

Other phase I studies are also under way. Leavitt et al. [42] administered recombinant human leukocyte A interferon to patients twice daily for 28 days without evidence of serious side effects.

Thus, now that several phase I studies are completed and still others are under way, efficacy data should soon follow. Eventually, double-blind studies will follow, making possible a quantitative assessment of native and recombinant interferons as antitumor agents.

IV. CONCLUSIONS

Shortly after the discovery of interferon in 1957, interest in the possibility that it might possess clinical utility was followed rapidly by a wave of unrealistic optimism: by the late 1960s and 1970s scientists from all over the world were experimenting with interferon as an antiviral and antitumor agent; few, if any, negative results were reported. Indeed, almost every laboratory finding provided further evidence that interferon was a very potent therapeutic material largely free from significant side effects. This wave of great hope continued into the late 1970s; during this entire period the glowing prospects of interferon were also tracked closely by the news media. Even while this fascinating scientific and medical progress was occurring, the only apparent obstacle—unavailability of sufficient material to conduct clinical trials—was being solved by the "genetic engineers." As molecular biologists, they succeeded in inserting the gene(s) that code for human interferon in bacteria. This feat allowed the production of inexpensive and plentiful interferon substances for clinical application. Thus, during the next few years, especially 1979-1982, a sizable number of clinical trials were either completed or well under way; however, these trials brought initial disappointments in that dramatic cures were not achieved. Subsequently, mounting concern was voiced that interferon might not be the "magic bullet" for cancer. First, prominent investigators delivered their caveats in the scientific press and then even newspapers and popular magazines featured articles stating that "interferon may not be a miracle drug" or "interferon may be no better than currently available cancer therapy." Not only scientists and doctors but even investors became pessimistic and probably overly critical. Large emotional peaks and valleys seem often to be part of the American experience regarding new advances in biomedicine.

The widespread public disappointment, however, has not been without some benefits. As a result of the disillusionment, many researchers intensified their analyses and we now have a much better understanding of how interferon works. Apparently, it does not by itself necessarily lyse tumor cells directly and thereby cause tumors to shrink. Rather, for example, interferon activates the immune system; specifically, it is now known that the NK (natural killer) cells are strongly activated by exquisitely small concentrations of interferon. With the insight that interferon may exert at least part of its antitumor activity by enhancing a component of the cellular immune system (e.g., the NK cells), it is not at all surprising that interferon did not work well in all cancer patients. Furthermore, the clinical significance of the fact that many of the patients who entered into the initial clinical trials were in a profound state of immunosuppression, either from their malignancy or the resultant chemotherapy, was more fully realized. This appreciation provided one explanation of why interferon might not be universally efficacious. Additionally, it became increasingly apparent that studies aimed at determining dose range or dose regimen had not yet been carefully and thoroughly developed. Thus, in retrospect, it was felt that certain patients were not only given an inappropriate dose of interferon, but may also have received it at an improper stage of their disease process. During treatment, the cellular immune system of many of the patients may have been so deranged that it was simply not possible for any immune modifier, interferon included, to mediate its effect.

On the brighter side of this complexity, we now have for the first time ample evidence that certain tumors in certain patients can respond to interferon remarkably well, for example, patients with juvenile laryngeal papillomatosis. Other cancers at particular stages also appear to respond to interferon treatment, such as malignant melanoma and breast cancer. Apparently, what is now required is a better understanding of the mechanism of interferon action and a means by which patients are preselected for capability to respond. The authors believe that such a time is not far away and that soon we will witness the compilation of powerful evidence clearly supporting interferon's utility for specific cancers. While these clinical data are being assembled, it is hoped that further refinements in knowledge of primary structure (amino acid sequence, location of disulfide bridges, and the role of the carbohydrate embellishment), along with studies of secondary and tertiary structure (identification of the active sites, etc.), will occur. These studies will strengthen both the existing programs in clinical pharmacology of interferons as well as open up new synthetic approaches to the production of interferon fragments which may exert only one of the spectra of biological activities resident in the entire interferon molecule. It is indeed possible that the quest for the "interferon cure" will be met by modern medicinal chemistry and the ability to synthesize an oligopeptide with a highly focused or targeted effect. Alternatively, the duplication or improvement of nature's process and product may prove elusive. In such a case, we may need to rely therapeutically on obtaining interferons from living human cells for a while longer while molecular studies actively continue.

REFERENCES

1. D. Gillespie, E. Piquignot, and W. A. Carter, in Handbook of Experimental Pharmacology: Interferons and Their Applications (P. E. Came and W. A. Carter, eds.), Springer-Verlag, Heidelberg, 1983, Vol. 71, pp. 45-63.
2. K. C. Zoon and R. Wetzel, in Handbook of Experimental Pharmacology: Interferons and Their Applications (P. E. Came and W. A. Carter, eds.), Springer-Verlag, Heidelberg, 1983, Vol. 71, pp. 79-97.

3. I. Gresser and M. G. Tovey, Biochim. Biophys. Acta, 516: 231-247 (1978).
4. W. E. Stewart, II, The Interferon System (W. E. Stewart, II, ed.), Springer-Verlag, New York, 1979, pp. 292-303.
5. I. Gresser, J. Coppey, and C. Bourali, J. Natl. Cancer Inst., 43: 1083-1089 (1969).
6. R. L. Kassel, Clin. Obstet. Gynecol., 13: 910-927 (1970).
7. P. E. Came and D. H. Moore, Proc. Soc. Exp. Biol. Med., 137: 304-305 (1971).
8. M. Krim and R. K. Sanders, in Interferons and Their Actions (W. E. Stewart II, ed.), CRC Press, Cleveland, Ohio, 1977, pp. 153-201.
9. P. Atanasiu and C. Chany, C. R. Acad. Sci., 251: 1687-1689 (1960).
10. H. Strander, in Report of the International Workshop on Interferon in the Treatment of Cancer, Sloan-Kettering Institute for Cancer Research, New York, 1975, p. 39.
11. A. Rabson, in Report of the International Workshop on Interferon in the Treatment of Cancer, Sloan-Kettering Institute for Cancer Research, New York, 1975, p. 39.
12. B. Caparros, G. Rosen, and S. Cunningham-Rundles, Am. Assoc. Can. Res. (1982), Abstr. 474.
13. T. C. Merigan, K. Sikora, J. H. Breeden, R. Levy, and S. A. Rosenberg, N. Engl. J. Med., 299: 1449-1453 (1978).
14. N. O. Hill, A. Kahn, E. Loeb, A. Pardue, C. Aleman, G. Dorn, and J. M. Hill, in Interferon and Properties and Clinical Uses (A. Kahn, N. O. Hill, and G. L. Dorn, eds.), Leland Fikes Foundation Press, Dallas, 1980, pp. 668-680.
15. J. U. Gutterman, G. R. Blumenchein, R. Alexanian, H. Y. Yop, A. U. Buzdar, F. Cabanillas, G. N. Hortobagyi, E. M. Hersh, S. L. Rasmaussen, M. Harmon, M. Kramer, and S. Pestka, Ann. Intern. Med., 93: 399-406 (1980).
16. S. Haglund, P. G. Lundquist, K. Cantell, and H. Strander, Arch Otolaryngol., 107: 327-332 (1981).
17. G. J. Pazin, M. Ho, H. W. Haverkos, J. A. Armstrong, M. C. Breining, H. L. Wechsler, A. Arvin, T. C. Merigan, and K. Cantell, Effects of Interferon on Human Warts, in press.
18. H. Strander and K. Cantell, in The Production and Use of Interferon for the Treatment and Prevention of Human Virus Infections (C. Waymouth, ed.), Tissue Culture Association, Rockville, Md., 1974, pp. 49-56.
19. H. Mellstedt, A. Ahre, M. Bjorkholm, G. Holm, B. Johansson, and H. Strander, Lancet, 1: 245-247 (1979).
20. E. F. Osserman, W. H. Sherman, R. Alexanian, J. U. Gutterman, and R. L. Humphrey, 11th Annu. UCLA Symp. Chem. Biol. Interferons: Relationship to Therapeutics, Squaw Valley, Calif., 1982, p. 93.
21. S. E. Krown, M. Burk, J. M. Kirkwood, D. Kerr, J. J. Nordlund, D. L. Morton, and H. F. Oettgen, in The Biology of the Interferon

System (E. DeMaeyer, G. Galasso, and H. Schellekens, eds.), Elsevier/North-Holland, Amsterdam 1981, pp. 394-400.
22. J. R. Quesada, J. U. Gutterman, D. Swanson, and A. Trindade, Am. Assoc. Cancer Res., Abstr. 562 (1982).
23. A. Billiau, P. DeSomer, V. G. Edy, E. DeClercq, and H. Hubertine, Antimicrob. Agents Chemother., 16: 56-63 (1979).
24. J. Horoszewicz, S. Leong, J. Dolan, M. Brecher, C. Tebbi, A. Freeman, W. Aungst, and E. Mirand, Int. Symp. New Trends Hum. Cancer Immunother., 1980, pp. 908-919.
25. M. J. Hawkins, S. E. Krown, E. C. Borden, F. Real, M. Krim, S. Cunningham-Rundles, H. Oettgen, R. W. Fox, C. C. Stock, and F. J. Rauscher, Jr., Am. Assoc. Cancer Res., Abstr. 973 (1982).
26. M. Ogawa and K. Ezaki, Conf. Clinical Potential of Interferon in Viral Diseases and Malignant Tumors (Japan Med. Res. Found., ed.), Oiso, Japan, 1980, pp. 41-42.
27. M. Shimoyama, T. Kitahara, M. Nakazawa, T. Ise, I. Adachi, S. Yoslinda, K. Nomura, and H. Ichikawa, Conf. Clinical Potential of Interferon in Viral Diseases and Malignant Tumors (Japan Med. Res. Found., ed.), Oiso, Japan, 1980, pp. 43-44.
28. K. Ishihara and K. Hayasaka, Conf. Clinical Potential of Interferon in Viral Diseases and Malignant Tumors (Japan Med. Res. Found., ed.), Oiso, Japan, 1980, pp. 52-53.
29. M. Nagai, T. Arai, S. Kohno, and M. Kohase, Conf. Clinical Potential of Interferon in Viral Diseases and Malignant Tumors (Japan Med. Res. Found., ed.), Oiso, Japan, 1980, pp. 54-55.
30. J. S. Horoszewicz, S. S. Leong, M. Ito, R. F. Buffet, C. Karakousis, E. Holyoke, L. Job, J. G. Dolen, and W. A. Carter, Cancer Treat. Rep., 62: 1899-1906 (1978).
31. G. P. Murphy, J. Surg. Oncol., 17: 99-111 (1981).
32. W. A. Carter, J. G. Dolen, S. S. Leong, J. S. Horoszewicz, A. O. Vladutiu, A. I. Leibowitz, and J. P. Nolan, Cancer Lett., 7: 243-249 (1979).
33. W. A. Carter and J. S. Horoszewicz, Cancer Treat. Rep., 62: 1897-1898 (1978).
34. G. M. Scott and Csonka, Bri. J. Vener. Dis., 55: 442-445 (1979).
35. L. Jacobs, J. O'Malley, A. Freeman, and R. Ekes, Science, 214: 1026-1028 (1981).
36. A. Billiau, J. Bloemmen, M. Bogaerts, H. Cleys, J. Van Damne, M. DeLey, P. DeSomer, A. Drochmans, H. Heremans, A. Kriel, J. Schetz, G. Tricot, C. Vermylen, R. Verwilghen, and M. Waer, Eur. J. Cancer, 17: 875-882 (1981).
37. P. K. Weck and P. E. Came, in Handbook of Experimental Pharmacology: Interferons and Their Applications (P. E. Came and W. A. Carter, eds.), Springer-Verlag, Heidelberg, 1983, Vol. 71, pp. 339-349.

38. S. Sherwin, S. Fein, J. Whisnant, and R. Oldham, 11th Annu. UCLA Symp. Chem. Biol. Interferons: Relationship to Therapeutics, Squaw Valley, Calif., 1982, p. 92.
39. N. B. Finter, G. Allen, K. H. Fantes, M. D. Johnson, T. Priestman, J. Toy, and J. G. Woodrooffe, 11th Annu. UCLA Symp. Chem. Biol. Interferons: Relationship to Therapeutics, Squaw Valley, Calif., 1982, p. 91.
40. J. U. Gutterman, S. Fine, J. Quesada, S. J. Horning, J. F. Levine, R. Alexanian, L. Bernhardt, M. Kramer, H. Spiegel, W. Colburn, P. Trown, T. Merigan, and Dziewanowski, Ann. Intern. Med., 96: 549-556 (1982).
41. S. J. Horning, J. F. Levine, R. A. Miller, S. A. Rosenberg, and T. C. Merigan, JAMA, 247: 1718-1722 (1982).
42. R. D. Leavitt, P. L. Duffey, P. H. Wiernik, S. Fein, D. Scogna, and R. Oldham, Am. Soc. Clin. Oncol., C-162 (1982).

INDEX